Race, Culture, and Disability

Rehabilitation Science and Practice

Edited by:

Fabricio E. Balcazar, PhD
University of Illinois at Chicago

Yolanda Suarez-Balcazar, PhD
University of Illinois at Chicago

Tina Taylor-Ritzler, PhD
University of Illinois at Chicago

Christopher B. Keys, PhD
DePaul University

JONES AND BARTLETT PUBLISHERS
Sudbury, Massachusetts
BOSTON   TORONTO   LONDON   SINGAPORE

World Headquarters

Jones and Bartlett Publishers
40 Tall Pine Drive
Sudbury, MA 01776
978-443-5000
info@jbpub.com
www.jbpub.com

Jones and Bartlett Publishers
Canada
6339 Ormindale Way
Mississauga, Ontario L5V 1J2
Canada

Jones and Bartlett Publishers
International
Barb House, Barb Mews
London W6 7PA
United Kingdom

Jones and Bartlett's books and products are available through most bookstores and online booksellers. To contact Jones and Bartlett Publishers directly, call 800-832-0034, fax 978-443-8000, or visit our website www.jbpub.com.

Substantial discounts on bulk quantities of Jones and Bartlett's publications are available to corporations, professional associations, and other qualified organizations. For details and specific discount information, contact the special sales department at Jones and Bartlett via the above contact information or send an email to specialsales@jbpub.com.

This publication is designed to provide accurate and authoritative information in regard to the Subject Matter covered. It is sold with the understanding that the publisher is not engaged in rendering legal, accounting, or other professional service. If legal advice or other expert assistance is required, the service of a competent professional person should be sought.

Production Credits
Publisher: David Cella
Acquisitions Editor: Kristine Johnson
Associate Editor: Maro Gartside
Editorial Assistant: Catie Heverling
Production Assistant: Ashlee Hazeltine
Senior Marketing Manager: Sophie Fleck
Manufacturing and Inventory Control Supervisor: Amy Bacus
Composition: Northeast Compositors
Art Rendering: George Nichols
Title Page and Cover Design: Scott Moden
Cover Image: African-American Woman: © Lucian Coman/Dreamstime.com
    African Textile: © Bonsa/Dreamstime.com
Printing and Binding: Malloy, Inc.
Cover Printing: Malloy, Inc.

Library of Congress Cataloging-in-Publication Data
Race, culture, and disability : rehabilitation science and practice / Fabricio E. Balcazar ... [et al.].
    p. ; cm.
  Includes bibliographical references and index.
  ISBN-13: 978-0-7637-6337-4 (pbk.)
  ISBN-10: 0-7637-6337-3 (pbk.)
  1. Medical rehabilitation—United States. 2. Minorities—Rehabilitation—United States. 3. Transcultural medical care—United States. I. Balcazar, Fabricio E.
  [DNLM: 1. Rehabilitation—organization & administration—United States. 2. Cultural Competency—United States. 3. Disabled Persons—rehabilitation—United States. 4. Healthcare Disparities—United States. 5. Outcome Assessment (Health Care)—United States. 6. Prejudice—United States. WB 320 R118 2010]
  RM930.5.U6R33 2010
  362.1089—dc22
                        2009008086

6048
Printed in the United States of America
13 12 11 10 09   10 9 8 7 6 5 4 3 2 1

To our children:
Faby, Daniel, Andres, Sylvia, Sophie, Benjamin, and
Daniel. May they inherit a world that honors diversity.

—Editors

Contents

SECTION II—The Nature of Disparities in Outcomes for Multicultural Populations with Disabilities 53

Contributing Authors

Reginald Alston, PhD
University of Illinois Urbana-Champaign
Champaign, IL

Francisco Alvarado, MD, MA
Illinois Department of Human Services
Springfield, IL

Juan Carlos Arango, PhD
Virginia Commonwealth University
Richmond, VA

Jeanie Castillo, MA
American Indian Disability Technical
    Assistance Center
Missoula, MT

Fong Chan, PhD, CRC
University of Wisconsin–Madison
Madison, WI

James Charlton, MA
Access Living Center for Independent
    Living, University of Illinois at Chicago
Chicago, IL

Julie Clay, MPH
Montana Department of Public Health and
    Human Services
Helena, MT

Judith A. Cook, PhD
University of Illinois at Chicago
Chicago, IL

William E. Cross Jr, PhD
University of Nevada at Las Vegas
Las Vegas, NV

Oscar A. Donoso, MA
DePaul University
Chicago, IL

Carlos Drazen, MA
University of Illinois at Chicago
Chicago, IL

Alo Dutta, PhD, CRC
Southern University
Baton Rouge, LA

Charisse Ewing, PsyD
Johns Hopkins Medical Institutions
Baltimore, MD

Glenn T. Fujiura, PhD
University of Illinois at Chicago
Chicago, IL

Teresa Garate, MEd
Chicago Public Schools
Chicago, IL

Jorge Garcia, PhD
The George Washington University
Washington, DC

Edurne Garcia-Iriarte, PhD
Trinity College Dublin
Dublin, Ireland

Carol J. Gill, PhD
University of Illinois at Chicago
Chicago, IL

Yanling Li Gould, MS, MA
University of Illinois at Chicago
Chicago, IL

Rooshey Hasnain, EdD
University of Illinois at Chicago
Chicago, IL

Brigida Hernandez, PhD
YAI/National Institute for People with
    Disabilities
New York, NY

Felicia Hill-Briggs, PhD, ABPP
Johns Hopkins Medical Institutions
Baltimore, MD

Elizabeth V. Horin, PhD
Hines VA Hospital
Hines, IL

Jessica A. Jonikas, MA
University of Illinois at Chicago
Chicago, IL

Erin Kelly, PhD
Shriner's Hospitals for Children–Chicago
Chicago, IL

Kennesha Kelly, BA
Johns Hopkins Medical Institutions
Baltimore, MD

Gary Kielhofner, DrPH, OTR
University of Illinois at Chicago
Chicago, IL

Leah Kinney, MA
HCSC/Blue Cross Blue Shield
Chicago, IL

**Madan M. Kundu, PhD, FNRCA, CRC,
    NCC, LRC**
Southern University
Baton Rouge, LA

Paul Leung, PhD
University of North Texas
Denton, TX

Allen N. Lewis, PhD, CRC
Virginia Commonwealth University
Richmond, VA

Rene Luna, BA
Access Living Center for Independent
    Living
Chicago, IL

Mary A. Matteliano, MS, OTR/L
University of Buffalo, State University of
    New York
Buffalo, NY

Gloria Morales-Curtin, MEd
El Valor Corporation
Chicago, IL

Angela Odoms-Young, PhD
University of Illinois at Chicago
Chicago, IL

Lisa A. Razzano, PhD, CPRP
University of Illinois at Chicago
Chicago, IL

Maria E. Restrepo-Toro, MS , CPRP
Boston University
Boston, MA

Juleen Rodakowski, MS, OTR/L
University of Illinois at Chicago
Chicago, IL

Holly Ruch-Ross, ScD
Independent Research and Evaluation
    Consultant
Evanston, IL

Anrea Saul, MA
DePaul University
Chicago, IL

Tom Seekins, PhD
University of Montana
Missoula, MT

Julissa Senices, PhD
Private Practice
Coral Gables, FL

Aisha Shamburger, MS, CRC
Virginia Commonwealth University
Richmond, VA

Dianne L. Smith, PhD, OTR/L
University of Missouri
Columbia, MO

John H. Stone, PhD
University at Buffalo, State University of
    New York
Buffalo, NY

Orville H. Townsend, MA
Iowa Vocational Rehabilitation Services
Iowa City, IA

Glen W. White, PhD
University of Kansas
Lawrence, KS

Felicia Wilkins-Turner, EdD
Mashantucket Pequot Tribal Nation
    Vocational Rehabilitation Program
Mashantucket, CT

Celestine Willis, MA
University of Illinois at Chicago
Chicago, IL

**Keith B. Wilson, PhD, CRC, NCC, ABDA,
LPC**
The Pennsylvania State University
University Park, PA

About the Editors

Fabricio E. Balcazar, PhD, is a professor in the Department of Disability and Human Development and director of the Center for Capacity Building on Minorities with Disabilities Research at the University of Illinois at Chicago. Dr. Balcazar is a community psychologist whose research interests include the promotion of culturally competent services and the empowerment of ethnically diverse populations with disabilities and their families.

Yolanda Suarez-Balcazar, PhD, is a professor and head of the Department of Occupational Therapy and codirector of the Center for Capacity Building on Minorities with Disabilities Research at the University of Illinois at Chicago. Dr. Suarez-Balcazar is a community psychologist interested in researching empowerment, participatory evaluation, and culturally competent interventions.

Tina Taylor-Ritzler, PhD, is project director of the Center for Capacity Building on Minorities with Disabilities Research at the University of Illinois at Chicago. Dr. Taylor-Ritzler's primary interest is in understanding individual, organizational, and societal factors that support and challenge the lives of people with disabilities and their families, in particular those from diverse cultural backgrounds.

Christopher B. Keys, PhD, is a professor and past chair of the Department of Psychology at DePaul University and professor emeritus and past chair of the Department of Psychology at the University of Illinois at Chicago. Dr. Keys's research interests include positive psychology and empowerment of people with disabilities and their families, with a special interest in members of diverse multicultural groups.

Acknowledgments

Support for this book was received in part by a grant from the National Institute on Disability and Rehabilitation Research (NIDRR), U.S. Department of Education, to the Center for Capacity Building on Minorities with Disabilities Research (Award #H1333A040007). Financial support was also provided by the Office of the Dean of the College of Applied Health Sciences, the Department of Disability and Human Development, and the Department of Occupational Therapy at the University of Illinois at Chicago. Additional financial support was provided by the Office of the Dean of the College of Liberal Arts and Sciences and the Department of Psychology at DePaul University.

We appreciate the valuable assistance of Kerry Maloney, Sarah Weaver, Juleen Rodakowski, Monica Ciukaj, and Edurne Garcia-Iriarte who assisted with the formatting and editing of the book. We also appreciate the clerical support of Ximena Melo-Bravo and Claudia Garcia. Finally, we thank Courtney Bates Everette and Antonio Vasquez for their contributions to the ideas presented in the Implications for Training Future Generations chapter. The opinions expressed in this book are those of the authors and not necessarily those of NIDRR or the other funding sources.

Foreword

"It is in the shelter of each other that the people live."

—Irish proverb

We are at a unique time in American history; a time in which there is an unprecedented opportunity for transformation related to race, ethnicity, and culture. One need look no further than the election of President Obama and his 2009 inauguration to see evidence of the potential for change. *Race, Culture, and Disability*, edited by Balcazar and colleagues, is a roadmap for that transformation as it relates to persons with disability and their families and caregivers. As with any good map, this text provides the reader with context, information, and direction. The direction comes in the form of multiple interdisciplinary perspectives. The four editors represent a collage of researchers and practitioners from the perspectives of disability studies and human development, occupational therapy, and psychology. They have assembled an equally diverse cast of contributors who provided 20 chapters dealing with topics in four major areas of interest: Conceptual Issues, Assessment Issues, Intervention and Service Issues, and a final section including Integrative Commentaries and Implications for Science and Practice.

In Chapter 1, the authors state that the book was developed with the purpose of informing researchers, graduate students, and practitioners in the field of rehabilitation about the status of current research and practice related to culturally diverse individuals with disabilities. The ensuing chapters include information highways outlining the conceptual themes, access to service issues, and cultural challenges that must be traversed and understood if we are to reach our ultimate destinations of cultural competence and reduced disability disparities. *Race, Culture, and Disability* is more than a roadmap describing the status of current research and practice; it is also an atlas to the (potential) future . . . a future in which the vision and goal of *Disability in America* (Pope & Tralov, 1991) will become a reality. The goal identified in 1991, to reduce the incidence and prevalence of disability in the United States, as well as the personal, social, and economic consequences of disability in order to improve the quality of life for individuals and families across all racial and ethnic groups remains relevant today. We can begin to transform this goal into a reality with the help of *Race, Culture, and Disability* and the commitment of the professionals, researchers, and consumers who will be informed and empowered by the knowledge this book contains.

—Kenneth Ottenbacher, PhD
University of Texas Medical Branch

REFERENCES

1. Pope AM, Tralov AR. Disability in America: Toward a National Agenda for Prevention. Washington, DC: National Academies Press; 1991.
2. WHO. ICF: International Classification of Functioning, Disability and Health. Geneva, Switzerland, World Health Organization; 2001.
3. Field MJ, Jette AM. The Future of Disability in America. Washington, DC: National Academies Press; 2007.

CHAPTER 1

Introduction
Examining the Nexus of Race, Culture, and Disability

Fabricio Balcazar, PhD.

INTRODUCTION

As the ethnic diversity of the population in the United States has increased, so has the number of individuals with disabilities from diverse ethnic backgrounds (Fujiura & Yamaki, 2000). Despite this increase, the topics of race, culture, and disability have rarely been examined together. *Race, Culture, and Disability: Rehabilitation Science and Practice* seeks to fill this void by bringing together the work of leading rehabilitation and disability scholars that focuses on individuals with disabilities from diverse cultural backgrounds. Prior to the publication of this book, researchers, students, and practitioners in the field of rehabilitation have sought to address questions such as: Do the experiences of people of color with disabilities differ from those of White people with disabilities? And, if so, in what ways? What factors are related to poor outcomes for people of color with disabilities receiving vocational rehabilitation (VR) services? What approaches may improve the training of new generations of culturally competent rehabilitation practitioners? What approaches might improve the services provided by practitioners already in the field? What are the next steps for research in the nexus of race, culture, and disability? Given these and other questions, this book was developed with the purpose of informing researchers, graduate students, and practitioners in the field of rehabilitation about the status of current research and practice related to culturally diverse individuals with disabilities. The book also examines conceptual themes and the nature of disparities regarding access to services and rehabilitation outcomes for people from various cultural backgrounds, offering suggestions for research, practice, and teaching.

One of the main challenges of American society as we enter the 21st century is addressing and bridging ongoing differences among our people and moving toward cooperation and solidarity. Americans need to retake the spirit that so impressed Alexis De Tocqueville when he made his observations in 1835. He saw democracy as an equation that balanced liberty and equality, and that had concern for the individual as well as for the community. On the other hand, De Tocqueville also saw the great injustices that permeated the social structure of this country when he considered the current and probable future condition of the three races that inhabited the territory of the United States at the time:

> *The first who attracts the eye, the first in enlightenment, in power and in happiness, is the white man, the European, man par excellence; below him appear the Negro and the Indian. These two unfortunate races have neither birth, nor face, nor language, nor mores in common; only their misfortunes look alike. Both occupy an equally inferior position in the country that they inhabit; both experience the effects of tyranny; and if their miseries are different, they can accuse the same author for them (De Tocqueville, 1835).*

Today, racial differences have been exacerbated by growing economic inequality, leaving poor and underserved communities with limited access to quality employment, education, healthcare, transportation, housing, and other services that impact people's lives. Religious and political differences continue to make it difficult for people to communicate with one another. The dominance of ableism marginalizes people with disabilities and limits their access to employment and other opportunities for full participation in society. Given these many challenges, individuals and service systems need to take greater responsibility for changing the ways in which they interact with individuals with disabilities from different cultural backgrounds.

Racism and its legacy have proven difficult to eradicate. To begin to eradicate racism, individual- and systems-level awareness and knowledge are needed. People of all races need to become aware of their role in maintaining and challenging the status quo. Kivel (2002) makes a good point when discussing the responsibility of White people in a racist society. He says, "You did not choose your skin color, native language, or culture. You are not responsible for being White or for being raised in a White-dominated, racist society. . . . You are responsible for how you respond to racism" (p.12). But White people are not the only ones who discriminate. People of all races, classes, and colors discriminate against each other. African Americans of darker skin color are often looked down upon by those with lighter skin. I grew up in a society, like many others, that discriminated against people on the basis of many different features, particularly social class. People could be discriminated against not only for the color of their skin, but for the brands of clothes they wore, which were a symbol of class status. People were also discriminated against because of the way they talked, the neighborhood they lived in, the brand of car they drove, or the school they attended. Almost any aspect of life—including last names—could be used to set people apart from others and make them endure differential treatment. Disability—especially if it was visible—was another source of discrimination and marginalization. So, it becomes apparent the importance of one's culture and its influence on how we interact with each other.

As pointed out by Talley and Donnell (2007), "culture impacts all aspects of our lives, from the way we perceive ourselves, others, and our environment, to the way that we assess and respond to the situations and individuals we encounter" (p. 71). In American society, culture has gained prominence as we struggle with the issue of cultural assimilation versus cultural pluralism. Sue raised several important questions about this issue: Should we advocate Americanization of new immigrants or should we allow ethnic customs, traditions, and diverse cultures to flourish? Is it advisable for immigrants to acculturate in order to enhance functioning? Or should we advocate pluralism, promoting the co-existence of distinct cultural groups in society? There are no simple answers to these questions. Sue (2003) concluded that the environment in which people function has a direct effect on how comfortable people feel about their culture and their interactions with individuals from other cultures.

The growing cultural and racial/ethnic diversity of our nation forces us to engage with individuals who are different from us. Our degree of familiarity with people from various racial/ethnic and cultural groups depends, in part, on our degree of exposure to diversity, our willingness to notice and learn from others who may be different from us, and our desire to enrich our own perspective and culture. We struggle with the term *minority* because it has been associated with the notions of inferiority and deficits. Sue (2003) argues that "the concept of minority implies that a majority exists, but one could argue that the United States has no real ethnic majority groups because Whites can be classified as a mix of many different ethnic groups and Whites are not the majority in the world." (p. xx). Sue emphasizes that the "minority" status of American Indians, African Americans, Asian Americans, and Latinos is not solely a function of their own cultures or of value discrepancies with mainstream Americans; rather, members of these groups have experienced historical and contemporary forms of prejudice and discrimination that led to their marginalization. Therefore, in this book we have used the terms "diverse" and "multicultural" to refer to the members of ethnic and racial groups in American culture.

Disability is another key human difference that has led to historical discrimination and marginalization. Devlieger, Rusch, and Pfeiffer (2003) indicated that people with disabilities have been portrayed and researched in many ways. These trends, they add, have been ideological, reflecting the role of history on the relationship between a universal phenomenon and a context from which the meaning of disability is constructed. Rehabilitation for individuals with disabilities is a process of helping them function as effectively as possible in their daily lives and helping them become independent and/or productive (Crabtree, Royeen, & Benton, 2006). To recognize that independence, we use the terms "person with a disability" or "people with disabilities." These terms recognize that the person is primary and thus more important than the disability and that the individual is an independent human being and not fundamentally in the role of a patient, client, or consumer. Crabtree et al. suggest that cultural proficiency in rehabilitation is necessary for practitioners in order to be able to effectively interact with individuals with disabilities from diverse ethnic/cultural groups and to be able to understand their personal wishes, beliefs, preferences, choices, expectations, and values. Crabtree et al. conclude the following:

> *At best, the potential lack of agreement on basic values, beliefs, or attitudes complicates the issues that must be addressed for successful outcomes and confounds the rehabilitation practitioner's efforts to provide competent and effective services. At worst, conflict between ethnic and cultural beliefs, values and attitudes undermine the best intentions of rehabilitation practitioners and the efforts of consumers to lead lives that for them are consistent with their own ethnic and cultural beliefs and values. (p. 4)*

Despite the complexities of the topics of race, culture, and disability in the United States, there are very few books that are dedicated to rehabilitation research and practice as they relate to these topics. This book attempts to help researchers, graduate students, and practitioners address theoretical, practical, and research-based questions by helping them ground their future work in what we currently know about the intersect of race, culture, and disability and its implications for rehabilitation science and practice.

OUTLINE OF THE BOOK

This book is the result of a process of engaging leading rehabilitation researchers in sharing their current work in a national conference organized by the Center for Capacity Building on Minorities with Disabilities Research at the University of Illinois at Chicago and held in Chicago in July, 2007. The conference brought together approximately 100 leading scholars in the field of rehabilitation of individuals with disabilities from diverse ethnic and/or cultural groups and related areas of study. The conference served as a working meeting in the preparation of the book as chapter authors engaged in discussion of their work. The resulting book is organized into four sections:

SECTION I: The Nature of the Scientific Research at the Nexus of Race, Culture, and Disability

This section sets up the conceptual framework for the discussion of issues related to the nexus of race, culture, and disability. It provides an overview of how rehabilitation researchers are addressing these issues and reviews the parallels between the development of African American identity and disability identity.

Fujiura and Drazen review the concept of research focused on the intersection of race and disability. Their analysis of the literature originated from a sense that disability and rehabilitation scholars have yet to engage in a systematic dialogue over the meaning of race and ethnicity in their research. The authors ask how research questions translate into different forms of thinking about the nexus of race, culture, and disability. This chapter examines in detail three possible responses to this question: (a) studies of the efficacy of an intervention on racial or ethnic minority samples; (b) studies in which race, disability, or a combination is implicitly framed as the independent variable; and (c) queries about how race, disability, or a combination moderates or mediates other cause and effect relationships.

Gill and Cross examine points of convergence, divergence, and interplay among racial/cultural identity development and disability identity development. The authors discuss three patterns of socialization and identity acquisition in the African American community (viz.,, traditional, conversion as resocialization, and recycling). These patterns are contrasted with current research on disability identity development. The authors conclude with ideas for practice suggested by links between disability identity and black identity (e.g., acknowledging diversity within the group; accepting that disability can be a stimulus of community-building, pride, and culture; and considering in-group representation and issues of power).

SECTION II: The Nature of Disparities in Outcomes for Multicultural Populations with Disabilities

This section has seven chapters, starting with analyses of issues that cross racial/ethnic cultural groups, like the appropriateness of psychological assessments for people of color, access to VR services for people of color, challenges for providing culturally appropriate care, and challenges in providing psychiatric care. The section ends with population specific issues, like employment challenges for Native Americans and women of color with disabilities, and the challenges in accessing VR services for Asian Pacific Americans with disabilities.

Hernandez et al. examine the appropriateness of four commonly used psychological tests when assessing people of color with disabilities [i.e., the Wechsler Adult Intelligence Scale (WAIS III); the Minnesota Multiphasic Personality Inventory (MMPI); the Rorschach Inkblot Test (RIT); and the Beck Depression Inventory (BDI)]. The authors consider the extent to which these tests have been standardized with culturally diverse populations and examine the reliability and validity of the instruments. The authors also review the empirical studies related to theses tests and the performance of multiethnic populations on the tests (namely African Americans, Asian Americans, Latinos, and Native Americans).

Wilson and Senices hypothesize that skin color could be a predictor of rehabilitation outcomes. In order to support their point, the authors examined data on Black Latinos' outcomes within the VR system. The authors discuss the implications of colorism in VR practice and research. They acknowledge the need to expand the research in this area, including more objective measures of people's skin color given that most studies utilize subjective measures (self reports) that could be unreliable.

Hill-Briggs et al. address issues that apply to the inpatient physical medicine and rehabilitation care of African Americans. First, they examine the challenges of diagnostic accuracy, appropriateness, and effectiveness of treatments with African Americans from the broader mental health literature. Second, they consider how to provide culturally proficient psychological care to African Americans in rehabilitation. Third, they offer three examples of promising health-related research directions leading to more effective assessment and intervention with African Americans. They suggest that these approaches can be adapted to rehabilitation settings serving people with disabilities. Finally, they propose a research agenda for further examining disparities and developing evidence-based practice for delivering effective care to African Americans in inpatient rehabilitation settings.

Cook et al. define cultural competence in the field of mental health and discuss six ways in which specific features of mental illness and its sociocultural context create challenges for mental health and rehabilitation professionals working with people with psychiatric disabilities from different cultures. These include: (a) cultural variations in the view of mental illness; (b) cultural diversity in help-seeking behaviors for mental health difficulties; (c) cultural variations in the use of language and verbal communication; (d) cultural attitudes toward the use of Western psychotropic medications; (e) lack of cultural diversity in the mental health workforce; and (f) use of indigenous healers for mental health problems. The authors argue that unless the fields of mental health and rehabilitation begin to address some of these issues specifically and concretely, attempts to assess and promote cultural competence will miss the mark and recovery of individuals with psychiatric disabilities will continue to lag behind that of individuals with other types of disabilities and medical conditions.

Clay et al. examine inadequacies in the infrastructure for supporting the employment of Native Americans and Alaska Natives with disabilities. They argue that these challenges must be addressed to create sufficient employment and rehabilitation opportunities for tribal members with disabilities. They propose that this can be accomplished through partnerships across tribal sectors but warn that solutions cannot be imposed from the outside. Rather, tribes need to address gaps in employment infrastructure, including utilizing technical assistance to develop solutions that fit their circumstances, which are culturally relevant and respect tribal sovereignty. The authors propose the Tribal Disability Actualization Process (TDAP), which is a model for self-directed disability and rehabilitation service development.

Smith and Alston argue that there is a dearth of research focusing on issues of employment and rehabilitation of women of color with disabilities. Their chapter presents information regarding employment issues of women with disabilities. Also explored are issues concerning women, ethnically diverse individuals with disabilities, and women with disabilities in general. The authors propose a supply and demand approach for employment of women of color with disabilities. Finally, the authors make some suggestions for rehabilitation professionals regarding how best to address some of the issues faced by women of color with disabilities in a culturally sensitive manner.

Hasnain and Leung present an overview of the issues experienced by Asian Pacific Americans in dealing with vocational and other rehabilitation service systems. They start by pointing out the complexity of this racial category, which includes multiple and diverse countries of origin, different migratory experiences over time, and multiple variations in culture and ethnic identification. The authors consider the reasons why this group is underserved, under-reached, and under-researched, despite or perhaps in part because of the misconceptions about being the "model minority group." They also examine cultural issues among these groups, such as beliefs about disability and perceptions of stigma and shame associated with it, reliance on the family for support, and the role of acculturation.

SECTION III: Models to Improve Rehabilitation Services for Multicultural Populations with Disabilities

This section includes six chapters divided into two subsections. The first subsection includes three chapters and refers to *Models for training rehabilitation providers in postsecondary and professional training programs.* This includes the formation of future rehabilitation professionals in university settings and the training of students and professionals on ethical issues.

Matteliano and Stone identify educational approaches that could be effective in preparing future service providers to work with clients from other cultures. They first review data on immigration trends and the ethnosocial composition within the rehabilitation profession, and then briefly review the definitions of cultural competence and some of the conceptual models that guide rehabilitation practice. The chapter also includes a brief review of measurement instruments of cultural competence, pointing out the scarcity of outcome measures in this area. The authors describe their approach for teaching cultural competence at the college level, which includes: (a) integrating cultural competency into existing courses; (b) developing a cultural competence curriculum that is profession-specific rather than generic; (c) utilizing multidisciplinary case studies for students to practice; and (d) making the materials widely available to instructors.

Lewis and Shamburger propose a three-factor model to help VR counselors determine what to consider in order to provide effective services to consumers who are culturally different from the counselor. The factors require counselors to consider: (a) the developmental stage of the consumer; (b) the stage of cultural identification of the consumer; and (c) the way in which the consumer defines optimal adjustment to the impairment. There are also some key activities that aid in establishing a positive relationship with the consumer by learning who the consumer is, and by determining the fit between the counselor and the consumer. The authors provide several strategies that counselors can use to implement the model with their current consumers and examples of model implementation with different consumer groups.

Garcia describes theoretical, ethical decision-making models and summarizes empirical research geared toward evaluating or testing these models from a multicultural perspective. The author discusses potential applications of these models, particularly the trans-cultural integrative model that he developed. He provides examples to illustrate how the model works and summarizes some of the main findings from an evaluation of the model with 60 VR counselors who participated in the study. Finally, the author addresses the implications of the current research for educators and practitioners, as well as the need to conduct research that expands knowledge about multicultural ethics.

The second subsection, *Models for rehabilitation practice,* also includes three chapters. These address models of cultural competence training of rehabilitation professionals in the field, a culturally and contextually grounded model for evaluation capacity building, and a systems approach to placement for culturally diverse individuals with disabilities.

Balcazar et al. provide a rationale for promoting cultural competence, analyze the various definitions of cultural competence, and conduct a systematic review of existing cultural competence models in the fields of health, counseling, and rehabilitation. The authors identified 18 cultural competence models and based on their analysis,

propose a model that synthesizes the most common components of the models identified in the literature. The authors also identified 23 factors that influence diversity
(both observable factors such as race, gender, age, appearance, or physical disability
and non-observable factors such as level of education, degree of acculturation,
socioeconomic status, etc). The authors conclude that cultural competence is a
process of "becoming" that implies both a desire and a professional obligation to
effectively serve individuals from different cultures.

Suarez-Balcazar et al. provide a culturally- and contextually-grounded framework of
evaluation intended to build the capacity of organizations to track outcomes for people with disabilities from diverse backgrounds. Based on an analysis of the literature,
the authors proposed a framework for evaluation capacity building that includes
organizational (viz.,., leadership, climate, learning, and resources) and individual
factors (viz.,,, readiness, motivation, and competence). These factors are grounded in
contextual and cultural factors (viz.,., cultural competence, funders' pressures for
evaluation, changes in consumer's needs, public opinion, and geographic location).
The authors present an example gleaned from a community-based organization
serving primarily Latino individuals with developmental disabilities. They conclude
that the framework allows individuals to recognize the complexity of the cultural
and sociopolitical environment that surrounds and influences the organization and
its evaluation activities.

Kundu and Dutta describe a contextually sensitive systems theory as it is applied to
the placement process of culturally diverse people with disabilities.. The process
gives credence to two instruments: A Systems Approach to Placement: Self-
Assessment by Students and Counselors (SAP: SASC) and the Systems Approach to
Placement: Intake Assessment and Outcome Evaluation (SAP: IAOE). The SAP:
SASC identifies the training needs of students and professionals of diverse backgrounds. The SAP: IAOE identifies the holistic service needs of individuals with
disabilities. It also assists in developing a functional individualized plan for employment for optimal service delivery, and increases the probability of long-term placement outcomes.

SECTION IV: Integrative Commentaries

This book is enriched by the perspectives of the scientists who conduct research, the
practitioners who work with people with disabilities from diverse backgrounds and
the students and recent graduates who have learned and want to learn more about
this area of work. These perspectives are presented in three commentaries.

Arango et al. consider the potential impact of the chapters on the directions for future research and theory development in the field of rehabilitation. They conclude by emphasizing the need to focus research on individual, system, and community level changes regarding the services and supports provided to individuals from diverse backgrounds.

Garate et al. examine the practical applications of the chapters from the perspective of a VR counselor, two Centers for Independent Living advocates, and a special educator. They emphasize the importance of helping service providers address the needs of culturally diverse individuals with disabilities.

Rodakowski et al. reflect on the previous chapters in discussing opportunities and challenges related to conducting research with culturally diverse populations with disabilities and examine the implications for the training of future researchers and practitioners in the field of rehabilitation.

Keys concludes by reflecting on how the science in this important intersection of race, culture, and disability has clearly demonstrated major disparities in service access, retention, and outcomes for people with disabilities from diverse backgrounds. He suggests that current research, training, and practice can be improved by adopting and building upon the work presented in this book. This work involves integrating the complexities of disability into the research to complement the developing complexities in our understanding of racial and ethnic diversity. It also concerns integrating cultural insights about race/ethnicity and disability into our educational, practice, ethical decision–making, and evaluation activities in rehabilitation.

This book identifies disparities in outcomes for ethnically diverse individuals with disabilities, a critical challenge facing rehabilitation systems and professionals today, and suggests strategies to improve rehabilitation services for this population. This book is of interest to current rehabilitation scholars and graduate students seeking to understand research and practical issues related to race, culture, and disability. It is also of interest to those looking to improve rehabilitation services for individuals with disabilities from ethnic minority backgrounds. The book serves as the leading source on the research knowledge for scholars, faculty teaching courses on diversity issues, graduate students, and professionals who seek to understand the nature of the disparities in outcomes between individuals with disabilities from diverse cultural backgrounds and strategies for addressing these disparities. It is our intent that this volume will move the field forward and contribute to improving the quality of life of people with disabilities from diverse backgrounds.

REFERENCES

Crabtree, J. L., Royeen, M., & Benton, J. (2006). Cultural proficiency in rehabilitation: An introduction. In M. Royeen & J. L. Crabtree, *Culture in rehabilitation: From competency to proficiency* Upper Saddle River, NJ: Pearson Prentice Hall.

De Tocqueville, A. (1835). *Democracy in America.* Retrieved October 12, 2008, from *http://xroads .virginia.edu/~HYPER/DETOC/1_ch18.htm*

Devlieger, P., Rusch, F., & Pfeiffer, D. (2003). Rethinking disability as same and different: Toward a cultural model of disability. In P. Devlieger, F. Rusch, & D. Pfeiffer (Eds.), *Rethinking disability: The emergence of new definitions, concepts and communities* (pp. 9–16). Antwerp, Belgium: Garant.

Fujiura, G. T., & Yamaki, K. (2000). Trends in demography of childhood poverty and disability. *Exceptional Children, (2),* 187–99.

Kivel, P. (2002). *Uprooting racism: How white people can work for racial justice.* Philadelphia, PA: New Society Publishers.

Sue, S. (2003). Foreword. In K. M. Chun, P. B. Organista, & G. Marin (Eds.), *Acculturation: Advances in theory, measurement, and applied research* (pp. xvii–xxi). Washington, DC: American Psychological Association.

Talley, W., & Donnell, C. (2007). Preparing culturally competent practitioners for rehabilitation and allied health. In P. Leung, C. R. Flowers, W. B. Talley, & P. R Sanderson (Eds.) *Multicultural issues in rehabilitation and allied health.* Linn Creek, MO: Aspen Professional Services.

The Nature of Scientific Research at the Nexus of Race, Culture, and Disability

CHAPTER 2

"Ways of Seeing" in Race and Disability Research

Glenn T. Fujiura, PhD and
Carlos Drazen, MS

INTRODUCTION

The following review presents a conceptual overview of race and disability research drawn from the fields of rehabilitation, education, history, cultural studies, public health, and medicine. Our focus is on the assumptions, rationales, and functions of research rather than the content or details of methodology. This approach emerges from a sense that rehabilitation and disability scholars have yet to engage in a systematic dialogue over the meaning of race and ethnicity in research. There is no single point of entry for researchers interested in the study of the intersection of race and disability. Rather, multiple disciplines representing an array of perspectives on inquiry have been employed in the body of work over the years. The intent of the review is to provide scholars, particularly new researchers, with a template for organizing how research problems have been conceptualized in this area. Despite all of the attention devoted to the topic, the ways in which race is relevant to the disability dialogue remain very much a matter of debate. In effect, have we really reflected on our constructions of race in the research questions we ask? In the following review we considered these constructions across three dimensions: (a) the traditions of research represented in the literature, (b) functions served by the research questions, and (c) the construction of the nexus in the questions. We conclude with an analysis and a summary of how these dimensions are represented across the body of contemporary research.

RESEARCH QUESTIONS AND TRADITIONS OF INQUIRY

During the 1980's, interest in alternative methodologies led to what has been called the "paradigm wars". These were debates focusing on the merits of alternative traditions of inquiry, and typically presented in terms of the relative merits of the quantitative and qualitative research traditions (Gage, 1989). Although the quantitative–qualitative distinction is still commonly applied, the dichotomy fails to reflect the true diversity of research on the nexus of race and disability.

Research texts were examined to learn more about the traditions of the paradigm wars. The search yielded a veritable forest of "isms" describing models, doctrines, philosophies, systems, or theories describing ways of knowing, including: constructivism, holism, interpretivism, phenomenologicalism, positivism, revisionism, relativism, structural-functionalism, technocentrism, and the assorted post-, pre-, and pseudo- variations. At some risk of oversimplification the central differences across perspectives can be reduced to three variations in emphasis: (a) postpositivism with its emphasis on objectivity and verifiable knowledge (the postpositivist, as opposed to the positivist, accepts the potentially biasing effects of the human researcher); (b) constructivism with its emphasis on meanings and other subjective representations; and (c) transformative inquiries, a hybrid term coined by Mertens (2005) to describe a class of approaches anchored on understanding the "social, political, cultural, economic, ethnic, gender, and disability values in the construction of reality" (Mertens, p. 23). These perspectives represent approaches sensitive to different facets of a given social phenomenon. Furthermore, differences among perspectives are often more a matter of degree rather than a matter of kind. To emphasize meanings and values in research, for example, is not necessarily tantamount to rejecting the importance of objectivity.

Postpositivist Constructions

Experimental, or causal, thinking is at the heart of research on race and disability. The process and logic of experimental concepts were developed by John Stuart Mill, the 19th century philosopher, and should be familiar to students of the social sciences. These concepts include: (a) causes precede effects in time; (b) when causes are present, effects will be present; (c) when causes are absent, effects are absent; and (d) when two phenomenons are observed to co-vary, they are associated in some manner (Campbell & Stanley, 1963; Dewey, 1931). The essence of experimental conceptualization is comparative: A variable that is being measured under two or more conditions is held constant, to the greatest extent possible, in all respects except for the variables being tested. Differences in the outcome are attributed to the differences in the independent variables. This basic scheme can be expanded into literally hundreds of design options.

The notion that experimental thinking is central to our conceptions of race and disability research may strike those familiar with the research as a serious misrepresentation; there are precious few studies involving direct manipulation of an independent variable by the researcher, or use of randomly assigned subjects to treatment and control conditions, which are key features of experimental methodology. Even the well-designed quasi-experimental efforts (i.e., studies not employing random assignment but capable of controlling most threats to internal validity) are rare. Nonexperimental methods such as surveys, interviews, archival analyses, and naturalistic observation, to name just a few, represent the dominant resources in the toolkits of researchers in the area. Nevertheless, experimental concepts very much affect our ways of thinking about the phenomenon of race and disability. Much, although not all, of the race and disability research has emerged from social science-based disciplines where the experimental method is held as the paragon for inquiry. Not coincidentally, the orientation dominates the research training curricula in most subdisciplines of the social sciences. Research coursework tends to emphasize experimental design, and statistical instruction largely focuses on the analysis of data derived from experimental studies. How does experimental thinking translate into questions about the nexus of race and disability? We observe three variations: (a) studies of the efficacy of an intervention on racial or ethnic minority samples; (b) studies in which race, disability, or a combination is implicitly framed as the independent variable; and (c) queries about how race, disability, or a combination moderates or mediates other cause and effect relationships.

The first group of studies is the most direct and appropriate application of experimental thinking in race and disability. They are experimental in intent and design. The questions are framed around the role of race in mediation intervention effectiveness (e.g., "Does the intervention efficacy interact with race and/or disability?"; Taylor, Baranowski, & Young, 1998), or are questions about the efficacy of interventions designed specifically for racial or ethnic minority groups or issues (Taylor-Ritzler et al., 2001). Causal inference is established by maximizing the similarity of the conditions via design controls, and then directly manipulating the intervention.

Not all causal questions are manifested in experimental designs. In the second form of questions, a broad array of dependent variables is compared across race or ethnic groups. Examples include employment rates (Meade, Lewis, Jackson, & Hess, 2004), health (Furner, Giloth, Arguelles, Miles, & Goldberg, 2004), relationships with rehabilitation professionals (Wintersteen, Mensinger, & Diamond, 2005), earnings and benefits (Lustig & Strauser, 2004), multiple sclerosis-associated disability (Marrie, Cutter, Tyry, Vollmer, & Campagnolo, 2006), and well-being after injury (Krause, Broderick, Saladin, & Broyles, 2006), among others. Implicit in the framing of each question is whether a disparity exists and if race or ethnic groups account, directly or indirectly, for the difference.

The third and largest variation in experimental frameworks is represented in queries about how race, disability, or combinations thereof are affected by other variables, or mediate other presumed causes. Study methodologies range from pre- and post-test designs using race as the group variable, to large scale cross-sectional surveys evaluated with multivariate statistical techniques. The concept of mediation is an old one in behavioral research (Baron & Kenny, 1986) and refers to a variable intervening between a presumed cause and the outcome variable of interest. Capella (2002), for example, critiqued much of the body of the rehabilitation outcome research for not accounting for the effects of other variables in addition to racial or ethnic groupings. While his analysis of vocational rehabilitation (VR) outcomes still found group differences, the degree of difference was affected by gender, age, and severity of the impairment. Similarly, Giesen, Cavenaugh, and Sansing (2004) found differences varying across forms of impairment, with greater access to the VR system among African Americans with visual impairments. In these studies, racial and ethnic group differences are mediated through other personal characteristics such as impairment, severity, or gender. Other examples of research questions directed to the mediating effect of racial groups include: (a) quality of care (Richardson, Anderson, Flaherty, & Bell, 2003); (b) pain-related disability (Edwards, Moric, Husfeldt, Buvanendran, & Ivankovich, 2005); (c) restrictiveness of school placement (Hosp & Reschly, 2002); and (d) VR outcomes (Moore, Feist-Price, & Alston, 2002; Warren, Giesen, & Cavenaugh, 2004).

Constructivist Approaches

Constructivism is employed here to represent a broad class of inquiry that embraces human subjectivity. The notion that an empirical reality exists apart from human consciousness is rejected. Silverman, Smola, and Musa's (2000) interviews with older African American and White research participants is prototypical of the approach. The essential question was one of "meanings" attached to the concept of "healthy" and "not healthy," and the potential effect of culture on these perceptions. The subjective experience of the participant was the point of the analysis. Other examples include King, Teplicky, King, and Rosenbaum's (2004) exploration of disability and religion in the Black church using interviews, or Dossa's (2005) case study of a female activist who was Muslim and disabled. Consider the character of their questions and the purposes served by their framing. King et al. asked how the Black church affected the disability experience of its disabled members; Dossa asked how overlapping identities relate to each other and their contexts. While the postpositivists frame questions in terms of a reduced set of variables in order to better control extraneous explanations and isolate causal effects, the constructivist embraces complexity and subjectivity. Reality is socially constructed and thus can only be understood through the experiences of those we study. The researcher does not attempt to control the internal world, but rather seeks to be an interpreter of human experience.

Transformative Applications

Mertens (2005) employs the "transformative label" to describe studies focused on examining social, cultural, and historical influences on our knowing. The classification provides an imperfect fit in the three-way taxonomy; research can readily overlap with constructivist and postpositivist perspectives, and does not do justice to the nuances of many forms of research falling under the transformative label, such as critical inquiry, or historical research. Nonetheless, the category is very useful for our analysis of race and disability research since an important core of work that has emerged over the past few decades has focused on challenging the basis of both our political and cultural understandings of disability and race.

An example of this concept is presented in Ferri and Connor's (2005) exploration of contemporary resistance to school inclusion for children with disabilities. The investigators portray the resistance as an extension of the racism seen in the efforts to desegregate schools in response to the Supreme Court's Brown decision. In their analysis of what they referred to as the "discourses of exclusion" (p. 468), Ferri and Connor argue that disability inclusion and racial desegregation are intimately related, with special education serving as a new institutional mechanism for maintaining the status quo. Balcazar, Garate-Serafini, and Keys' (2004) application of an empowerment intervention for low-income minority youths with disabilities provides a wonderful juxtaposition of perspectives. Although seemingly constructed as a standard pre- and post-test intervention study, the study question, intervention design, and study purpose were anchored in the framework of social oppression (Freire, 1970). The intervention and study purpose focused on shifting power relationships, and the role of the investigators was explicitly framed in terms of agents of social change. This is a far cry from the public persona of the researcher as the detached observer.

Summary: Research Questions and Traditions of Inquiry

The thematic threads of the different traditions, and the overlap in their applications should suggest a continuum along which all forms of inquiry lie. The study of race and disability must be a broadly conceived effort such that our interpretations of the phenomenon under study are not confounded with the methods employed in studying it. The human visual system is an excellent metaphor for the research task. Our visual system does not *see* so much as *reconstruct* a visual representation of the external world; much like the research enterprise, images are complementary parts of the whole.

The vast majority of studies are experimental in construction, although exploratory in intent. Their purpose is to identify disparities across groups, or to better understand how differences across racial groupings interact with other collateral variables such as impairment or economic status. This approach makes sense, at least from the perspective that our efforts remain at a very early stage of development: The studies attempt to impose conceptual order on phenomena not well understood. Although this is an extremely important heuristic function, it is merely the outer shell of inquiry. The fact of differences across groups defined by race and/or ethnicity is only the starting point.

This is an important perspective to maintain when evaluating the body of literature. For example, Helms, Jernigan, and Mascher (2005) cogently argue for the replacement of racial categories in research designs with other more meaningful variables than race such as identity or social categories. And while we agree that race is an imperfect and often irrelevant variable, their recommendation for alternative groupings is only a partial solution to the study of race and disability. Our brief summary of approaches, broadly labeled as post-positivist, constructivist, and transformative work, should illustrate how the framing of problems as group differences is only one facet of the phenomenon.

This is not a critique of the experimental approach, but rather a cautionary note about framing the research question. Attempts to identify differences based on group identity or to isolate the most important predictor may not lead to the most relevant research question. The answers drawn from studying such research questions should be interpreted for what they are—efforts to isolate patterns of relationships amidst a noisy environment of unknown complexity. The critical point is that the researcher acknowledges both the complexity of the phenomenon under study, and the limitations of the particular question addressed.

THE FUNCTIONS SERVED BY RESEARCH QUESTIONS

For those interested in the broad view of disability and race, the better question may be what functions the questions serve. Among the various taxonomies employed in the research literature, a very broad three-way taxonomy modified from Lieberson (1985) is particularly useful: (a) description and fact-finding; (b) identifying patterns; and (c) theory testing. Excluded here from Lieberson's taxonomy is his fourth function, suggesting policy, since relevance to policy in the body of disability research arguably is implied in virtually all disability research efforts.

Description and Fact-Finding

Fact-finding is one of the most common forms of inquiry and is organized around the systematic documentation of differences between racial and ethnic groups. A consistent theme in disability and race research is the ongoing effort to measure and report population size or group status on various indicators relevant to disability policy: educational achievement (Bound, Burkhauser, & Nichols, 2001), employment (Meade et al., 2004), poverty (Fujiura & Yamaki, 2000), prevalence (Manton & Gu,

2001), and many others. Many of the basic comparative studies cited in the previous section can also be described as serving the fact-finding function. The associated question is simple: Is there a difference on some indicator between groups defined by race and ethnicity? Although the question is simple, the implications are potentially profound. Consider the visibility given to annual poverty statistics. Prior to the development of the poverty line in the 1960s and the description of the proportion of Americans living in poverty, the issue was largely invisible in the national policy deliberations and politics (Batchelder, 1966). Basic description serves a foundational role in identifying needs and isolating issues to be addressed through additional research. Thus, the question represents the first and foundational form of inquiry. While debates over the validity of racial categories are an important scientific issue (Helms et al., 2005), racial groupings remain a potent category for the purposes of policy and politics, and statistical descriptions of these groups serve to inform the debates.

Patterns

The second function the research focus shifts to is the identification of patterns: associations among variables or regularities that might be invoked as explanatory mechanisms to account for the phenomenon of interest (the word, explanatory, is employed here in its most common denotation). As noted in the previous section, the vast majority of studies of race and disability typify this approach. The identification of patterns encompasses an admittedly wide range of research questions, ranging from ethnographically-oriented descriptive studies (Devlieger & Albrecht, 2000) to direct tests of relationships predicted by formal models (Adams & Boscarino, 2005). In Devlieger and Albrecht's qualitative narrative of African Americans with disabilities in Chicago for example, they explored the disability identity in the context of inner-city life, noting common themes and relating them to identification. The intent of the study was to obtain a more simple description; the authors attempted to develop possible explanatory mechanisms for understanding the cultural basis of disability identity. Here, the descriptive question can be viewed as serving a hypothesis discovery function in which the raw data of description is used to identify associations among variables in an area of inquiry relatively unknown. The distinction between the gathering of facts and hypothesis discovery is subtle and arguably more conceptual than real since a subordinate objective for most fact-finding researchers is the identification of themes and the proposal of causal models. Indeed, all of the examples of descriptive research cited in the preceding section could reasonably be employed as examples here.

At the other end of the continuum are studies that are essentially exploratory but within the limits of a theoretical structure. In Adams and Boscarino's (2005) analysis of the relationship between race and posttraumatic stress disorder (PTSD), a widely used stress process model was employed to frame the question and guide variable selection (Thoits, 1995). The model suggests that demographic or social resources can affect stress reactions, and subsequently predicts greater PTSD among minorities. Thus, the researcher brings to bear upon the exploration an a priori model and explanatory template. Adams and Boscarino employed past research and theoretical rationale to strategically constrain a potentially vast variable set. Theory helped to organize the inquiry; however, the adequacy of the theory was of only secondary interest. The authors did not bother to comment on the adequacy of the model, despite finding no differences between racial and ethnic groups with PTSD.

Theory Testing

The distinction between the theory-testing function and questions articulated in the framework of formal models is again one of degree rather than kind. The distinguishing feature is the centrality of theory to the study's purpose. Unfortunately, we cannot bring to bear a study on race and disability whose research question is defined in both construction and intent by an underlying theoretical framework. Although theoretically driven, theory-testing research is not necessarily bound to any specific research methodology; it is most closely associated with the experimental method. Deductive logic begins with testable propositions derived from theory, and facts are marshaled in direct tests of theoretical expectations. This is the paradigm of the physical sciences so often held as the exemplar for social inquiry. The relationship between experimental logic and the theory-testing functions of research is a close one because both are essentially reductionist and explanatory in character. Ironically, it is Hernandez's (2005) qualitative study of disability identity among young men with acquired spinal cord injury that comes closest to a theory-testing question. Organized around Gill's (1997) model of disability identity development, Hernandez identified in her findings support for Gill's model as well as points of inconsistencies.

Summary: Functions Served by Research Questions

The purpose of this brief discussion is to make explicit what should be apparent from even casual inspection of the literature on disability and race, that research serves multiple and equally valuable functions. No doubt, the vast majority of scholars engaged in the field would agree. It is not a new or radical idea that inquiry has many forms and basic assumptions. The point of the foregoing discussion is not to denigrate or promote one approach over the other. Rather, researchers must carefully consider the purposes of the inquiry and connect them in an optimal manner to the different ways of knowing represented in different methodological approaches.

THE CONSTRUCTION OF QUESTIONS AROUND DISABILITY AND RACE

Both disability and race are contested concepts (Fujiura & Rutkowski-Kmitta, 2001; Omi, 2001); their intersection certainly overlays nuance onto complexity. The range of relevant domains and disciplines is daunting. In the absence of disciplinary boundaries, one is confronted with the task of connecting ideas across multiple domains of inquiry, each operating within its own conceptual framework. The utility of race in research remains embroiled in controversy, most notably in terms of its relationship to health and medicine (Anderson & Nickerson, 2005; Freeman, 1998; Lee, Mountain, & Koenig, 2001). The essential critique revolves around the disjuncture between public policy and the underlying biology of race, which suggests the lack of biological utility in race groupings. There are, of course, significant medical and health status disparities across racial lines, and virtually all critics of race as a basis of classification acknowledge these differences. The fact that race exists as a social rather than a biological construct does not lessen the reality of how it articulates with the basic indices of well-being in American society (Omi). Minow's (1990) reference to the "dilemma of difference" is relevant to our discussion here. Attention to the construct of race may facilitate movement toward equity or result in greater stigmatization, and thus the "racialization" of research is not to be taken lightly. Great thought must be given to the conceptual construction of research. The design and analysis of studies using racial groupings can be relatively straightforward, but the real challenge is in how the interpretations are managed.

How have researchers approached the nexus of race with disability? Employing a concept mapping approach (Trochim, 1989), we evaluated published articles incorporating the themes of race and disability from the fields of rehabilitation, education, history, cultural studies, public health, and medicine, among others. Excluded from consideration was a very large body of research in which race was included as a variable but was incidental to the core purpose of the research. Although racial groupings often figure prominently in these types of analyses, the inclusion of racial or ethnic groups was primarily to assess generalization (Clark, Stump, & Wolinsky, 1997; Jaffee et al., 2005) or to control for potential confounds related to racial status. Concept mapping is a general approach to the generation and organization of a topic or construct rather than a specific set of techniques (Trochim, 2001); for our purposes the mapping was based on an iterative series of structured evaluations of studies. Each review involved developing a label describing: (a) the study function, (b) how the author(s) conceptualized the nexus of race and disability in the study's research question, and (c) the tradition of inquiry represented in the study methodology. For some studies, discussion was required to reach consensus on the label. Labels were revised where necessary when subsequent reviews revealed new perspectives, and preliminary pictorial representations, or maps, were drawn identifying each of the labels and their hypothesized interrelationships. A final map was arrived at relatively quickly and subsequent reviews were employed to challenge the adequacy of the map as a classification tool (see Figure 2-1). The intent was not to exhaustively review the literature but rather to identify a comprehensive taxonomy to describe the construction of research questions. Each study was evaluated on the basis of this question: How do the investigators construct the nexus of race and disability in their research questions? In effect, research questions represent our raw data.

Three core constructions were identified through which the interaction of race and disability is interrogated: (a) What is the nature of disparity?; (b) What is the role of culture?; and (c) What is the meaning of race and disability? Within each of these broad lines of inquiry, questions cluster around a larger number of research sub-themes. The identification and analysis of disparities was the dominant basis for research and includes the group comparison studies and meditational research described in the foregoing sections. Culture is an admittedly broad construct and includes such diverse efforts as evaluations of culturally competent behaviors and attitudes as they relate to access, and range from studies of individuals to entire

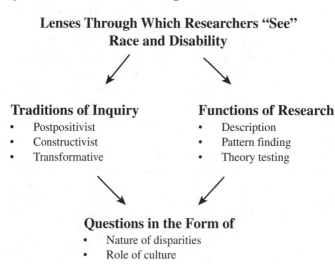

Figure 2-1

systems. A third variant is a hybrid category and represents a broad class of questions seeking to better contextualize the nexus of race and disability through the lens of critical social analysis or phenomenology. Phenomenological studies fall into one of three lines of research that look at self-identity or the disability experience as mediated by cultural consciousness.

The review now turns to an analysis of each of the themes.

The Nature of Disparity

The study of differences across groups defined by race or ethnicity is far and away the largest body of research in disability and race. While there are numerous variations, all studies are constructed on the core logic that differences between racial and ethnic groups must be identified to be corrected, or that the differences serve as explanations for other indicators of disparity. It should not be surprising that much of the research on race and disability is represented within this general class. As was noted in the preceding review of race and disability research, social constructions of civil rights and equality have framed the empirical enterprise throughout the latter half of the 20th century. A principal dynamic of society, in particular American society, are the interchanges between groups formed by the demographics of gender, class, geography, and race, among other status variables. Three basic lines of inquiry emerged from our review of the disparity literature and are organized around the themes of: (a) descriptions of status variable differences, (b) differences in access, and (c) mediators of disparity. One of the most common forms of inquiry is organized around the systematic documentation of differences between racial and ethnic groups on basic status variables, which account for the dominance of the group comparison studies described earlier. Disparity research can be viewed as an ongoing effort to find *real* differences on some indicator—employment status, health, identity, etc. The fundamental challenge in formulating questions about group differences is that racial and ethnic status carries conceptual baggage. Observed differences may be attributable not to the racial or ethnic groupings but to other characteristics such as educational or economic differences that are collateral to group membership. Thus, much of the work on disparities can be summarized as the identification of differences in status, access, and other dynamics with the critical caveat. This caveat, expressed through covariates and controls, is race and ethnicity-related differences at root may not be racially or ethnically based but rather reflect other differences associated with race at this time in this society (e.g. socioeconomic differences). What explains the persistence of these comparisons across racial groups in light of the "superficial differences" that race represents (Pasamanick & Knobloch, 1957)? We suspect that race per se, is not the point of the research, but rather the need to draw attention to the continued existence of educational, economic, vocational, housing, health service access, and other inequities linked to minority status.

The Role of Culture

Culture and its corollary, competence, define an enormous agenda for the field because they reflect not just a constituency of people, but skills, attitudes, policies, statutes, and practice (Roberts et al., 1990). A casual review of materials related to race, ethnicity, and disability will reveal nearly ubiquitous references to culture in various flavors: cultural diversity, cultural pluralism, culture and diversity, cultural competence, cultural sensitivity, multiculturalism, and transculturalism, among other flavors of culture. The succinct and understated caveat of Triandis and Suh (2002) is heeded here: "the conceptualization of culture is by no means a simple matter" (p. 135). We will not venture into the analysis of the concept of culture. Rather, we will focus superficially on applications of the concept, however defined, in the construction of research questions.

The primary line of inquiry emerging from our review of the interrogation of culture in the race and disability literature was the query about culture as an explanatory variable. Invoking culture as an explanatory variable is actually one of the oldest applications in race and disability research. The debates over diagnosis and assessment that were linked to the series of court cases in the early 1970s were challenges regarding cultural biases in educational placement tests: Diana v. State Board of Education (1970), Larry P. v. Riles (1971), PASE v. Hannon (1980), and Marshall et al. v. Georgia (1984), among others. The issue of bias, or unfair assessment, has been evaluated in terms of cultural effects, linguistic barriers, and class bias, and the debate continues across education, health services, rehabilitation, and other related fields (Clark et al., 1997; Harry, 1994; Kilbourne, Haas, Mulsant, Bauer, & Pincus, 2004; Parker & Philp, 2004). The focus of these questions was never simply about disparities in the accuracy of assessment but about the intersection of disability and culture and thus the validity of our disability conceptions (Guskin & Spicker, 1968; Kirk, 1964). Harry's analysis began with consideration of bias in assessment and ended in a discussion of strands that "combine into a complex and mutually inextricable force to place poor and, in particular, minority students at a disadvantage" (p. 65). Other examples of the use of culture variables as an explanatory variable have been in studies of the Black church (King, 1998), health perceptions (Silverman et al., 2000), pain (Edwards et al., 2005), and quality of life (Brown, McCauley, Levin, Contant, & Boake, 2004). A large number of investigations falling within the theme of cultural investigations involve questions focused on the role of cultural competence. As commonly applied in the literature, studies have focused on the roles that knowledge, behaviors, attitudes, and other characteristics play in traditional service-oriented contexts. Studies range from evaluations of individual competencies (Alston & McCowan, 1994; Nufer, Rosenberg, & Smith, 1998; Rosenthal, Wong, Moore Blalock, & Delambo, 2004) to evaluations of the competencies of entire systems (Alston, 2004; Pugach & Seidl, 1996; Sapon-Shevin & Zollers, 1999; Whaley, 2004).

The study of disability in a historical or cross-national context has long been used by scholars as a tool for interrogating various aspects of culture and, in like fashion, culture is used to frame questions about the intersections of race and disability (Edgerton, 1968; Manion & Bersani, 1987). To the extent that race and ethnicity are merely visible proxies for the more substantive differences represented in cultural differences, culture as an explanatory variable is an obvious and potent avenue of study.

The Meaning of Race and Disability

There is little question that the nexus of race and disability is undeveloped and little understood. In Kuhn's (1970) paradigmatic perspective, paradigms define the problems and methods of a research field. A mature paradigm would be characterized by commonly accepted theories, measurements, and procedures. According to Kuhn, paradigms evolve in subtle ways, often through minor changes in the language of scientific communities, in the framing of problems, and in the selection of phenomenon to study. In this section, we include research efforts focused on expanding the boundaries of our language about the study of race and disabilities. Like the preceding areas we reviewed, this third thrust of inquiry is not bounded by discipline or methodology. Studies tend to come from the transformative inquiry tradition since the work is, by definition, an attempt to challenge the status quo. In the same manner that Ferri and Connor (2005) asserted that special education was a form of institutional control for minorities, Molina's (2006) study of Mexican immigration in the early 20th century asks us to "blur the boundaries between the categories of race and disability" in the study of marginalized groups." (p. 33) Other forms of inquiry are represented as well. Dossa's (2005) case study of Mehrun, a Ugandan refugee with polio, is an example of a constructivist question that directly expands the boundaries of the existing paradigms of disability, gender, and race identity. In assuming the vantage point of Mehrun, the investigator describes these intersecting identities in the course of daily life. Identities converge in some contexts but are separated in others, and Dossa argues that organizing paradigms predicated on only one identity cannot inform her daily reality. Fujiura (2000) and Block, Balcazar, & Keys (2002), working from a more traditional social science perspective, argue for a reframing of race and disability issues into one of economic inequity and political power.

Summary: The Objects of Our Knowing

The preceding review, simplified as it is, provides some context for our exploration of the epistemology of the race and disability question. Each of these threads of inquiry touch upon core dynamics in the basis of our knowing: the exploration of inequity via identification of disparities, of systems of belief and behavior that mediate group differences, or the phenomenology of personal meanings.

SUMMARY AND CONCLUSION

In Burke's (1935) wide-ranging analysis of human communication, he noted that "a way of seeing is always a way of not seeing" (p. 70). As applied to our topic, the quote serves as a cautionary note for academics where success requires specialization and the disciplines are often divided along traditions of inquiry. What should be apparent from the preceding review is that while many investigators study race and disability, they do so in different ways and with different questions, often isolated from each other.

Three thematic elements have been emphasized in this review: (a) the diversity of forms of inquiry used in race and disability research, and the subtle bias toward reductionist questions; (b) the diversity of research functions; and (c) the complexity and expansiveness of questions related to the nexus of race and disability. What does this review reveal for the researcher planning to contribute to the extant body of work? The review reveals that disability and race are lodged in the interaction of virtually all spheres of human experience and activity; one does not readily compartmentalize such phenomenon. The circuitous route of our review across traditions of inquiry, functions, and questions encompasses everything from the social and political, to the physical environment and the psychology of experience. This kind of route serves as a cautionary note that there are no simple methods for characterizing this research. With respect to method, function, and question, we advocate no approach over another and set no topical priorities. All efforts are complementary. From each form of question a different piece of the portrait of the phenomenon is revealed; the intersection of race and disability will be best reconstructed through a combination of different perspectives. The experimental comparison of interventions across groups formed by race cannot be disentangled from a critical analysis of federal employment and income policies, or from the neighborhood the individuals live in, or from the meanings and experiences of the individuals as they navigate an often indifferent or hostile culture.

The central issue is to carefully frame the question to achieve the research goal, while remaining fully cognizant of the strengths and limits of any given question. The manner of the interactions between race and disability and the ways in which they are relevant remain very much a matter of debate and considerable mystery. The lesson of the short history of race and disability research is that, while we all understand in very general terms the profound influence of race, we truly do not understand its consequences for disability (Fujiura, 2000). We must be open to its consequences, many of them as yet unknown, and look deeply into its construction within our research paradigms. To paraphrase Burke (1935), do not be blinded by "ways of not seeing" (p. 70). A researcher's task is to appreciate the limitations of method—the distortions and incomplete images yielded by different lines of inquiry—and to focus on the very difficult challenge of using these images to illuminate the larger reality of race and disability.

REFERENCES

Adams, R. E., & Boscarino, J. A. (2005). Differences in mental health outcomes among Whites, African Americans, and Hispanics following a community disaster. *Psychiatry, 68(3),* 250–265.

Alston, R. J. (2004). African Americans with disabilities and the Social Security Administration's return-to-work incentives. *Journal of Disability Policy Studies, 14(4),* 216–221.

Alston, R. J., & McCowan, C. J. (1994). Aptitude assessment and African American clients: The interplay between culture and psychometrics in rehabilitation. *Journal of Rehabilitation, 60(1),* 41–46.

Anderson, N. B., & Nickerson, K. J. (2005). Genes, race, and psychology in the genome era: An introduction. *The American Psychologist, 60(1),* 5–8.

Balcazar, F. E., Garate-Serafini, T. J., & Keys, C. B. (2004). The need for action when conducting intervention research: The multiple roles of community psychologists. *American Journal of Community Psychology, 33(3),* 243–252.

Baron, R. M., & Kenny, D. A. (1986). The moderator–mediator variable distinction in social psychological research: Conceptual, strategic, and statistical considerations. *Journal of Personality and Social Psychology, 51(6),* 1173–1182.

Batchelder, A. B. (1966). *The economics of poverty.* New York: John Wiley & Sons.

Block, P., Balcazar, F. E., & Keys, C. B. (2002). Race, poverty and disability: Three strikes and you're out! Or are you? *Social Policy, 33(1),* 34–38.

Bound, J., Burkhauser, R. V., & Nichols, A. (2001). *Tracking the household income of SSDI and SSI applicants.* Ann Arbor: Michigan Retirement Research Center, University of Michigan.

Brown, S. A., McCauley, S. R., Levin, H. S., Contant, C., & Boake, C. (2004). Perception of health and quality of life in minorities after mild-to-moderate traumatic brain injury. *Applied Neuropsychology, 11(1),* 54–64.

Burke, K. (1935). *Permanence and change: an anatomy of purpose.* New York: New Republic Press.

Campbell, D. T., & Stanley, J. C. (1963). *Experimental and quasi-experimental designs for research on teaching.* Chicago: Rand McNally.

Capella, M. E. (2002). Inequities in the VR system: Do they still exist? *Rehabilitation Counseling Bulletin, 45(3),* 143.

Clark, D. O., Stump, T. E., & Wolinsky, F. D. (1997). A race- and gender-specific replication of five dimensions of functional limitation and disability. *Journal of Aging and Health, 9(1),* 28–42.

Devlieger, P. J., & Albrecht, G. L. (2000). Your experience is not my experience: The concept and experience of disability on Chicago's near west side. *Journal of Disability Policy Studies, 11(1),* 51–60.

Dewey, J. (1931). Social science and social control. *New Republic, 67,* 276–277.

Dossa, P. (2005). Racialized bodies, disabling worlds "they [service providers] always saw me as a client, not as a worker." *Social Science & Medicine, 60(11),* 2527–2536.

Edgerton, R. B. (1968). Anthropology and mental retardation: A plea for the comparative study of incompetence. In H. J. Prehm, L. A. Hamerlynck & J. E. Crosson (Eds.), *Behavioral research in mental retardation* (Monograph No. 1). Eugene: University of Oregon Press.

Edwards, R. R., Moric, M., Husfeldt, B., Buvanendran, A., & Ivankovich, O. (2005). Ethnic similarities and differences in the chronic pain experience: A comparison of African American, Hispanic, and White patients. *Pain Medicine, 6(1),* 88–98.

Ferri, B. A., & Connor, D. J. (2005). Tools of exclusion: Race, disability, and (re)segregated education. *Teachers College Record, 107(3)*, 453–474.

Freeman, H. P. (1998). The meaning of race in science—considerations for cancer research. *Cancer, 82(1)*, 219–225.

Freire, P. (1970). *Pedagogy of the oppressed* (M. B. Ramos, Trans.). New York: Continuum.

Fujiura, G. T. (2000). The implications of emerging demographics: A commentary on the meaning of race and income inequity to disability policy. *Journal of Disability Policy Studies, 11(2)*, 66–75.

Fujiura, G. T., & Rutkowski-Kmitta, V. (2001). Counting disability. In G. Albrecht, K. Seelman, & M. Bury (Eds.), *Handbook of disability studies* (pp. 69–96). Thousand Oaks, CA: Sage.

Fujiura, G. T., & Yamaki, K. (2000). Trends in demography of childhood poverty and disability. *Exceptional Children, 66(2)*, 187–99.

Furner, S. E., Giloth, B. E., Arguelles, L., Miles, T. P., & Goldberg, J. H. (2004). A co-twin control study of physical function in elderly African American women. *Journal of Aging and Health, 16(1)*, 28–43.

Gage, N. L. (1989). The paradigm wars and their aftermath: A "historical" sketch of research on teaching since 1989. *Educational Researcher, 18(7)*, 4–10.

Giesen, J. M., Cavenaugh, B. S., & Sansing, W. K. (2004). Access to vocational rehabilitation: The impact of race and ethnicity. *Journal of Visual Impairment & Blindness, 98(7)*, 410–419.

Gill, C. J. (1997). Four types of integration in disability identity development. *Journal of Vocational Rehabilitation, 9*, 39–46.

Guskin, S. L., & Spicker, H. H. (1968). Educational research in mental retardation. In N. R. Ellis (Ed.), *International review of research in mental retardation* (pp. 217–278). New York: Academic Press.

Harry, B. (1994). *The disproportionate representation of minority students in special education: Theories and recommendations.* (Project FORUM, Final Report). Alexandria, VA: National Association of State Directors of Special Education. (ERIC Document Reproduction Service No. ED374637)

Helms, J. E., Jernigan, M., & Mascher, J. (2005). The meaning of race in psychology and how to change it: A methodological perspective. *The American Psychologist, 60(1)*, 27–36.

Hernandez, B. (2005). A voice in the chorus: Perspectives of young men of color on their disabilities, identities, and peer-mentors. *Disability & Society, 20*, 117–133.

Hosp, J. L., & Reschly, D. J. (2002). Predictors of restrictiveness of placement for African-American and Caucasian students. *Exceptional Children, 68(2)*, 225–238.

Jaffee, K. D., Liu, G. C., Canty-Mitchell, J., Qi, R. A., Austin, J., & Swigonski, N. (2005). Race, urban community stressors, and behavioral and emotional problems of children with special health care needs. *Psychiatric Services, 56(1)*, 63–69.

Kilbourne, A. M., Haas, G. L., Mulsant, B. H., Bauer, M. S., & Pincus, H. A. (2004). Concurrent psychiatric diagnoses by age and race among persons with bipolar disorder. *Psychiatric Services, 55(8)*, 931–933.

King, S., Teplicky, R., King, G., & Rosenbaum, P. (2004). Family-centered service for children with cerebral palsy and their families: A review of the literature. *Seminars in Pediatric Neurology, 11(1)*, 78–86.

King, S. V. (1998). The beam in thine own eye: Disability and the Black church. *Western Journal of Black Studies, 22(1)*, 37.

Kirk, S. A. (1964). Research in education. In H. A. Stevens & R. Heber (Eds.), *Mental retardation: A review of research* (pp. 57–99). Chicago: University of Chicago Press.

Krause, J. S., Broderick, L. E., Saladin, L. K., & Broyles, J. (2006). Racial disparities in health outcomes after spinal cord injury: Mediating effects of education and income. *Journal of Spinal Cord Medicine, 29(1),* 17–25.

Kuhn, T. S. (1970). The structure of scientific revolutions (2nd ed.). Chicago: University of Chicago Press.

Lee, S. S., Mountain, J., & Koenig, B. A. (2001). The meanings of "race" in the new genomics: Implications for health disparities research. *Yale Journal of Health Policy, Law, and Ethics, 1,* 33–75.

Lieberson, S. (1985). Making it count: The improvement of social research and theory. Berkeley: University of California Press.

Lustig, D. C., & Strauser, D. (2004). Employee benefits for individuals with disabilities: The effect of race and gender. *Journal of Rehabilitation, 70(2),* 38–46.

Manion, M. L., & Bersani, H. A. (1987). Mental retardation as a western sociological construct: A cross-cultural analysis. *Disability, Handicap and Society, 2(3),* 231–45.

Manton, K. G., & Gu, X. (2001). Changes in the prevalence of chronic disability in the United States Black and Nonblack population above age 65 from 1982 to 1999. *Proceedings of the National Academy of Sciences, USA, 98(11),* 6354–6359.

Marrie, R. A., Cutter, G., Tyry, T., Vollmer, T., & Campagnolo, D. (2006). Does multiple sclerosis-associated disability differ between races? *Neurology, 66(8),* 1235–1240.

Meade, M. A., Lewis, A., Jackson, M. N., & Hess, D. W. (2004). Race, employment, and spinal cord injury. *Archives of Physical Medicine and Rehabilitation, 85(11),* 1782–1792.

Mertens, D. M. (2005). *Research and evaluation in education and psychology: Integrating diversity with quantitative, qualitative, and mixed methods* (2nd ed.). Thousand Oaks, CA: Sage.

Minow, M. (1990). *Making all the difference: Inclusion, exclusion, and American law.* Ithaca, NY: Cornell University Press.

Molina, N. (2006). Medicalizing the Mexican: Immigration, race, and disability in the early-twentieth-century United States. *Radical History Review, 2006(94),* 22–37.

Moore, C. L., Feist-Price, S., & Alston, R. J. (2002). VR services for persons with severe/profound mental retardation: Does race matter? *Rehabilitation Counseling Bulletin, 45(3),* 162–67.

Nufer, Y., Rosenberg, H., & Smith, D. H. (1998). Consumer and case manager perceptions of important case manager characteristics. *Journal of Rehabilitation, 64(4),* 40–46.

Omi, M. A. (2001). The changing meaning of race. In N. J. Smelser, W. J. Wilson, & F. Mitchell (Eds.), *America becoming: Racial trends and their consequences* (Vol. 1, pp 243–263). Washington, DC: National Academies Press. Parker, C., & Philp, I. (2004). Screening for cognitive impairment among older people in Black and minority ethnic groups. *Age and Ageing, 33(5),* 447–452.

Pasamanick, B., & Knobloch, H. (1957). Race, complications of pregnancy, and neuropsychiatric disorder. *Social Problems, 5(3),* 267–278.

Pugach, M. C., & Seidl, B. L. (1996). Deconstructing the diversity-disability connection. *Contemporary Education, 68(1),* 5–8.

Richardson, J., Anderson, T., Flaherty, J., & Bell, C. (2003). The quality of mental health care for African Americans. *Culture, Medicine and Psychiatry, 27(4),* 487–498.

Roberts, R., Barclay-McLaughlin, G., Cleveland, J., Colston, W., Malach, R., Mulvey, L., et al. (1990). *Workbook for developing culturally competent programs for families of children with special needs.* Washington, DC: Georgetown University Child Development Center.

Rosenthal, D. A., Wong, D., Moore Blalock, K., & Delambo, D. A. (2004). Effects of counselor race on racial stereotypes of rehabilitation counseling clients. *Disability and Rehabilitation, 26(20),* 1214–1220.

Sapon-Shevin, M., & Zollers, N. J. (1999). Multicultural and disability agendas in teacher education: Preparing teachers for diversity. *International Journal of Leadership in Education, 2(3),* 165–90.

Silverman, M., Smola, S., & Musa, D. (2000). The meaning of healthy and not healthy: Older African Americans and Whites with chronic illness. *Journal of Cross-Cultural Gerontology, 15(2),* 139–156.

Taylor, W. C., Baranowski, T., & Young, D. R. (1998). Physical activity interventions in low-income, ethnic minority, and populations with disability. *American Journal of Preventive Medicine, 15(4),* 334–343.

Taylor-Ritzler, T., Balcazar, F. E., Keys, C. B., Hayes, E., Garate-Serafini, T., & Espino, S. R. (2001). Promoting attainment of transition-related goals among low-income ethnic minority students with disabilities. *Career Development for Exceptional Individuals, 24(2),* 147–67.

Thoits, P. A. (1995). Stress, coping, and social support processes: Where are we? What next? *Journal of Health and Social Behavior, Spec No. 53,* 53–79.

Triandis, H. C., & Suh, E. M. (2002). Cultural influences on personality. *Annual Review of Psychology, 53(1),* 133–160.

Trochim, W. M. K. (1989). An introduction to concept mapping for planning and evaluation. *Evaluation and Program Planning, 12(1),* 1–16.

Trochim, W. M. K. (2001). *The research methods knowledge base* (2nd ed.). Cincinnati, OH: Atomic Dog Publishing.

Warren, P. R., Giesen, J. M., & Cavenaugh, B. S. (2004). Effects of race, gender, and other characteristics of legally blind consumers on homemaker closure. *Journal of Rehabilitation, 70(4),* 16–21.

Whaley, A. L. (2004). Ethnicity/race, paranoia, and hospitalization for mental health problems among men. *American Journal of Public Health, 94(1),* 78–81.

Wintersteen, M. B., Mensinger, J. L., & Diamond, G. S. (2005). Do gender and racial differences between patient and therapist affect therapeutic alliance and treatment retention in adolescents? *Professional Psychology: Research and Practice, 36(4),* 400–408.

CHAPTER 3

Disability Identity and Racial-Cultural Identity Development: Points of Convergence, Divergence, and Interplay

Carol J. Gill, PhD and
William E. Cross, Jr., PhD

INTRODUCTION

Disability and *Blackness* are signifiers for two groups historically linked to social oppression, discrimination, marginalization, and stigmatization—conditions encumbering other socially defined groups, such as gay and lesbian people, Native Americans, Chicanos, etc. In the 1960s and 1970s, each group took turns finding ways to intrude, disrupt, and irritate the status quo. The ultimate aim was to reshape mainstream sensibilities and make the inclusion of individuals often regarded as strangers, deviants, or damaged people possible. Consciousness-raising, a key characteristic of these movements, stimulated in-group affiliation, attachment, and advocacy, thereby laying a foundation for group identity development. In its early evolution, the discourse on disability identity borrowed heavily from the discourse on racial-cultural identity in general and Black identity development in particular. Over time, notions of identity multiplicity and intersectionality surfaced in both the disability identity literature and the work of racial-cultural theorists, extending the complexity and relevance of both frameworks.

The organization of this chapter reflects the theoretical interplay between the discourses on racial-cultural identity development and disability identity development. The chapter starts with a rationale that links the dynamics, or the "work," of racial-cultural identity and disability identity. *Part One* moves to a summary of current trends in the racial-cultural identity literature. *Part Two* shifts the focus to disability identity. *Part Three* examines the usefulness as well as the problems of bridging blackness and disability in the context of identity. Finally, the chapter ends in a discussion of potential directions for research and practice.

PART ONE: SUMMARY OF RACIAL-CULTURAL IDENTITY DEVELOPMENT

Race, Culture, and Existentialism

Concern for racial-cultural identity development can be found among persons whose humanity has been *racialized* by the larger society at five levels: (a) individual-biological, (b) individual-psychological, (c) group, (d) community, and (e) culture. There is the general misperception that race is a biological construct fundamentally wedded to a genetic classification system; however, the originators of the discourse always spoke of a *hybrid* concept linking race and culture. Henri Count Boulainvilliers, of 17th century France, is credited with being the first to coin the phrase *discourse on race*, and his definition was, to say the least, flexible. He thought the aristocracy was a superior race ordained to rule commoners whom he viewed to be another, albeit inferior, race (Guthrie, 2003). Two centuries later, Joseph Count Gobineau (1816–1882), another French thinker, gave birth to the so-called modern *scientific* racial classification system that divides humankind into various racial categories (White, Yellow, and Black). Gobineau's categorization of humankind made use of physical markers such as body-type, hair texture, lip size, facial features, etc. (Guthrie). However, the inventors of race always understood it to be a *signifier of culture*. It was not simply that Europeans were White and others were of a different color and physiognomy; the concept of race stretched to mean anything cultural or otherwise associated with each race (i.e., individual, family, kin, group, community, religion, society). In fact, Gobineau believed race *created* culture (Guthrie, 2003).

As a heuristic, the concept of race has constantly vacillated between notions of physicality and culture, resulting over the course of history in conceptual ambiguity. Here in the United States, the strong association of race with human physical features has caused many observers to overlook the racial plasticity played out in other settings. *Race has been, and can be, interpreted to mean just about anything physical or cultural.* In the genocidal encounters resulting in the Holocaust, the Slaughter of Armenians at the turn of the 20th century, the recent mass killing madness that was Rwanda, and the calamity of "ethnic cleansing" called Bosnia, the differences between exterminators and victims were not physical but imagined or actual cultural, religious, political and ideological differences, all falling under the rubric "race." In using race to explain everything—from the biological to the psychological and cultural—in the end nothing is explained. What can be said is that race is perhaps the most diabolic yet efficacious concept of *stigma* invented by humankind. Its efficacy is derived not from scientific validity and "proofs" but in the power of one group to impose race-based stigma upon another.

Stigma imposition engenders an *existential dilemma*—if not crisis—within target-group members, compelling them to devote psychological energy that engages, dismisses, enacts, transacts, and, where possible, transcends the constraints of stigma. Combined with cultural elements derived from the target group's history and collective experience, stigma management can drive group identity and meaning-making. In developing, sustaining, and refining stigma management competencies as well as in using culture as a shield, source of motivation, and anchor for meaning-making, the discourses on racial-cultural identity and disability identity find common ground. Although the content or social representation for each discourse is descriptively distinctive, latent dynamics are similar. The purpose of the range of identities (i.e., there is no one disability identity or one racial-cultural identity) associated with each target group is similar: *To live a meaningful life in the face of macro and micro aggressions linked to stigma and to absorb, protect, and perhaps contribute to the social group's culture and general welfare.*

Epiphany, Conversion, and Resocialization

The Black Social Movement of the 1960s and 1970s had two phases: (a) a civil rights phase that took flight in reaction to the 1954 Supreme Court School Desegregation Decision and was all but grounded in the aftermath of riots following the murder of Martin Luther King, Jr. in 1968; and (b) a Black power phase that first emerged during the Watts Riots in 1965 and peaked in influence between King's murder and the mid-to-late 1970s. The modern discourse on Black identity (circa 1960s to the present) has its origins in the psychological experiences of young and middle-aged Black adults who were participants in the Black power phase. However, many of the Black power participants had their psychological roots in phase one activities in the 1950s and early 60s (civil rights). Consequently, their participation in phase two activities (Black power) necessitated an identity change captured in the phrase: Negro-to-Black-conversion (Cross, 1971).

Not surprisingly, a major psychological dynamic of the Black power phase was identity conversion, and theorizing conversion led to the psychology of nigrescence or simply *Nigrescence Theory* (Cross, 1971). The psychology of nigrescence explored a five-stage phenomenological model of identity conversion that took as its starting point a person holding an otherwise functional and healthy identity that discounted the significance of race (*Pre-encounter*). Subsequently, the Pre-encounter identity is challenged in thunderbolt-like fashion by an epiphany compelling the person to seek personal change (*Encounter*). The person submits to oceanic, true believer, and total-commitment attitudes fueled by a war between the old and new self, taking place just beneath the surface (*Immersion-Emersion*). The process culminates in identity habituation, psychological homeostasis, and worldview reformulation (*Internalization*). In the end, a pre-existing and fully formulated adult identity is transformed or reformulated through conversion. In its earliest iteration (Cross, 1971), Nigrescence Theory was linear and subject to prototypical depictions, as one identity type was associated with each stage.

In 1991 (Cross), Nigrescence Theory was expanded to account for the fact that persons entering the process (at the Pre-encounter identity stage) hold a wide *range* of identity constellations. However, the multiple expressions of Pre-encounter shared the tendency to accord limited importance to race and Black culture. Pre-encounter is the identity belief system held by Black people, who, beyond the fact that they are nominally Black, make meaning of themselves and the world around them through attitudes, philosophies, values, and worldviews that accord limited significance to race and Black culture. The stance is not necessarily negative but dismissive (low salience).

Several negative identity attitudes are also included in the revision of Pre-encounter, such as miseducation and racial-self-hatred. *Miseducation* attitudes reflect the tendency information about Black people and Black culture as factual, when in reality such information is stereotypical. Such negative stereotypes are "compartmentalized" by the person making it possible to embrace them as "truths" about the group but not the self, even though the person is a member of the disparaged group. *Racial-self-hatred* is the tendency to experience self-loathing, unworthiness, and self-hatred as a consequence of the person having internalized powerful negative ideas, feelings, and beliefs about being Black at both the collective and *personal* levels.

Just as the revised theory (Cross, 1991, 1995) reconfigures Pre-encounter to account for identity variability at the front end of the process, identity diversity is also incorporated into the dynamics of identity resolution. To the extent that the original model linked a *single identity type* with Internalization, the revised theory associates advanced identity development with not one, but a broad range, or "cluster," of identity configurations. To make explication of the theory manageable, the following identity exemplars are highlighted throughout the revised theory: (a) Afrocentric (race and Black culture salience expressed as a monocultural orientation); (b) Bicultural (synthesis of being Black and American, identity duality, fusion, and shared salience); (c) Multicultural (a sense of Blackness fused with two or more additional cultural reference points); and (d) Intersectional (an extension of the multicultural exemplar where the additional reference points are social class, sexual orientation, disability identity, and/or religious perspective, etc., as in a person who is Black, female, lesbian, disabled, and poor). Moderate-to-high salience for race and Black culture is common to all exemplars (none of the exemplars reflect low salience or negative salience) but the *configuration* of salience can be expressed monoculturally, biculturally, multiculturally, or intersectionally. Any and all of these identity exemplars are the result of socialization processes (Cross & Fhagen-Smith, 2001; Cross & Cross, 2007), and three patterns of socialization have been highlighted.

Pattern A: Traditional Socialization and Identity Acquisition

The inculcation of some *variant* of Blackness through traditional socialization (infancy across early adulthood) is called Pattern A. The emphasis on variant makes clear that cutting edge discussions of traditional socialization of Black youth result not in one, but in a range, of identities with the common attribute of according moderate-to-high salience to race and Black culture. From this perspective Afrocentric (high-*singular* salience), Bicultural (*dual*-cultural salience), Multicultural (a sense of Blackness fused with *multiple* points of cultural salience), and Intersectional (a sense of Blackness fused with a range of *additional identity* concerns such as being Black, disabled, lesbian, and female) are all possible outcomes of traditional socialization.

On the other hand, Tatum (2003) points out that not all Black parents subscribe to the centrality of race. Some raise their children in the opposite direction; striving, instead, to inculcate a positive identity that accords limited salience to race and Black culture, as in an *Assimilated* identity or *Color-Blind-Humanist* frame of reference. One could also add the so-called *Cosmopolitan* identity (Appiah, 2006) that fuses elements of assimilation, passing, and a yearning to be invisible. From the vantage point of the Cosmopolitan, discourses on racial-cultural and disability identity are trivialized and treated as passé, and to engage in such discourses is said to perpetuate one's own oppression (Davis, 2007). Consequently, a comprehensive life span perspective on racial-cultural socialization (Cross & Fhagen-Smith, 2001; Cross & Cross, 2007) maps the unfolding of both race and culturally salient expressions of Blackness (i.e., Afrocentric, Bicultural, Multicultural and Intersectional) as well as low-salient stances (Assimilationist, Color-blind, Cosmopolitan, and Humanist oriented). As to the latter, Cross and Cross label positive but low-salient identity patterns as *Alternate* identities.

Every variant of Black identity is understood to emerge as a consequence of *generic* psychological processes. However, due to space limitations, we will only highlight a process germane to the period covering pre-adolescence and early adulthood. For example, the general literature on human development shows that youth enter pre-adolescence with ideas and feelings about themselves and the world shaped, in large measure, by their parents and significant others. In a general sense—keeping the focus within Western societies—identity proclivities expressed by pre-adolescents have been constructed and inculcated but not critically self-examined. However, when they enter the more autonomous spaces of middle school and especially high school, identity exploration, contestation, and experimentation become commonplace. By late adolescence and early adulthood, scrutiny gives way to identity habituation and internalization, revealing a young adult who has taken ownership of the self. Marcia (1966) refers to these three developmental points—drawn from the writings of Erik Erikson—as identity statuses wherein pre-adolescent identity is equated with a formulated but relatively unexamined identity status known as *Foreclosed,* the exploration-testing dynamics of adolescence as *Moratorium,* and the point of self-acceptance, habituation, and self-ownership as *Achievement.*

Grafting Marcia's perspective to a discussion of Black identity development, Cross and Fhagen-Smith (2001) state that regardless of the type of Black identity being tracked across the life span—Afrocentric, Assimilated, Bicultural, etc.—each will be the object of the *same* psychological processes. Thus, the development of an Afrocentric variant of Black identity will be no more or less subject to Foreclosed, Moratorium, or Achieved experiences than the unfolding of any other type of Black identity. The same is true for the development of positive (Alternate) identity options that accord limited salience to race and Black culture (i.e., Assimilated or Humanist). As an aside, the trajectory need not be linear because a teen may enter Moratorium with an Assimilationist stance and exit with a frame dominated by Bicultural attitudes and/or some other frame; in another instance, a young girl may enter Moratorium with an intense Afrocentric gaze only to emerge at early adulthood with an openly lesbian focus.

Pattern B: Conversion as Resocialization

The successful acquisition of a variant of Black identity through Pattern A may preclude having to go through a conversion experience (Pattern B) later in life, with several important *exceptions*. First, a parent may raise a child such that race and culture issues are downplayed or treated as trivial. Thereby, a self-concept is fashioned deriving little, if any, meaning from race and Black culture (e.g., Assimilationist and Humanist stances). Such a child may emerge as an adult with the type of identity that places her/him at risk for a racial-cultural epiphany. Here we use "risk" to connote frame vulnerability, not pathology. A person operating with a frame of reference that accords limited salience to race and Black culture is at risk of encountering a race and culture-loaded experience for which the person's ongoing frame of reference has no answer. If the encounter takes on the force of an epiphany, it may trigger a full-blown conversion. Additionally, should too much internalized racism leak through socialization resulting in miseducation—or worse—elements of racial self-loathing, the stage is set for Pattern B as a corrective for self-negativity. A conversion takes place after the results of traditional socialization have taken hold; consequently, a conversion experience involves psychological *re-socialization*.

Pattern C: Recycling

For the sake of argument, let us presume that in a random sampling of 10,000 Black people between the ages of 15 and 30, 85% arrived at their sense of racial-cultural identity through Pattern A and the remainder through identity conversion, or Pattern B. In a manner of speaking, this *foundational* identity can be achieved through either pathway. Independent of whether a foundational identity is the result of Pattern A or Pattern B, *how is continued growth and possible expansion of the foundational identity explained?* The possibility of growth beyond either Patterns A or B has been considered by Parham (1989), the distinguished Black psychologist, Afrocentric philosopher, and past president of the Association of Black Psychologists. He refers to this added growth as identity recycling, and Cross and Fhagen-Smith (2001) label it Pattern C. According to Parham, a person with a well-developed core identity encounters a *racial-cultural-related* question/challenge tied to personal, family, and employment contexts. The immediate solution may not be obvious—literally throwing the person for a loop. In working through and processing the "challenge," the person's foundational or core identity is *enhanced* in the sense that the person is now able to incorporate into her/his narrative what it is like to be confronted with, and live through, the challenge in question. As life involves a constant series of such challenges, a person is afforded various opportunities to develop a view of life that is thick, deep, rich, and complicated. In this example we are stressing how a sense of wisdom can develop. Of course, life's microaggressions can have a reverse effect leading to pain, bitterness, depression, alienation, and hatred, but in the limited space we have available here, we err toward the positive progression across the life span.

> . . . *Nigrescence Recycling begins with an adult* Foundational Black Identity, *and in response to a* Life Span Encounter, *a person discovers a minor or major gap in his or her thinking about Blackness. Should the person take the encounter seriously, a state of Immersion-Emersion is entered as a way to resolve the challenges posed by the life span encounter. Following the transition phase,* Internalization of the Enhancement *becomes evident. Finally, the overall developmental outcome is an* Enhanced Foundational Identity. . . . *Consequently, whether a person has achieved a Black identity through* Nigrescence Pattern A *(identity development through the formative socialization process during infancy, childhood, preadolescence, and adolescence) or* Nigrescence Pattern B *(Black identity development achieved through identity conversion), he or she will likely be subject to continued growth through* Nigrescence Pattern C. *(Parham's concept of Nigrescence Recycling; Cross & Fhagen-Smith, 2001, pp. 266)*

The Black Identity as a Lived Experience

The last element of Nigrescence Theory that shows promise in dialogue with the discourse on disability identity is an analysis of how race and Black culture are transacted in everyday life. Boykin's (1986) Triple Quandary Theory suggests that Black people must learn to negotiate three "worlds" or types of experiences: (a) the world of marginalization, insult, discrimination, and racism; (b) the world of the mainstream; and (c) the world that constitutes the Black community itself. Building on Boykin's perspective, Strauss and Cross (2005) identified five transactional modalities that operationalize identity as a lived experience in everyday life: (a) *Buffering* (transacting racism and discrimination), (b) *Code-switching* (moving in and out of the mainstream), (c) *Bridging* (transacting friendships across social categories), (d) *Bonding and Attachment* (transacting relationships within the Black community), and (e) *Individuality* (transacting one's sense of individuality). In this model, the five forms of expressiveness connote not five different identities within the same person, but a coherent identity that reticulates a *repertoire* of expressions. The person is said to be the same person from one situation to the next (identity coherence); however, the demand characteristics of the situation determine what form of identity expression (or mix of expressions) the person will apply.

Contrary to its depiction as a theoretical dead-end and political Neanderthal (Davis, 2007), Black identity theory has evolved into a cutting edge perspective. It supports a rich, complex, and relevant discussion of stigma management and culture engagement, and offers directives for counseling–clinical applications. It can even help comprehend Alternate identity options such as Color-blind, Assimilated, Humanist, and Cosmopolitan. Given this capacity for handling complex expressions of identity within a heterogeneous group, Black identity theory may offer useful insights for research and practice regarding disability identity.

PART TWO: OVERVIEW OF DISABILITY IDENTITY

Background and State of Scholarship on Disability Identity

As has been true for African Americans and other groups engaged in social justice movements, the civil rights activism of Americans with disabilities sets the stage for their heightened concern with questions of personal and group identity. This interest in self-definition was bolstered by the language and spirit of the 1990 Americans with Disabilities Act (ADA). The ADA recognized that people with a wide range of disability types and social backgrounds compose "a discrete and insular minority:" subject to social discrimination. However, little empirical research has addressed identity issues affecting people with disabilities, in contrast to the large body of research from the 1970s to the 1990s linking ethnic, gender, and sexual minority identity to such benefits as high self-esteem and resilience to prejudice (Anspach, 1979; Cross, 1971; Goffman, 1963; Marcia, 1966).

One possible reason for this lag in research is that, historically, the dominant paradigm in disability research has been medical or remedial, that is, pathology-focused. Instead of viewing disability as a social/political/cultural phenomenon and regarding people with disabilities as a distinct social group, researchers have traditionally perceived people with disabilities as a dysfunctional sector of the general population, defined by deviant biology. Consequently, researchers who investigated self-concept in persons with disabilities have tended to focus on individual adjustment clinically measured against norms. Disabled people's identity thus has not been considered worthy of study in its own right as a cultural or subcultural phenomenon.

Medical models that frame disability as a disruption of normal experience have several severe limitations for explaining aspects of disability identity formation, either as a conversion experience or as a developmental process:

1. They treat the process as a problem of individual adjustment, failing to address the social and cultural forces acting on the individual, such as discrimination.
2. They focus only on the potential negative impact of disability rather than viewing disability in terms of potential personal enrichment, community, and culture.
3. They have little to say about the development of self in persons who have been disabled all their lives; therefore, they have few positive guidelines about "normal" disability identity development to offer counselors, teachers, etc.
4. They pay very little attention to within-group variation or intersections of identity based on gender, race, sexual orientation, etc.

Another possible barrier to research on disability identity is that, until recently, researchers in the disability fields have rarely been persons with disabilities. Much of the empirical work on identity models for other nondominant cultural communities (racial, ethnic, women, and gay/lesbian) has been led by scholars indigenous to those communities. The personal interest and direct experience derived from group membership may be significant in motivating, energizing, and guiding identity research efforts.

A third barrier may be ambivalent feelings of group members toward embracing a devalued identity. In written autobiographical accounts and research interviews, persons with disabilities commonly report having absorbed from society and its prime messengers—family, teachers, and health professionals—the sense that their disabled parts are inferior and should be transcended. Drawing from the discussion of negative racial identity in the previous section (Cross, 1991, 1995), this phenomenon can be viewed as a prime example of miseducation paving the way to disability self-hatred. Since most people with disabilities live in families with nondisabled members, they have few of the opportunities for direct intergenerational transmission of positive identity that women and ethnic/racial minority members experience

(Gill, 1994). Consequently, until the past two decades, researchers may have detected little interest among disabled people in issues of identity.

That is no longer true. After two generations of disability rights and independent living activism, many Americans with disabilities have expressed a significant shift in attitude about their group, their place, and who they are in society (Longmore, 2003). A disability historian, Longmore refers to this shift of interest to questions of identity as the "second phase" of the disability rights movement, contrasting it with the political struggle for antidiscrimination laws that marked the "first phase." In some ways this shift parallels the transition from "civil rights" to "Black power" discussed earlier in the section on racial-culture identity.

Growing interest in disability identity is now evident in many forums: autobiographical books and memoirs (e.g., Hockenberry, 1995); disability studies texts (Davis, 2003; Siebers, 2008); online disability discussion groups and advocacy websites; festivals, parades, art exhibits, and performances focusing on disability culture and pride; panels addressing identity at disability studies conferences; and journal articles analyzing the existence, trajectory, form, value, and even risks of disability identity. Furthermore, broader interdisciplinary efforts exploring politicized or minority identity have started to invite work from disability studies scholars, most notably the series of seminars and books generated by the Future of Minority Studies project at Cornell and partner universities across the country.

Most of the scholarship on disability identity, however, is conceptual, with scattered efforts to validate empirically some of this work. Goffman's (1963) classic work on stigma and spoiled identity has been particularly influential and widely cited. Goffman had much to say about the impact of social forces on the self-image of persons with disabilities, particularly the devastating impact of prejudice. Written before the contemporary disability rights movement, however, his analysis reflects little recognition of persons with disabilities as active agents in constructing positive personal identities bolstered by identification with a stigmatized but nonetheless vital and powerful minority group (Anspach, 1979). As an "outside" observer, his work reflects none of the affirmative tone or dynamism of the models offered by Cross (1971), or of Boykin (1986) and colleagues for other socially marginalized groups.

Current Debates Regarding Disability Identity

Along with increased political and intellectual interest in disability identity, challenging critiques have emerged as well. Some disability scholars agree with the general postmodern criticism of minority identity (discussed earlier in relation to *Cosmopolitan* identity expression) that identity politics is an outmoded and destructive project (Davis, 2003). They argue that collective cultural identity re-inscribes oppression by substantiating arbitrary categories imposed by the dominant culture (Galvin, 2003). This process, they say, imposes a restrictive mythology of common experience on individuals simply because they share a physical or mental characteristic. Why, they might ask, would a woman professor who has been blind from birth have much in common with a war veteran who has recently sustained a brain injury? They assert that it is essentialist to believe that any biological feature, including skin color or functional impairment, is a valid basis for identity. A related criticism of identity politics is that it holds members of a group hostage to the pain of social injury, a dynamic that seems antithetical to empowerment.

Alongside these general criticisms of group identity is a critique that focuses on disability in particular. Some disability scholars argue that the idea of disability identity establishes impairment as the foundation of one's identity. Thereby, it bolsters the medical model of disability and imposes an arbitrary binary distinction of disabled/nondisabled upon the continuum of human variation (Davis, 2003; Galvin, 2003). This criticism recalls the concern discussed earlier that Black identity validates biological markers such as skin color as a basis for distinguishing human difference. Critics also argue that disability is an unstable category with more permeable boundaries than other minority group parameters. Anyone can become disabled, and one's functional status is highly context dependent. Therefore, they maintain, it makes no sense to view persons with disabilities as sharply distinct from persons without disabilities. Following from the potentially encompassing nature of disability as a category, it is also argued that the disability population is extraordinarily diverse and, therefore, the idea of a common disability identity isolates disability artificially from intersecting identities related to race, gender, sexuality, class, age, and other axes of social significance (Galvin).

In addition to rejecting disability identity as a construct, some scholars criticize any effort to compare or analogize race and disability. They argue that it is inaccurate and disrespectful to impose parallels on phenomena that are different in so many ways, including their history, social dynamics, personal and group experience, forms of violence, and impacts. Additionally, there is a concern that such comparisons may reenact the conflation of race with biological deficiency, a notion that has historically fueled discrimination against African Americans (Baynton, 2001).

An interesting recent development in group identity discourse addresses some of these criticisms of disability identity. It comes from minority studies scholars working in a critical realist framework who engage with postmodern critics to defend the honor of minority identity (Alcoff, Hames-García, Mohanty, & Moya, 2006). They agree that simplistic notions of group identity can be divisive or can tether a person's sense of self to biological markers on one hand or social injury on the other hand. Nonetheless, they assert that unjust treatment predicated on embodied difference is a social reality for many people, whether the "difference" is skin color or atypical body functioning. Arguably, such treatment shapes disabled people's experience in ways that link them, regardless of the nature of their individual impairments, motivating collective forms of resistance.

This realist perspective can be helpful in evaluating and responding to criticisms of disability identity. Although people with disabilities are a heterogeneous collective (and what social minority group is not heterogeneous?), and although disability is an unstable arbitrary category (and what socially defined category is stable?), people categorized as disabled in our society do have resultant experiences in common that potentially connect them. Perhaps it is time to ponder some larger questions, such as: Why must linkages between persons who share stigma be constraining rather than empowering? Why can collective identity not expand to embrace and celebrate heterogeneity rather than downplay it? In other words, in the spirit of Cross's (1991, 1995) Multicultural and Intersectional identities, why can there not be a grown-up version of identity politics? A wise form of identity politics encompasses diversity and cultural intersections as givens and encourages affirmative community-building as well as coalition-building without the constriction and separation that is associated with its earlier forms. For example, Der-Karabetian and Ruiz's (1997) research on Latino identity indicates it is possible to have a strong minority identity while concurrently celebrating one's place in the majority culture. Or as a disability rights teeshirt from the 1980s eloquently proclaimed, "I want it all!"

PART THREE: BLACK IDENTITY THEORY AS INSPIRATION TO EXPLORE DISABILITY IDENTITY

Black Identity Theory and Implications for Disability Identity

We seek to demonstrate that Black identity theory may inform ideas and theory-building around disability identity; however, it is not our intention to argue for or to present an exhaustive explication of the fit between the two discourses. In concluding this discussion of racial-cultural identity and disability identity, we list some elements of Black identity theory that seem particularly relevant to disability identity development:

1. *Black identity as meaning-making:* Central to the discourse on Black identity is not physicality per se but the existential encounter with society's categorization of oneself as a member of a stigmatized social group. Independent of stigma, the meaning one may derive from the culture of the group is also of core importance. In parallel, disability identity is first and foremost a discourse driven by meaning-making and interpretation in response not necessarily to one's physical/cognitive difference but to society's categorization of people perceived as different.

2. *Black identity and patterns of socialization:* Black identity theory and ideas about disability identity first crossed paths in the early and late 1970s. Adults and in some cases adolescents narrated the way epiphanies lead to identity conversions or identity resocialization. The stage-model approach sprang from these explorations. Today both communities are concerned with the socialization of youth. Black identity theory is instructive in showing that there are multiple socialization pathways across the life span and patterns of analysis potentially applicable to disability identity.

3. *Multiple Black identities:* Black identity theory embraces the perspective that there is no singular expression of Black Identity. Around the identity-nodes of low, moderate, high, and negative salience are clustered multiple exemplars that help explain the range of meaning-making systems to be found in the Black community. The need to codify identity variability within the disability identity discourse is critical, including the task of deconstructing notions of Assimilation, Passing, Humanism, and Cosmopolitan. A multifaceted identity model that accounts for variability in identity expression is consistent with the ontological and experiential complexity of disability.

4. *Identity as enactments:* The move toward an activity theory approach to Black identity—that is the *doing* of identity in everyday life—is a major breakthrough. In place of static personality states, traits, and categories, the discourses on Black and disability identity can now stress the *enactment* or expression of identity in everyday life, as transacted across a range of contexts. The transactional categories of Buffering, Code-switching, Bridging, Bonding, and Individuality may be particularly useful in understanding various strategies of social interaction adopted by disabled persons across varying contexts.

Ideas for Research on Disability Identity Suggested by Black Identity

As indicated earlier, systematic research on disability identity is meager and has not flourished in a climate that is skeptical of politicized cultural identity. There have been some studies that attempt to formulate or validate theories of disability identity but few have looked at the intersection of disability and other group identities, including Black identity. Gill, Taylor, Nepveux, Ritchie, & Weeber (2007) are engaged in qualitative research that has begun to explore these intersections. Recurrent themes in the data thus far include the following:

- Disabled persons commonly report experiences of isolation and silence in families regarding disability. Except for instances in which disability has been openly discussed as a negative element in family life, it is rarely addressed at all.

In terms of Black identity theory, these conditions may contribute to a legacy of miseducation about disability.

- There is a positive relationship between disability identity and positive contact with disability groups. Possibly, per Cross (1971, 1995), Immersion and Bonding/Attachment are important correlates of a positive disability identity, as they are for Black identity.
- A variety of negative and positive encounters can initiate the development of disability identity. For example, a disturbing *encounter* with disability discrimination can prod someone toward a disability identity but so can meeting a romantic partner who demonstrates appreciation for the disabled individual "just the way she/he is!"
- It is critically important to most people with disabilities to be recognized as full and complex human beings. They differ in how important they think disability is in shaping who they are. Some worry that any focus on their disability status will prevent others from recognizing their full humanity. Perhaps they are leaning toward a disability version of humanist or cosmopolitan identity expression or are invested in passing or assimilating to the nondisabled world. Others feel that they can never feel fully accepted if they downplay their disability, suggesting a more disability-salient identity analogous to the Afrocentric outcome in Black identity theory (Cross, 1971).
- There is no simple relationship between race and disability. Some people of color with disabilities have prioritized their identification and affiliation with persons who share their cultural/racial heritage and have had little contact with disability groups. They tend to see disability in terms of limitation rather than identity. Race has high salience but disability has low salience in their expressions of identity. Other people of color have had substantial contact with disability groups. They are more likely to identify as *disabled* and to reference parallels between race and disability. For example, some say that their experiences of race-based oppression have prepared them to understand disability as a social minority experience. Race and disability are both highly salient for them, suggesting intersectional expressions of identity.

Looking at such findings in the context of Cross' racial-cultural identity work is interesting yet challenging. Regarding the developmental issues crucial to Pattern A identity formation, for example, disability, unlike race, may not even factor into an individual's life experience until well into adulthood. A large proportion of individuals have developed stable identities as nondisabled persons before becoming disabled, and the fact of disablement itself, then, constitutes an abrupt encounter event. An interesting research question is, does this new encounter with disability trigger a new Pattern A identity quest befitting a new person with a disability, or does it resemble more a dramatic variant of the Pattern B conversion? Furthermore, after reaching some form of psychological resolution subsequent to becoming disabled, individuals may experience additional events, both positive and negative, that shake their identity moorings. These events may stimulate them to develop a disability identity or to revise their inaugural effort at incorporating the disability experience into their core identity. Does this process have features in common with the Pattern C *recycling* process described by Cross and Fhagen-Smith (2001)?

For persons disabled early in life, there are particular barriers to Pattern A development of a disability identity. Family taboos about acknowledging disability may compound the isolation of a child raised in a family where few, if any, individuals have disabilities. Ironically, the isolation may continue through the school years if disabled children are the beneficiaries of progressive school inclusion policies that mainstream them into "regular" education classrooms where there may be no other disabled children. It is understandable, then, that many children with disabilities develop adult identities in which disability has low salience and low positive valence. Research on the disability identity issues of disabled children raised in the mainstream would help illuminate the hazards and opportunities of inclusion. For example, studies of parents' and teachers' communications about disability may uncover some interesting dynamics between identity formation and the messages about disability that surround children as they develop. Another important aspect of development is the nature of reference groups for identification. Do children with disabilities who have opportunities to "hang out" with other children with disabilities develop different identities, or more or less robust identities, than children who are embedded in a largely nondisabled world?

The relationship between salience and positiveness or negativeness of disability in identity certainly calls for further empirical investigation. Does a low-salient but negative disability configuration underlie the identity of the "overcomer" or of the exceptionally assimilated disabled person who pursues membership in the dominant nondisabled culture and avoids contact with disabled peers? Does a high-salient negative disability configuration characterize the disabled person with internalized low self-expectations? Additionally, it would be interesting to know if low-salient disability identities are more likely for some types of impairments. For example, is disability generally less salient for persons with learning disabilities than for wheelchair-users because the impairment of the former group is less immediately apparent during everyday social interactions? Are persons with less apparent impairments more likely to seek assimilation or to attempt "passing" (as nondisabled) than are individuals with obvious impairments? If so, to what effect? Another set of questions concerns the ways in which salience or identity patterns are influenced by historical context. There have been dramatic changes in public life between 1970 and the present. Not only are social systems and values different but the media that deliver cultural messages have changed. For example, how does online communication shape or possibly homogenize individual and group orientation to identity, pushing toward Humanist and Assimilationist stances? How do such media encourage group identity building by enabling communication among those with similar statuses who previously had more difficulty getting and staying in contact?

Another interesting research question is how assimilation responses of disabled children raised in their primarily nondisabled families compare to assimilation responses in cultural minority children adopted by dominant culture families. In this regard, children with disabilities may be viewed as bicultural or as transcultural "adoptees," bridging the world of disability and the nondisabled world (Gill, 1994). Do disabled children, like transracial adoptees, benefit from exposure to adult peers to instill pride in their differences from their adoptive families and to teach them strategies for addressing their marginalization in the mainstream?

The disability rights and disability pride movements have helped inspire a new breed of parent who views disability in sociopolitical terms (Gill). Such parents are conscious of the social marginalization that their disabled children will confront. They take steps to ensure that their kids form bonds with strong role models with disabilities, engage in disability-positive cultural activities, and learn strategies from disability advocates. There are also persons with disabilities who are raising children with disabilities in a milieu of disability activism and culture (Gill). There is no longitudinal research tracking the development of such "encultured" children to date. However, it would not be surprising to find that these children end up with a Pattern A identity in which disability is salient and positive. Similarly, persons who acquire disabilities as adults, have contact with strong disability groups, and have had exposure to disability pride and culture activities may be more likely to see disability as an important and valuable aspect of identity. Therefore, they may be more likely to achieve a positive, salient disability identity through Patterns B or C.

In terms of identity transactions in daily life, disability again presents complex scenarios to study. Regarding bridging, for example, many persons with disabilities form relationships with both disabled and nondisabled persons. However, depending on the salience and positiveness of disability in their identity configuration, one or the other type of relationship may be deeper or more desired. An interesting bridging phenomenon unique to many disabled people is their relationship to nondisabled personal assistants, interpreters, and readers. Often these relationships develop a depth and cross-cultural trust that cannot be characterized simply as a service provision. For example, such assistants may be given entree into disability or deaf community activities and may learn the language, culture, and codes of those communities. Regarding bonding, the rapidly expanding disability art and culture movement has been drawing disabled people into connection with other disabled people whom they might have formerly avoided for fear of reinforcing stigma. Through enjoying art and performance by disabled artists, by learning about disability history, and by celebrating disability pride, many persons with disabilities are acknowledging a new sense of belonging and community that they did not expect to have in their lifetimes. These under-investigated phenomena provide important opportunities for research that can expand our understanding of variations in the identity formation process.

Ideas for Practice Suggested by Links between Disability Identity and Black Identity

The discussion of links between the discourses on Black identity and disability identity highlights several points to consider in providing counseling and other services to persons with disabilities:

1. *Diversity within the group*: Although most socially defined "minority" groups are heterogeneous, the complexity of the disability category is underacknowledged in service delivery. Disability status intersects with multiple axes of diversity and marginalization, including race, gender, sexuality, class/caste, and age. Moreover, varieties of impairment—physical, sensory, learning, psychiatric—contribute to disabled people's diversity of experience and perspectives. Disability does not trump all other human differences; neither should it be dismissed as inconsequential.

2. *Disability affirmative approaches*: Part of acknowledging that disability is a social category is realizing that despite its legacy of oppression, disability can be a stimulus of community-building, pride, and culture. Professionals who understand the sociopolitical nature of disability are less apt to convey messages that disability is inherently tragic and limiting. Informed professionals can support clients in seeking information and support from the disability community, in seeking action against injustice, and in discovering the emerging disability culture.

3. *Developmental variations*: It may be helpful for professionals to recognize the developmental aspects of disability identity. Clients will differ in the manner and timeframe by which they integrate disability into their sense of self. For example, an individual disabled since childhood may have little trouble accepting disability (Pattern A acquisition), but may not have had many opportunities to develop a positive identity foundation. In contrast, a person disabled later in life may have developed a strong, elaborated identity but may harbor lifelong stereotypes that suggest disability is antithetical to a positive self (which could foreclose the unfolding of a Pattern B conversion). Another individual might be revisiting identity concerns late in life after encountering a challenge to an achieved disability identity (Pattern C recycling). Exploring where the individual is in the trajectory toward disability identity (and her/his concurrent identities) and not expecting uniformity among clients may help determine the kind of supports that will be most helpful.

4. *Expressive variations*: Similarly, professionals cannot expect all people with disabilities to end up with one particular identity configuration. Variations in the salience and positiveness of one's disability experience may result in a multiplicity of disability identity and alternate expressions across individuals. Furthermore, the shape of disability identity for a particular client may fluctuate across time and contexts as she/he enacts different styles for different situational demands. Again, professionals who are prepared for these variations in identity may be better positioned to support individuals with disabilities who, for example, need to Code-switch and project Assimilationist or Cosmopolitan qualities during a job interview yet may seek Bonding/Attachment to a disability community for affirmation after a grueling week on the job market.

5. *In-group representation and power issues*: Acknowledging disability as a sociopolitical category as well as a potential site for identity development urges professionals to increase their awareness of issues of power and representation.

Understanding that people with disabilities report a long history of oppressive treatment in service systems may help professionals respect a client's wariness or pessimism regarding the service relationship. Professionals who convey awareness of this history and of the sociopolitical aspects of disability may seem particularly trustworthy. Such professionals are often better at relating in a way that reduces power inequities between service provider and receiver and signals a genuinely collaborative approach. They convey respect for who the client is as an individual and as a member of a stigmatized group. Whether or not the service provider has a disability may also affect rapport and trust in work with a disabled client. Such issues of group representation matter to many disabled persons just as they often matter to members of other marginalized groups.

CONCLUDING THOUGHTS

The future of disability identity is full of potential. As Black identity theory posits, stigma management can drive group identity and meaning-making. In the case of disability, the need to buffer the pain and material consequences of stigma can precipitate a quest for a strong disability identity. But the very permeability of the disability category and its potential applicability to any human being pushes the agenda beyond individual identity toward a social mission of redefining humanity and acceptable human differences. The idea of a strong, positive disability identity contradicts the judgment of functional limitation as tragic and as "other," leading logically and emotionally to a drive to make the world more universally open.

As universal design and inclusion practices take hold, there is a commonly expressed hope that the full range of human functional variation will be accepted and planned for and that disability will become an obsolete category. The same hope has been expressed with respect to race. However, it is not necessarily the people living under those categories who harbor that hope, nor is it clear that disability oblivion, any more than "color blindness" would be ideal. Some disability activists may prefer a world that respects the value of life with disability, that honors the contributions of the disability culture, and that supports a disability-centric identity. Others with disabilities might hope for a world that accepts them as people first and that encourages a Cosmopolitan identity. Others yet may want it all: a neutral acknowledgement from society that human differences exist, as well as social conditions that support an endless variety of identity outcomes based on individual proclivities rather than restrictive categories. We do not yet have data to confirm the relative benefits of these different identity pathways.

Nonetheless, some young parents and professionals are encouraging children with disabilities to internalize a universal humanistic ideal, hoping, like Black parents who downplay the salience of race (Tatum, 2003), that these children will accept their differences but will view them as fundamentally unimportant. It will be fascinating to see the kinds of identities these children of the universe grow up to have. Will they end up with the strongest sense yet of their own value as disabled people, or will they find themselves ill-equipped to deal with the social and political vicissitudes awaiting them? Time will tell and, hopefully, researchers, service professionals, and activists alike will study and learn from what unfolds.

REFERENCES

Alcoff, L. M., Hames-García, M., Mohanty, S. P., & Moya, P. M. L. (2006). *Identity politics reconsidered*. New York: Palgrave Macmillan.

Anspach, R. R. (1979). From stigma to identity politics: Political activism among the physically disabled and former mental patients. *Social Science & Medicine, 13A*, 765–773.

Appiah, K. A. (2006). *Cosmopolitanism*. New York: W. W, Norton.

Baynton, D. (2001). Disability and the justification of inequality in American history. In P. K. Longmore & L. Umansky (Eds.), *The new disability history: American perspectives* (pp. 33–57). New York: New York University Press.

Boykin, A. W. (1986). The triple quandary and the schooling of Afro-American children. In U. Neisser (Ed.), *The school achievement of minority children* (pp. 57–92). Hillsdale. NJ: Lawrence Erlbaum.

Cross, W. E., Jr., (1971). The Negro-to-Black conversion experience. *Black World, 21*, 13–27.

Cross, W. E., Jr., (1991). *Shades of Black*. Philadelphia: Temple University Press.

Cross, W. E., Jr., (1995). The psychology of nigrescence: Revising the Cross model. In J. S. Ponterotto, J. M. Casa, L. A. Suzuki, & C. M. Alexander (Eds.), *Handbook of multicultural counseling* (93–122). Newbury Park, CA: Sage.

Cross, W. E., Jr., & Cross, T. B. (2007). Racial-ethnic-cultural identity development (REC-ID): Theory, research, and models. In C. McKown & S. Quintana (Eds.), *Handbook of race, racism, and the developing child* (pp. 154–181). Hoboken, NJ: Wiley.

Cross, W. E., Jr., & Fhagen-Smith, P. (2001). Patterns of African American identity development: A life span perspective. In C. L. Wijeyesinghe & B. W. Jackson (Eds.), *New perspectives on racial identity development: A theoretical and practical anthology* (pp. 243–270). New York: New York University Press.

Davis, L. J. (2003). *Bending over backwards: Disability, dismodernism, and other difficult positions.* New York: New York University Press.

Davis, L. J. (2007). Deafness and the riddle of identity. *The Chronicle of Higher Education,* pp. B6–B8.

Der-Karabetian, A., & Ruiz, Y. (1997). Affective bicultural and global-human identity scales for Mexican-American adolescents. *Psychological Reports, 80,* 1027–1039.

Galvin, R. (2003). The paradox of disability culture: The need to combine versus the imperative to let go. *Disability & Society, 18,* 675–690.

Gill, C. J. (1994). A bicultural framework for understanding disability. *Family Psychologist, 10,* 13–16.

Gill, C. J., Taylor, R., Nepveux, D., Ritchie, H., & Weeber, J. (2007). *Family life and relationships: Perspectives from adults with disabilities.* Poster session presented at the annual meeting of the Society for Disability Studies, Seattle, WA.

Goffman, E. (1963). *Stigma: Notes on the management of spoiled identity.* Englewood Cliffs, NJ: Prentice Hall.

Guthrie, R. V. (2003). *Even the rat was white: A historical view of psychology* (2nd ed.). Boston: Allyn and Bacon.

Hockenberry, J. (1995). *Moving violations—War zones, wheelchairs, and declarations of independence—A memoir.* New York: Hyperion.

Longmore, P. K. (2003). *Why I burned my book and other essays on disability.* Philadelphia: Temple University Press.

Marcia, J. E. (1966). Development and validation of ego identity status. *Journal of Personality and Social Psychology, 3,* 551–558.

Parham, T. A. (1989). Cycles of psychological nigrescence. *The Counseling Psychologist, 17*(2), 187–226.

Siebers, T. (2008). *Disability theory.* Ann Arbor: University of Michigan Press.

Strauss, L. C., & Cross, W. E., Jr. (2005). Transacting Black identity: A two-week daily-diary study. In G. Downey, J. S. Eccles, & C. M. Chatman (Eds.), *Navigating the future: Social identity, coping, and life tasks* (pp. 67–95). New York: Russell Sage.

Tatum, B. D. (2003). *Why are all the Black kids sitting together in the cafeteria?: Conversations about race.* New York: Basic Books.

The Nature of Disparities in Outcomes for Multicultural Populations with Disabilities

CHAPTER 4

Psychological Testing and Multicultural Populations

Brigida Hernández, PhD;
Elizabeth V. Horin, PhD;
Oscar A. Donoso, MA; and
Andrea Saul, MA

INTRODUCTION

As the United States has become increasingly diverse, much attention has been paid to the cultural competence of educators, practitioners, and researchers. Cultural competence has been defined as the ability to provide services that are perceived by clients as relevant to their problems and helpful for intervention outcomes (Dana, 1993). Culturally competent abilities involve the acknowledgment and acceptance of cultural differences; appreciation of one's culture on thinking and behavior; and recognition of culturally prescribed communication, etiquette, and problem solving approaches. A tripartite model of cultural competence has been proposed by Sue, Arredondo, and McDavis (1992) that emphasizes: (a) awareness of biases, values, and assumptions, (b) understanding of the worldviews of culturally diverse clients, and (c) development of skills to implement and create culturally sensitive intervention strategies.

Recognizing the significance of cultural competence, the American Psychological Association (APA) has called for psychologists to strengthen their skills in this domain. Of particular interest for this chapter, the APA has highlighted the importance of providing culturally competent services when conducting psychological assessments. Specifically, the APA Ethics Code (American Psychological Association, 2002) includes two standards that address test bias. In selecting tests, Standard 9.02b stipulates that it is incumbent upon psychologists to determine whether a particular test can be used reliably and validly, given a client's population characteristics such as race, ethnicity, culture, language, gender, age, or disability. If reliability or validity data do not exist (or if psychologists use tests without established norms for the individual being assessed), psychologists should include the strengths and limitations of using such tests in their report of interpretations and recommendations. Standard 9.02c emphasizes the need to take an individual's language preference and competence into account when selecting an assessment method.

The purpose of this chapter is threefold. First, this chapter examines the appropriateness of four commonly used psychological tests when assessing multicultural populations in order to illustrate the complexities involved. The extent to which tests are or are not standardized with culturally diverse individuals may impact the appropriateness of the norms and test reliability and validity. Second, this chapter highlights implications of our test review for rehabilitation psychologists and counselors. As both generators and consumers of psychological reports, they play critical roles in how test data are interpreted and used. Third, this chapter provides approaches to consider when testing multicultural groups, as it is recognized that psychological testing has the potential to provide valuable information to assist individuals with disabilities seeking and receiving vocational rehabilitation (VR) services.

PSYCHOLOGICAL TESTING AND THE VR SYSTEM

Many people with disabilities seeking VR services undergo psychological testing to determine eligibility and subsequent services. In a three-year longitudinal study of 8500 VR clients, Hayward and Schmidt-Davis (2003a, 2003b) found that 35% received cognitive/psychological assessment services and 39% had records of cognitive/psychological assessments obtained. The psychological assessment phase of the VR process often involves the administration of tests within the domains of cognitive/intellectual and personality/social-emotional functioning (Cutler & Ramm, 1992).

Although the VR system aims to help people with disabilities, research has shown that multicultural populations tend to receive inequitable treatment at various points in the VR process (Bellini, 2003; Capella, 2002; Dziekan & Okocha, 1993; Hayward & Schmidt-Davis, 2003b; Kundu, Dutta, & Walker, 2006; Moore, 2001; Moore, Feist-Price, & Alston, 2002; Moore, Giesen, & Cavenaugh, 2005; Thomas, Rosenthal, Banks, & Schroeder, 2002; Wilson, 2000). For example, racial/ethnic minorities are less likely to be accepted into VR programs (Atkins & Wright, 1980; Capella, 2002; Dziekan & Okocha, 1993; Herbert & Martinez, 1992; Wilson, 2000) and more likely to be placed on waiting lists (Zea, García, Belgrave, & Quezada, 1997) when compared to Caucasians. Given these disparities and the weight of psychological evaluations for VR eligibility and service delivery, we review four well-established psychological tests to illustrate the complexities when testing adults of racially/ethnically diverse backgrounds.

Review of Commonly Used Psychological Tests for Adults of Diverse Backgrounds

The Wechsler Adult Intelligence Scale (WAIS-III), Minnesota Multiphasic Personality Inventory (MMPI), Rorschach Inkblot Test (RIT), and Beck Depression Inventory

(BDI) have been around for several decades and are among the most widely used standardized tests (Camara, Nathan, & Puente, 2000). To varying degrees, each is considered a "gold" standard as they are known to provide critical information related to identifying cognitive and social-emotional strengths and weaknesses. Along with their noted value, there are concerns when using these and other similar measures with individuals of diverse backgrounds. We discuss some of these concerns by examining the composition of the standardization samples in order to determine if people from multicultural populations were adequately included when establishing test norms, reliability, and validity. Then we review empirical studies germane to these four standardized tests and the performance of African Americans, Asian Americans, Latinos, and Native Americans. Although a number of databases were used for this chapter (i.e., ArticleFirst, ERIC, MedLine, Mental Measurements Yearbook, Periodical Abstracts, PsycInfo, and Social Sciences Abstracts), it is important to note that our review of empirical studies was not exhaustive. Table 4-1 provides an overview of the WAIS-III (WAIS-III Tulsky & Zhu, 1997), MMPI, Second Edition (MMPI-2, Hathaway & McKinley, 1989), RIT (Exner, 2003), and BDI, Second Edition (BDI-II, Beck, Steer, & Brown, 1996), along with our key findings.

The Wechsler Adult Intelligence Scale (WAIS-III)

Most test batteries include an assessment of cognitive and intellectual functioning to help in providing an overview of a person's strengths and weaknesses. Typically, such assessments are individualized and assist in the development of practical recommendations. Among clinical psychologists, the Wechsler scales have reigned supreme within this domain (Camara et al., 2000). It is noteworthy that the standardization sample of WAIS-III[1] included 2450 individuals, was based on the 1995 U.S. Census, and was stratified by age, sex, race/ethnicity, geographic region, and educational level (Psychological Corporation, 1997). However, when examining the racial/ethnic makeup across designated age groups, some degree of fluctuation is evident. For instance, the percentage of African Americans ranged from 5% for the 85–89 age group to 17% for the 18–19 age group, while the percentage of Latinos ranged from 2% for the 75–79 age group to 13% for the 20–24 age group. Of concern, Asian Americans and Native Americans were collapsed into an "other" category, which included bi- and multiracial individuals (Psychological Corporation).

For the most part, the WAIS-III performance of various racial/ethnic groups is limited to data collected for its standardization. When adjusted for age, gender, and education, Caucasians obtained higher Verbal IQ (VIQ), Performance IQ (PIQ), and

---

[1]Published in 2008, the WAIS-IV is the latest version of this instrument. Given its recent publication, it was not included in this chapter.

Table 4-1 Overview of Four Commonly Used Psychological Tests

Test	Purpose	Standardization sample	Scale/Factor names	General findings	Non-English version cited
WAIS-III	Assesses cognitive abilities of adults ages 16 to 89 years	2,450 individuals aged 16 to 89 years	Full Scale IQ Verbal IQ Performance IQ	Support when using with: African Americans and Latinos (Psychological Corporation, 1997) Concerns when using with: • Asian Americans and Native Americans (Psychological Corporation, 1997) • African Americans (Kaufman & Lichtenberger, 2006) • Latinos (Kaufman & Lichtenberger, 2006) • Native Americans (Guilmet, 1975; Kaufman & Lichtenberger, 2006; Neisser et al., 1996)	WAIS: Chinese version (Okazaki & Sue, 2000); Spanish version (Wechsler, 1968) WAIS-Revised: Japanese and Hindi versions (Okazaki & Sue, 2000); Chinese version (Gong, 1983) WAIS-III: Chinese version (Wechsler, Chen, & Chen, 2002); Spanish version (Psychological Corporation, 2008) Wechsler Bellevue: Korean adaptation (Okazaki & Sue, 2000)
MMPI-2	Assesses psychopathology of adults ages 18 and over	2,600 individuals aged 18 to 64 years	3 validity scales (L, F, K) 8 clinical scales (hysteria, depression, hypochondriasis, psychopathic deviance, psychasthenia, paranoia, schizophrenia, hypomania)	Support when using with: • African Americans (Arbisi et al., 2002; Hall et al., 1999; Freuh et al., 1997; McNulty et al., 1997; Timbrook & Graham, 1994) • Latinos (Cabiya et al., 2000; Hall et al., 1999; Whitworth & McBlaine, 1993; Whitworth & Unterbrink, 1994)	Chinese (Cheung, Song, & Zhang, 1996)* Hmong (Deinard, Butcher, Thao, Vang, & Hang, 1996)* Japanese (Shiota, 1990)* Korean (Han, 1996)* Thai (Pongpanich, 1996)* 2 Spanish versions (Garcia-Peltoniemi & Azan Chaviano, 1993; Lucio et al., 1994)

Table 4-1 Overview of Four Commonly Used Psychological Tests (continued)

Test	Purpose	Standardization sample	Scale/Factor names	General findings	Non-English version cited
MMPI-2			2 non-clinical scales (masculinity-femininity, social introversion)	Support when using with: • Native Americans (Greene et al., 2003) Concerns when using with: • African Americans (Hall & Phung, 2001; McNulty et al., 1997; Timbrook & Graham, 1994) • Latinos (Graham, 2006; Lucio et al., 2001) • Asian Americans (Graham, 2006; Kwan, 1999; Shiota et al., 1996; Stevens et al., 1993; Tsai & Pike, 2000) • Native Americans (Graham, 2006; Pace et al., 2006; Robin et al., 2003)	
Rorschach Inkblot Test	Assesses psychopathology and personality of individuals ages 5 and over	600 adult non-patients	Not applicable	Concerns when using with: • African Americans (Frank, 1992; Meyer, 2002) • Latinos (Bachran, 2002; Frank, 1993) • Native Americans (Dana, 1983; Thomason, 1999)	Not applicable

Table 4-1 Overview of Four Commonly Used Psychological Tests (continued)

Test	Purpose	Standardiza-tion sample	Scale/Factor names	General findings	Non-English version cited
BDI-II	Assesses depressive symptoms of individuals ages 13 and over	500 adult outpatients and 120 college students	2 factors (cognitive and somatic)	Support when using with: • African Americans (Dutton et al., 2004; Grothe et al., 2005) • Asian Americans (Okazaki, 1997) • Latinos (Carmody, 2005; Contreras et al., 2004; Novy et al., 2001) Concerns when using with: • Native Americans (Allen, 1998; Thomason, 1999)	Chinese version of the original BDI (Zheng et al., 1988) Spanish version (Wiebe & Penley, 2005)

Note. * indicates as cited in Butcher et al. (2003).

Full Scale IQ (FSIQ) scores than African Americans, with discrepancies ranging from 11 to 13 points (Kaufman & Lichtenberger, 2006). Although the discrepancies were smaller, Caucasians also obtained higher scores than Latinos, with Latino means ranging from 96 to 99. Such gaps have led to longstanding, controversial debates about differential cognitive abilities based on racial/ethnic group membership (Rushton & Jensen, 2005) and the inadequacy of tests to accurately measure the cognitive abilities of culturally diverse individuals (Samuda, 1998).

Acculturation may also play an important role in the scores obtained by various racial/ethnic groups. In a preliminary study of acculturation and WAIS-III performance, Harris, Tulsky, and Schultheis (2003) examined data from 151 participants, representing 37 countries of origin from the standardization sample. The authors found that language preference and acculturation contributed to cognitive performance beyond the more common demographic variables of interest (viz. age and education). As a result, the authors highlighted the need for further research in this area and the importance of assessing acculturation when testing the cognitive/intellectual abilities of individuals of culturally diverse backgrounds.

Outside of the United States, there have been numerous attempts to translate and standardize earlier versions of the WAIS-III (i.e., Wechsler Bellevue, WAIS, and WAIS-Revised). Of interest for the testing of Asian Americans, there are Japanese and Hindi versions of the WAIS-Revised, a Chinese version of the original WAIS, and a Korean adaptation of the Wechsler Bellevue (Okazaki & Sue, 2000). It is not clear whether these adapted instruments are available and/or used in the United States, although some research has been conducted with the WAIS-Revised for China (WAIS-RC; Gong, 1983). Specifically, Ryan, Dai, and Paolo (1995) examined the VIQs and PIQs of the standardization samples of the WAIS-R and WAIS-RC and found relatively similar performances across both groups. Furthermore, Chan, Lee, and Luk (1999) reported on the development and refinement of the Chinese Vocabulary subtest for the WAIS-RC, and found that it loaded reasonably well on the verbal construct and demonstrated strong reliability. In a more recent study of the Chinese version of the WAIS-III (Wechsler, Chen, & Chen, 2002), Yao, Chen, and Tam (2007) found support for the four-factor structure of the instrument (Verbal Comprehension, Perceptual Organization, Working Memory, and Processing Speed) among individuals with and without schizophrenia.

Until recently, the Escala de Inteligencia de Wechsler para Adultos (EIWA; Wechsler, 1968), a Spanish version of the WAIS, was readily available and used. Its standardization sample included over 600 Puerto Ricans who had limited levels of formal education and were primarily rural residents. Given its publication year and distinct normative group, ongoing use of this instrument has warranted much attention and concern. Using standardization data from the EIWA and WAIS manuals, Gomez, Piedmont, and Fleming (1992) found evidence for a two-factor structure (Verbal and Performance domains). However, they also noted the need for additional research with a more heterogeneous sample of Latinos. Demsky, Gass, and Golden (1998) reanalyzed the standardization data as well, and found that the threshold for meaningful VIQ and PIQ differences on the EIWA differed from the WAIS and WAIS-R. Thus, scores from these measures were not comparable. Similarly, Lopez and Romero (1988) and Melendez (1994) examined the scoring procedures and conversion of raw scores to scale scores and found that EIWA scores were not directly comparable to WAIS scores because of significant scoring differences for similar responses. In 2008, the EIWA-III was published by the Psychological Corporation as a Spanish adaptation of the instrument for use with Puerto Rican clients. With updated norms and a factor structure that is consistent with the WAIS-III, it will likely represent a marked improvement over its predecessor.

Studies addressing the WAIS performance of Native Americans are limited and have indicated a tendency for VIQ mean scores to be lower than PIQ mean scores (as cited in Kaufman & Lichtenberger, 2006; Neisser, Boodoo, Bouchard, Boykin, Brody, et al., 1996). Guilmet (1975) cautioned against interpreting such gaps in scores as better developed performance (nonverbal) abilities, given the lack of culturally-sensitive verbal tests and testing in native languages.

In sum, there are a number of issues to consider when using the WAIS. First, the overall standardization sample of the WAIS-III was large, based on the U.S. Census, and stratified by age, sex, race/ethnicity, geographic region, and educational level. Although the makeup of the overall standardization sample is impressive, when examining specific age groups, racial/ethnic representations varied with some groups having better representation than other groups. Second, attention is needed when using the WAIS-III with African Americans, given that their mean IQ scores tend to be significantly lower than Caucasians. Such low scores may be misinterpreted as low intellectual abilities, thereby underestimating the potential impact of cultural factors. Third, use of the original EIWA with Spanish-speaking clients is problematic, given its publication date and lack of representation of Latino groups. The newly published EIWA-III holds some promise for the testing of Puerto Rican clients. Fourth, the Chinese version of the WAIS-III also shows promise when examining its factor structure among individuals with and without schizophrenia; however, more research is needed with different populations. Fifth, Native Americans tend to perform better with nonverbal tasks of the WAIS when compared to verbal tasks. Caution should be used when interpreting this gap, given that verbal tasks load on both culture and language.

Lastly, the construct of intelligence as measured by the WAIS adheres to a narrow and Euro-American conceptualization that may differ in other cultures. For instance, some Eastern cultures view intelligence as encompassing knowledge of social roles, while some African cultures consider cleverness, social responsibility, and practical thinking as important aspects of intelligence (as cited in Benson, 2003).

The Minnesota Multiphasic Personality Inventory (MMPI)

Frequently, psychological evaluations are conducted to assess for psychological disorders such as depression, anxiety, bipolar disorder, and schizophrenia. When used appropriately, results from such evaluations help establish appropriate vocational plans. Camara et al. (2000) found that among a variety of personality and social-emotional tests available, the MMPI, RIT, and BDI were ranked highly in terms of usage.

The Minnesota Multiphasic Personality Inventory, Second Edition (MMPI-2; Hathaway & McKinley, 1989) is a self-report measure designed to assess psychopathology. According to Butcher and Graham (1989), the original version of the MMPI has more than 115 recognized translations. On the clinical scales, a T-score at or above 65 is indicative of symptomology, and a 5-point or greater difference is needed for clinical significance when making group comparisons. The standardization sample of the MMPI-2 included 1138 men and 1462 women, of which 126 (11.1%) were African American men, 188 (12.9%) were African American women, 35 (3.1%) were Latino men, 38 (2.6%) were Latina women, 38 (3.3%) were Native American men, 39 (2.7%) were Native American women, 6 (0.5%) were Asian American men, and 13 (0.9%) were Asian American women (Hathaway & McKinley). Although this racial/ethnic diversity is an improvement over the original MMPI, it is apparent that the MMPI-2 does not adequately represent Latinos, Asian Americans, and Native Americans given current population estimates (U. S. Census Bureau, 2001). In addition, numerous studies have examined the MMPI-2 scores of African Americans and Latinos; in contrast, fewer have examined the scores of Asian Americans and Native Americans (Hall & Phung, 2001).

In a meta-analysis that examined 31 years of MMPI and MMPI-2 research, no substantive differences were found between African Americans, Latinos, and Caucasians on the validity or clinical scales (Hall, Bansal, & Lopez, 1999). Similarly, when examining data from the standardization sample and scores obtained by African Americans and Caucasians, Timbrook and Graham (1994) found that mean differences on the clinical scales were less than the five points needed to represent a meaningful difference. However, findings indicated that the Psychasthenia scale tended to under-predict anxiety symptomology in African American women.

When examining profiles of African Americans and Caucasians who were psychiatric inpatients, significant T-score differences were found, with African American men scoring higher on a validity (F) and four clinical (Psychopathic Deviate, Paranoia, Schizophrenia, and Hypomania) scales and African American women scoring higher on the Paranoia and Hypomania scales (Arbisi, Ben-Porath, & McNulty, 2002). However, further analyses led the authors to conclude that the MMPI-2 scores were not highly moderated by racial group membership. Frueh, Gold, de Arellano, and Brady (1997) found no differences in the MMPI-2 profiles of

African American and Caucasian patients with Posttraumatic Stress Disorder (PTSD). Findings were more mixed with other African American and Caucasian subgroups. Specifically, African American men in forensic settings scored lower on the Psychopathic Deviate scale and African American men in substance abuse settings scored lower on the Psychasthenia scale than their Caucasian counterparts (Hall & Phung, 2001). In a study of African American and Caucasian outpatients, for whom MMPI-2 and therapist rating data were available, no significant differences were found in the correlations of the two measures (McNulty, Graham, Ben-Porath, & Stein, 1997). However, African American women scored higher on the MMPI-2 Hypomania scale but not on the relevant therapist-reported measure. It is unclear whether this difference reflected test bias or actual differences, given that the sample of African American women was not substantially large.

A few studies have indicated that MMPI-2 differences among Latinos and Caucasians tend to be minimal; however, most of these studies have involved college students. Specifically, minimal differences were found in a study of MMPI-2 profiles of Mexican, Puerto Rican, and United States college students (Cabiya, Lucio, Chavira, Castellanos, Gomez, et al., 2000) and Hispanic American and Caucasian college students (Whitworth & McBlaine, 1993; Whitworth & Unterbrink, 1994). In contrast, with the MMPI-2 standardization sample, clinically significant differences (five T-score points or greater) were found between Latinas and Caucasian women on a validity scale (F) and several clinical scales (Hypochondriasis, Psychopathic Deviate, Psychasthenia, Schizophrenia, and Hypomania; Graham, 2006). Lucio, Ampudia, Duran, Leon, and Butcher (2001) also found numerous clinically significant differences when United States norms were applied, with Mexican men scoring clinically higher on a validity (L) and clinical (Hypochondriasis) scale, and Mexican women scoring clinically higher on a validity (L) and several clinical (Hypochondriasis, Depression, and Schizophrenia) scales. Moreover, the authors suggested that participants seemed to respond in ways to present themselves favorably and differed on items that related to morality rather than psychopathology. These cultural differences may incorrectly pathologize individuals, if context is not considered. Thus, the authors recommended the development of Mexican norms for Mexicans and Mexican Americans (Lucio et al., 2001). The MMPI-2 profiles of Latinos may also be impacted by acculturation. A study of Mexican American college students found evidence of the impact of ethnic identity and acculturation on the L and K validity scales (Canul & Cross, 1994). However, a second study focusing on the impact of acculturation did not replicate this finding (Lessenger, 1997).

A number of studies have examined Spanish versions of the MMPI-2, and overall findings have supported their utility. Fantoni-Salvador and Rogers (1997) used a Spanish version of the MMPI-2 with patients whose preferred language was Spanish and found that MMPI-2 profiles were significantly related to diagnoses of depression and schizophrenia, but not anxiety and substance abuse disorders. A Spanish version of the MMPI-2 (Lucio, Reyes-Lagunes, & Scott, 1994) was developed and administered to Mexican college students. In general, their profiles were similar to the United States college normative sample. The authors suggested that higher scores on the validity (L) and Depression scales among Mexican male respondents may have been more indicative of Mexican culture than symptomotology. Thus, the Spanish version of the MMPI-2 was considered appropriate to use with college populations, although further research was needed to determine its usefulness with other Mexican and Latin American populations. In a study of Mexican, Venezuelan, and Colombian college students and adult community residents (Boscan, Penn, Velasquez, Reimann, Gomez, et al., 2000), two Spanish versions of the MMPI-2 were administered: Inventario Multifasico de la Personalidad 2-Minnesota (Garcia-Peltoniemi & Azan Chaviano, 1993) and MMPI-2 for Mexico (Lucio et al., 1994). It was determined that both measures were adequate translations and may have applicability with Latino college students from these countries (Boscan et al.).

In a review of the literature, Kwan (1999) found that nontreatment Asian American respondents tended to have more elevated MMPI-2 profiles than their Caucasian counterparts, with higher scores on the Depression and Schizophrenia scales. Stevens, Kwan, and Graybill (1993) also found that Chinese female students scored higher than their Caucasian counterparts on a validity scale (L), perhaps indicating a presentation of virtuosity. Shiota, Krauss, and Clark (1996) cautioned that MMPI-2 elevations among Asians may be indicative of cultural differences and not necessarily psychopathology. In particular, elevations on the Depression scale may reflect cultural norms of modesty, restraint, and imperturbability. Moreover, given that there are many subgroups within the Asian community, findings from one subgroup may not be applicable for another (Butcher, Cheung, & Lim, 2003; Kwan; Sue et al., 1992; Tsai & Pike, 2000). In addition, Graham (2006) noted it was not appropriate to make conclusions about differences between Asian Americans and Caucasians from the standardization sample, given the small sample of Asian Americans.

Similar to Latinos, acculturation may impact the MMPI-2 profiles of Asian Americans. Kwan (1999) found that less acculturated Chinese respondents obtained significantly higher scores than their more acculturated counterparts. Further, Tsai and Pike (2000) found that low-acculturated Asian Americans obtained clinically elevated scores on the Schizophrenia scale; however, for recent immigrants, this scale may be capturing experiences of cultural alienation and social estrangement rather than psychopathology.

Both the MMPI-2 and its predecessor (MMPI) have been widely translated and adapted into various Asian languages including Chinese, Hmong, Japanese, Korean, and Thai (Butcher et al.). For this chapter, we focus on the Chinese MMPI-2 and response patterns among Chinese and Chinese Americans. The Chinese MMPI-2 has demonstrated translation equivalence, test-retest reliability, consistency of the factor structure, and validity with clinical samples (Butcher et al., 2003). However, Cheung

(1995) found that when Chinese norms were used, the profiles of Chinese psychiatric patients were not as elevated as with United States norms. Using the United States norms, elevations were noted on a validity scale (F) and two clinical scales (Depression and Schizophrenia). Consequently, a lower T-score of 60 instead of 65 has been suggested as the cutoff with the Chinese norms, as well as use of both United States and Chinese norms (Cheung).

With great tribal diversity, Native Americans were inadequately represented in the MMPI-2 standardization sample and clinically significant differences (five T-points or greater) were evident when their profiles were compared to Caucasians (Graham, 2006). Differences were also apparent in a study conducted by Robin, Greene, Albaugh, Caldwell, and Goldman (2003) that compared the MMPI-2 profiles of the Southwestern and Plains American Indian tribal members with overall scores from the standardization sample. Although no meaningful differences were found for any MMPI-2 scales between the two Native American tribes, differences were found between the combined tribal groups and the standardization sample (with the combined group obtaining higher scores on two validity scales [L and F] and the Psychopathic Deviate, Schizophrenia, and Hypomania scales).

In a follow-up study, Greene, Robin, Albaugh, Caldwell, and Goldman (2003) examined whether identified differences reflected test bias or actual differences by comparing the MMPI-2 elevations with responses on the Schedule for Affective Disorders and Schizophrenia-Lifetime. The elevated scores among the Native American group appeared to reflect substantial differences in symptoms when compared with the criterion group. Therefore, the authors found preliminary support for use of the MMPI-2 with Native Americans, and cautioned clinicians against dismissing elevations on these scales as test bias. Despite evidence supporting use of the MMPI-2 with Native Americans, participants of the Greene et al. study represented only 2 of more than 500 recognized Native American tribes. Additional concerns with Native Americans include the lack of focus on culturally specific aspects of functioning and pathology, existence of norms built upon cultural uniformity, and assumptions that elevated scores are maladaptive in specific contexts (Allen, 1998; Dana, 1986; Thomason, 1999).

Lastly, Pace, Robbins, Choney, Hill, Lacey, et al. (2006) examined the normative validity of the MMPI-2 with two distinct Native American tribes (Eastern Woodland Oklahoma and Southwest Plains Oklahoma). Similar to the Robin et al. (2003) study, for both groups clinically significant elevations were found on two validity scales (L and F) and four clinical scales (Hypochondriasis, Psychopathic Deviate, Schizophrenia, and Hypomania). Of note, members of the Eastern Woodland Oklahoma tribe with lower acculturation scores tended to score higher on the F and Schizophrenia scales than their counterparts. As a result, the authors suggested that MMPI-2 elevations among Native Americans may not necessarily reflect psychological distress but rather different ideologies or worldviews.

Overall, the MMPI-2 may pose some challenges for practitioners testing for the VR system. On the one hand, when used in conjunction with other test data, this popular measure may provide critical information to help determine VR eligibility and establish appropriate vocational goals. There is a body of research supporting its use with African Americans, Latinos, and Native Americans. In some cases, MMPI-2 elevations among multicultural groups were not clinically meaningful; in other cases, elevations appeared to reflect actual symptomology (Arbisi et al., 2002; Cabiya et al., 2000; Greene et al., 2003; Hall et al., 1999; Timbrook & Graham, 1994; Whitworth & McBlaine, 1993; Whitworth & Unterbrink, 1994). However, it is also important to note that use of the MMPI-2 with multicultural populations has raised some concerns. Specifically, the inadequate representation of Latinos, Asian Americans, and Native Americans in the standardization sample calls into question the cultural appropriateness of this measure. Second, there are studies cautioning that elevated scores may be less indicative of psychopathology and more indicative of cultural factors. This point is particularly evident when one considers how certain items related to depression, schizophrenia, and the potential for "faking good" may have different interpretations for members of various racial/ethnic groups. The Diagnostic and Statistical Manual of Mental Disorders (APA, 2000) acknowledges that culture-specific syndromes may not be indicative of a particular diagnostic category. Complicating item interpretation further is the role that acculturation may play on responses. Finally, when considering MMPI-2 responses among Latinos, Asian Americans, and Native Americans, it is imperative to keep in mind the heterogeneity of these groups.

The Rorschach Inkblot Test (RIT)

The Rorschach Inkblot Test (RIT) is another measure that has ranked highly among clinical psychologists (Camara et al., 2000). Similar to the MMPI-2, it is a measure of psychopathology; however, it is considered by many to be projective in nature. The RIT is particularly useful for assessing concerns with perceptual and psychotic processing. Over the decades, a number of scoring systems have been developed for RIT responses (Exner, 2003). In an attempt to integrate these systems, Exner developed the Comprehensive System, which is now commonly used. Exner's normative sample included 493 (82%) Caucasians, 60 (10%) African Americans, 36 (6%) Latinos, and 11 (2%) Asian Americans. Native Americans were not identified. Given current population estimates, it is evident that Latinos, Asian Americans, and Native Americans were not adequately represented.

With regards to the performance of various racial/ethnic groups, in a presentation at the International Rorschach Society (as cited in Ritzler, 2001), data of non-patients from eight countries (viz.,., Argentina, Belgium, Finland, Japan, Peru, Portugal,

Spain, and the United States) indicated consistency on most of Exner's coding variables. However, studies conducted within the United States using Exner's system have raised concerns. Specifically, Frank's (1992) review found that RIT profiles of African Americans reflected limited self-disclosure (i.e., fewer responses overall). Similarly, Meyer (2002) found that African Americans gave fewer responses and a high proportion of pure "form" responses, which are also suggestive of limited self-disclosure. However, when individuals were matched on education, inpatient status, gender, marital status, and age, differences were no longer apparent.

For Latinos, Exner's (2003) norms may be problematic. Bachran (2002) found that Latino clinical patients reported fewer "popular" responses when compared to Exner's clinical and nonclinical normative groups; "popular" responses are indicative of perception and social conventionality. Also expressing concern, Frank (1993) highlighted the need for additional research with Latinos, focusing on the development of culture specific norms and assessment of acculturation. Two theoretical discussions with Native Americans and the RIT were identified. Dana (1983) argued that the cross-cultural application of the RIT with this group was difficult due to the complexity of disentangling specific cultural effects. In a similar vein, Thomason (1999) noted that the RIT relied on a culturally influenced scoring system that was potentially inappropriate with members of non-literate societies or those with different worldviews. Thomason also highlighted the need for flexible interpretation, given evidence of sparse protocols (e.g., few responses) when the RIT was used with some Native American populations. No empirical studies specific to the RIT and Asian Americans were identified.

As a whole, there are a number of items to consider when using the RIT, including a normative sample that is not highly diverse and limited research examining the performance of multicultural populations. The few studies and discussions that were identified stressed the potential impact of culture on responses. In particular, response style and limited self-disclosure may influence scores (e.g., African Americans giving fewer responses overall). Furthermore, Latinos' limited exposure to United States mainstream culture may impact important scoring variables, and the RIT's cross-cultural applicability with Native Americans may be inadequate. It is clear that additional research is needed to better understand the utility of the RIT with racial/ethnic groups.

The Beck Depression Inventory (BDI)

A popular self-report measure of depressive symptoms, the Beck Depression Inventory, Second Edition (BDI-II; Beck, Steer, & Brown, 1996) included an outpatient standardization sample with the following racial/ethnic groups: 454 (91%) Caucasian, 21 (4%) African American, 18 (4%) Asian American, and 7 (1%) Latino.

The comparative group consisted primarily of 120 Caucasian college students. Given current United States population estimates, these figures indicate that multicultural populations were not adequately represented in either the standardization or comparison groups. However, a number of BDI-II studies have indicated that it may be an appropriate instrument to use with some groups.

Among African American primary care patients, BDI-II scores showed correspondence with depressive diagnoses as obtained from screening interviews (Dutton, et al., 2004). Using the same sample, Grothe, et al. (2005) found adequate fit for the proposed model of cognitive and somatic factors, and adequate criterion validity with patients who had a current diagnosis of major depression.

When examining the BDI-II scores of Asian American and Caucasian university students, Okazaki (1997) found that scores for the Asian American group were significantly higher than previously reported. However, score differences between the two groups were no longer evident after controlling for other factors (e.g., social anxiety). A Chinese version of the original BDI is available (Zheng, Wei, Lianggue, Guochen, & Chenggue, 1988), and its internal reliability and concurrent validity were deemed adequate with a sample of inpatients and outpatients from 24 hospitals in China. However, its construct validity was unsatisfactory, leading the authors to suggest that the Chinese BDI may not correspond well with Chinese culture and may lack sensitivity for screening depression. In contrast, Yeung, et al. (2002) found that the Chinese BDI had adequate sensitivity and specificity, along with positive and negative predictive value among Chinese American primary care patients. Of significance, respondents seemed more open to participating in this study when the measure was administered verbally by research assistants as opposed to the traditional paper-and-pencil format.

A large scale study of Latino and non-Latino United States college students found minor significant differences between the mean BDI scores of both groups, strong internal consistency for the measure, and support for its factor structure (Contreras, Fernandez, Malcarne, Ingram, & Vaccarino, 2004). Another study of ethnically diverse college students also found evidence for the internal consistency of the BDI-II, although there was a main effect for ethnicity, with Caucasian students reporting higher irritability and worthlessness than Latino students (Carmody, 2005). In a study of clinically anxious Latinos, Novy, Stanley, Averill, and Daza (2001) found strong internal consistency and convergent and discriminant validity with the BDI-II. Wiebe and Penley (2005) explored the internal consistency and factor structure of the English and Spanish versions of the BDI-II among undergraduates. The authors found strong internal consistency and adequate test-retest reliability for both language versions, with no significant language effects. In addition, a confirmatory factor analysis revealed an adequate fit between the Spanish instrument and the BDI-II's factor structure.

Research with the BDI and Native Americans is limited, with Horan and Cady (1990) using the measure for program planning. However, Thomason (1999) noted that there was insufficient evidence to recommend use of the BDI with Native Americans. Similarly, Allen (1998) highlighted that studies of depressive symptoms among Native Americans were challenging because of the western conceptualization of depression. For example, a lack of conceptual equivalence was found among Hopi tribe members and their understanding of depression (Mason, Shore, & Bloom, 1985, as cited in Allen, 1998), with most participants indicating that they thought no word or phrase for depression existed in their language.

Taken together, although racial/ethnic minorities are not highly represented in the outpatient standardization and comparative samples of the BDI-II, it appears to be an adequate measure for screening depression among African Americans and Latinos. However, for Asian Americans (and perhaps those who are less acculturated to United States mainstream culture), response style may impact scores. Moreover, the western conceptualization of depression as reflected in the BDI-II items may lack the sensitivity to screen depression among Asian Americans and Native Americans.

IMPLICATIONS OF THE TEST REVIEW FOR PRACTICE

For many people with disabilities seeking VR services, a psychological assessment is essential to determine eligibility into the system. Results from such an assessment are also used to guide vocational goals and work plans. It is recognized that much useful information can be garnered from testing, particularly when identifying the strengths and weaknesses in one's cognitive and social-emotional functioning. It is also important to consider that there has been some debate regarding the utility of psychological assessments when testing racial/ethnic minorities (Dana, 1993; Padilla, 1995; Sue et al., 1992).

This chapter presented information on four commonly used psychological tests to illustrate the complexities involved when testing African Americans, Asian Americans, Latinos, and Native Americans. From our review, we learned that despite the popularity and longevity of the WAIS-III, MMPI-II, RIT, and BDI-II, to varying degrees their standardization samples tended to lack adequate representation of multicultural populations. This was particularly true for Asian Americans and Native Americans. Even when groups were represented in the standardization sample, some empirical studies found differential performance based on race/ethnicity. In some cases, these differences were clinically meaningful; in other cases, these differences seemed to reflect the limitations of tests when assessing multicultural groups.

Given information presented in this chapter, we recommend that practitioners testing for the VR system keep the following in mind as they conduct assessments with diverse groups:

1. When selecting psychological tests, *review the composition of the standardization sample* and *existing research* to assess their appropriateness for various multicultural groups. With such information in hand, practitioners will be in a better position to select tests and interpret results.

2. Concerns have been raised with the *universality of western constructs* when discussing intelligence and psychological disorders (e.g., depression, anxiety, and schizophrenia). Given that tests have been developed with western constructs in mind, validity may not be adequate when testing multicultural populations (Sternberg & Grigorenko, 2001).

3. There is much *heterogeneity within racial/ethnic groups*. This point is quite evident when one considers the diversity of Asians, Pacific Islanders, Native Americans, Alaska Natives, and Latinos (Bureau of Indian Affairs, 2003; Lee, Lei, & Sue, 2001; U.S. Census Bureau, 2001). With such vast within-group heterogeneity, the noble task of having all racial/ethnic groups represented during test development and standardization becomes nearly impossible (Lee et al.).

4. In addition to within-group heterogeneity, members of many racial/ethnic groups differ when one considers levels of *language proficiency, immigration status, generation status, duration of stay in the United States, acculturation, and cultural values* (Allen, 1998; Cervantes & Acosta, 1992; Kwan, 1999; Lee, et al. 2001; Okazaki, 1997; Thomason, 1999). Such socio-cultural variables may influence psychological test results.

5. Socio-cultural variables may also impact how multicultural populations *approach and respond to psychological tasks*. Baker and Taylor (1995) highlighted several sources of potential bias when conducting psychological testing with African Americans, including linguistic differences, the social situation of the test, potential distrust of the examiner and the environment, and contextual match between cognitive performance and sociocultural experiences. Alston and McCowan (1994) noted similar concerns (e.g., testing response style, performance motivation, and language usage), and suggested that these variables may account for the poor success rate of African Americans with disabilities in VR settings.

6. A number of empirical studies have examined the testing performance of multicultural populations by *sampling college and university students*. It has been argued that such findings may have limited interpretation and external validity because undergraduates are not representative of the general population (Sears, 1986). Researchers need to be aware of this bias and design studies with results that have increased generalizability.

APPROACHES TO CONSIDER WHEN CONDUCTING ASSESSMENTS WITH MULTICULTURAL GROUPS

To help professionals conduct culturally-competent assessments within the VR system, we present three approaches to testing that embody the need for individualization and comprehensiveness. First, the Biocultural Model of Assessment proposed by Armour-Thomas and Gopaul-McNicol (1998) encourages a four-tier approach, with the first tier focusing on standardized testing and quantitative scores. The second tier incorporates testing of the limits to better understand scores obtained, particularly with cognitive tests. Testing of the limits may include suspending time limits, providing paper and pencil to perform tasks, and offering multiple-choice responses. The third tier is an ecological assessment that includes an assessment of health, language, acculturation level, education, social-emotional history, familial and community support, and performance at school, home, and community. Lastly, the fourth tier includes examining other forms of "intelligence" such as those proposed by Gardner (1983): linguistic, musical, logical-mathematical, spatial, bodily-kinesthetic, interpersonal, and intrapersonal. These four tiers provide quantitative and qualitative information in order to prepare assessments that account for clients' unique characteristics and histories.

Second, Dana (2005) proposed nine ingredients that aim to promote ethical multicultural assessment practice.

1. The Multicultural Assessment-Intervention Process (MAIP) is recommended, whereby a sequential flowchart of culturally relevant issues is considered when testing people of diverse backgrounds.
2. The language skills of both the client and assessor are evaluated to determine the adequacy of communication between the parties and to select appropriate tests.
3. Four areas of cultural competence are highlighted including (a) awareness, knowledge, and skills of multicultural populations; (b) appraisal and understanding of one's own culture/race; (c) critical understanding of multicultural research standards; and (d) culture-specific service delivery in order to elicit valid and reliable assessment data.
4. The client's cultural and racial identities are evaluated to determine the appropriateness of standardized tests.
5. The use of standardized and culture-specific tests is based on the adequacy of test construction, standardization, and norms for multicultural populations.
6. Cultural formulations and culture-bound disorders are considered when determining the appropriateness of diagnoses and interventions.
7. The applicability of standardized tests for diverse groups is considered when engaging in test interpretation.

8. When preparing psychological reports, clients are presented as cultural beings and the potential limitations of testing are discussed.
9. Clients are presented with test feedback in a culturally appropriate manner.

Lastly, Allen (2007) proposed a series of eight knowledge and skill areas pertinent to competent multicultural assessment.

1. Assessors are expected to possess knowledge of measurement theory and test construction.
2. The assessment process is viewed as a collaborative process.
3. Interviewing techniques are congruent with clients' social expectations.
4. Acculturation and identity status are assessed using interview and self-report measures.
5. Acculturation is considered when interpreting results.
6. When the impact of acculturation and identity status on standardized tests is unknown, clinical experience and local cultural norms are considered when interpreting results.
7. Written reports are expected to (a) address the quality of the client/assessor relationship; (b) incorporate cultural data; (c) describe confounds that contribute to possible bias; and (d) summarize findings, recommendations, and limitations.
8. If adaptations (nonstandardized) are made during testing, assessors need to acknowledge the ethical dilemmas associated with the adaptations.

CONCLUSION

As our nation becomes increasingly diverse, it is likely that we will see a large number of racial/ethnic minorities seeking VR services. From our review, it is evident that race and ethnicity are important variables to consider throughout the assessment process (i.e., test selection, test administration, data interpretation, and writing of reports). In addition, it is critical that professionals be informed about and incorporate assessment approaches that aim to adequately reflect clients' intellectual and social-emotional functioning. In the end, assessment approaches that strive for cultural competence may help multicultural populations with disabilities realize their vocational rehabilitation and employment goals.

REFERENCES

Allen, J. (1998). Personality assessment with American Indians and Alaskan Natives: Instrument considerations and service delivery style. *Journal of Personality Assessment, 70,* 17–42.

Allen, J. (2007). A multicultural assessment supervision model to guide research and practice. *Professional Psychology: Research and Practice, 38,* 248–258.

Alston, R. J., & McCowan, C. J. (1994). Aptitude assessment and African American clients: The interplay between culture and psychometrics in rehabilitation. *Journal of Rehabilitation, 60,* 41–46.

American Psychiatric Association. (2000). *Diagnostic and Statistical Manual of Mental Disorders,* Text Revision (4th ed.). Washington, DC: APA.

American Psychological Association. (2002). Ethical principles of psychologists and code of conduct. *American Psychologist, 57,* 1060–1073.

Arbisi, P. A., Ben-Porath, Y. S., & McNulty, J. (2002). A comparison of MMPI-2 validity in African American and Caucasian psychiatric inpatients. *Psychological Assessment, 14,* 3–15.

Armour-Thomas, E., & Gopaul-McNicol, S. (1998). *Assessing intelligence: Applying a bio-cultural model.* London: Sage.

Atkins, B. J., & Wright, G. N. (1980). Three views: Vocational rehabilitation of Blacks: The statement. *Journal of Rehabilitation, 46,* 40–46.

Bachran, M. A. (2002). Latinos' perceptions of the Rorschach inkblots: An examination of the popular response. In E. Davis-Russell (Ed.), *The California school of professional psychology handbook of multicultural education, research, intervention, and training,* (pp. 151–161). San Francisco: Jossey-Bass.

Baker, C. K., & Taylor, D. W. (1995). Assessment of African American clients: Opportunities for biased results. *Vocational Evaluation and Work Adjustment Bulletin, 28,* 46–51.

Beck, A., Steer, R., & Brown, G. (1996). *Beck Depression Inventory II Manual.* San Antonio, TX: Psychological Corporation.

Bellini, J. (2003). Counselors' multicultural competencies and vocational rehabilitation outcomes in the context of counselor-client racial similarity and difference. *Rehabilitation Counseling Bulletin, 46,* 164–173.

Benson, E. (2003). Intelligence across cultures. *Monitor on Psychology, 34,* 56–58.

Boscan, D. C., Penn, N. E., Velasquez, R. J., Reimann, J., Gomez, N., Guzman, M. et al., (2000). MMPI-2 profiles of Colombian, Mexican, and Venezuelan students. *Psychological Reports, 87,* 107–110.

Bureau of Indian Affairs. (2003). American Indian population and labor force report 2003. Retrieved March 25, 2008, from *http://www.doi.gov/triballaborforce2003.pdf*

Butcher, J. N., Cheung, F. M., & Lim, J. (2003). Use of MMPI-2 with Asian populations. *Psychological Assessment, 15,* 248–256.

Butcher, J. N., & Graham, J. R. (1989). *Topics in MMPI-2 interpretation.* Minneapolis: Department of Psychology, University of Minnesota.

Cabiya, J. J., Lucio, E., Chavira, D. A., Castellanos, J., Gomez, F. C., & Velasquez, R. (2000). MMPI-2 scores of Puerto Rican, Mexican, and U.S. Latino college students: A research note. *Psychological Reports, 87,* 266–268.

Camara, W. J., Nathan, J. S., & Puente, A. E. (2000). Psychological test usage: Implications in professional psychology. *Professional Psychology: Research and Practice, 31,* 141–154.

Canul, G. D., & Cross, H. J. (1994). The influence of acculturation and racial identity attitudes on Mexican-Americans' MMPI-2 performance. *Journal of Clinical Psychology, 50,* 736–745.

Capella, M. E. (2002). Inequities in the VR system: Do they still exist? *Rehabilitation Counseling Bulletin, 45,* 143–153.

Carmody, D. P. (2005). Psychometric characteristics of the Beck Depression Inventory-II with college students of diverse ethnicity. *International Journal of Psychiatry in Clinical Practice, 9*, 22–28.

Cervantes, R. C., & Acosta, F. X. (1992). Psychological testing for Hispanic Americans. *Applied & Preventive Psychology, 1*, 209–219.

Chan, D. W., Lee, H. B., & Luk, C. (1999). Developing a Chinese vocabulary test as a WAIS-R subtest for adults in Hong Kong. *Psychologia, 42*, 89–100.

Cheung, F. M. (1995). *Administration manual of the Minnesota Multiphasic Personality Inventory (MMPI) Chinese edition.* Hong Kong: The Chinese University Press.

Cheung, F. M., Song, W. Z., & Zhang, J. X. (1996). The Chinese MMPI-2: Research and applications in Hong Kong and the People's Republic of China. In J. N. Butcher (Ed.), *International adaptations of the MMPI-2: A handbook of research and applications* (pp. 137–161). Minneapolis: University of Minnesota Press.

Contreras, S., Fernandez, S., Malcarne, V. L., Ingram, R. E., & Vaccarino, V. R. (2004). Reliability and validity of the Beck Depression and Anxiety Inventories in Caucasian Americans and Latinos. *Hispanic Journal of Behavioral Sciences, 26*, 446–462.

Cutler, F., & Ramm, A. (1992). An introduction to the basics of vocational evaluation. In J. M. Siefker (Ed.), *Vocational evaluation in private sector rehabilitation* (pp. 31–66). Menomonie, WI: Materials Development Center.

Dana, R. H. (1983, March). Assessment of Native Americans: Guidelines and a format for test interpretation. In R. H. Dana (Chair), *Psychological assessment of Native Americans.* Symposium conducted at the meeting of the Society for Personality Assessment, San Diego, CA.

Dana, R. H. (1986). Personality assessment and Native Americans. *Journal of Personality Assessment, 50*, 480–500.

Dana, R. H. (1993). *Multicultural assessment perspectives for professional psychology.* Needham Heights, MA: Allyn & Bacon.

Dana, R. H. (2005). *Multicultural assessment: Principles, applications and examples.* Mahwah, NJ: Erlbaum.

Demsky, Y. I., Gass, C. S., & Golden, C. J. (1998). Interpretation of VIQ-PIQ and intersubtest differences on the Spanish version of the WAIS (EIWA). *Assessment, 5*, 25–29.

Dutton, G. R., Grothe, K. B., Jones, G. N., Whitehead, B. S., Kendra, K., & Brantley, P. J. (2004). Use of the Beck Depression Inventory-II with African American primary care patients. *General Hospital Psychiatry, 26*, 437–442.

Dziekan, K. I., & Okocha, A. A. G. (1993). Accessibility of rehabilitation services: Comparison by racial-ethnic status. *Rehabilitation Counseling Bulletin, 36*, 183–189.

Exner, J. E. (2003). *The Rorschach: A comprehensive system. Basic foundations and principles of interpretation* (4th ed.). New York: Wiley.

Fantoni-Salvador, P., & Rogers, R. (1997). Spanish versions of the MMPI-2 and PAI: An investigation of concurrent validity with Hispanic patients. *Assessment, 4*, 29–39.

Frank, G. (1992). The response of African Americans to the Rorschach: A review of the research. *Journal of Personality Assessment, 59*, 317–325.

Frank, G. (1993). The use of the Rorschach with Hispanic Americans. *Psychological Reports, 72*, 276–278.

Frueh, B. C., Gold, P. B., de Arellano, M. A., & Brady, K. L. (1997). A racial comparison of combat veterans evaluated for PTSD. *Journal of Personality Assessment, 68*, 692–702.

Garcia-Peltoniemi, R., & Azan Chaviano, A. (1993). *MMPI 2: Inventario Multifasico de la Personalidad-2 Minnesota.* Minneapolis: University of Minnesota Press.

Gardner, H. (1983). *Frames of mind: The theory of multiple intelligences.* New York: Basic Books.

Gomez, F. C., Piedmont, R. L., & Fleming, M. Z. (1992). Factor analysis of the Spanish version of the WAIS: The Escala de Inteligencia Wechsler para Adultos (EIWA). *Psychological Assessment, 4,* 317–321.

Gong, Y. X. (1983). Revision of Wechsler Adult Intelligence Scale in China. *Acta Psychologica Sinica, 15,* 362–369.

Graham, J. R. (2006). *Assessing personality and psychopathology* (4th ed.). New York: Oxford University Press.

Greene, R. L., Robin, R. W., Albaugh, B., Caldwell, A., & Goldman, D. (2003). Use of the MMPI-2 in American Indians: II. Empirical correlates. *Psychological Assessment, 15,* 360–369.

Grothe, K. B., Dutton, G. R., Jones, G. N., Bodenlos, J., Ancona, M., & Brantley, P. J. (2005). Validation of the Beck Depression Inventory-II in a low-income, African American sample of medical outpatients. *Psychological Assessment, 17,* 110–114.

Guilmet, G. M. (1975). Cognitive research among the Eskimo: A survey. *Anthropologica, 17,* 61–84.

Hall, G. C. N., Bansal, A., & Lopez, I. R. (1999). Ethnicity and psychopathology: A meta-analytic review of 31 years of comparative MMPI/MMPI-2 research. *Psychological Assessment, 11,* 186–197.

Hall, G. C. N., & Phung, A. H. (2001). Minnesota Multiphasic Personality Inventory and Millon Clinical Multiaxial Inventory. In L. A. Suzuki, J. G. Ponterotto, & P. J. Meller (Eds.), *Handbook of multicultural assessment: Clinical, psychological, and educational applications* (pp. 307–330). San Francisco: Jossey-Bass.

Harris, J. G., Tulsky, D. S., & Schultheis, M. T. (2003). Assessment of the non-native English Speaker: Assimilating history and research findings to guide clinical practice. In D. S. Tulsky, D. H. Saklofske, G. J. Chelune, R. K. Heaton, R. J. Ivnik, R. Bornstein, et al. (Eds.), *Clinical Interpretation of the WAIS-III and WMS-III* (pp. 343–390). San Diego, CA: Academic Press.

Hathaway, S. R., & McKinley, J. C. (1989). *Manual for the Minnesota Multiphasic Personality Inventory-2 (MMPI-2).* Minneapolis, MN: University of Minnesota Press.

Hayward, B. J., & Schmidt-Davis, H. (2003a). *Final report 1: How consumer characteristics affect access to, receipt of, and outcomes of VR services.* Report prepared under Contract Number HR92-022-001 for the Rehabilitation Services Administration, U.S. Department of Education. Research Triangle Park, NC: Research Triangle.

Hayward, B. J., & Schmidt-Davis, H. (2003b). *Final report 2: VR services and outcomes.* Report prepared under Contract Number HR92-022-001 for the Rehabilitation Services Administration, U.S. Department of Education. Research Triangle Park, NC: Research Triangle.

Herbert, J. T., & Martinez, M. Y. (1992). Client ethnicity and vocational rehabilitation case service outcome. *Journal of Job Placement, 8,* 10–16.

Horan, K., & Cady, D. C. (1990). Psychological evaluation of American Indians. *Arizona Counseling Journal, 15,* 6–12.

Kaufman, A. S., & Lichtenberger, E. O. (2006). *Assessing adolescent and adult intelligence.* Hoboken, NJ: John Wiley & Sons.

Kundu, M. M., Dutta, A., & Walker, S. (2006). Participation of ethnically diverse personnel in state-federal vocational rehabilitation agencies. *Journal of Applied Rehabilitation Counseling, 37*, 30–37.

Kwan, K. (1999). MMPI and MMPI-2 performance of the Chinese: Cross-cultural applicability. *Professional Psychology: Research & Practice, 30*, 260–268.

Lee, J., Lei, A., & Sue, S. (2001). The current state of mental health research on Asian Americans. *Journal of Human Behavior in the Social Environment, 3*, 159–178.

Lessenger, L. H. (1997). Acculturation and MMPI-2 scale scores of Mexican American substance abuse patients. *Psychological Reports, 80*, 1181–1182.

Lopez, S., & Romero, A. (1988). Assessing the intellectual functioning of Spanish-speaking adults: Comparison of the EIWA and the WAIS. *Professional Psychology: Research & Practice, 19*, 263–270.

Lucio, E., Ampudia, A., Duran, C., Leon, I., & Butcher, J. N. (2001). Comparison of the Mexican and American norms of the MMPI-2. *Journal of Clinical Psychology, 57*, 1459–1468.

Lucio, G. M. E., Reyes-Lagunes, I., & Scott, R. L. (1994). MMPI-2 for Mexico: Translation and adaptation. *Journal of Personality Assessment, 63*, 105–116.

McNulty, J. L., Graham, J. R., Ben-Porath, Y. S., & Stein, L. A. R. (1997). Comparative validity of MMPI-2 scores of African American and Caucasian mental health center clients. *Psychological Assessment, 9*, 464–470.

Melendez, F. (1994). The Spanish version of the WAIS: Some ethical considerations. *Clinical Neuropsychologist, 8*, 388–393.

Meyer, G. J. (2002). Exploring possible ethnic differences and bias in the Rorschach Comprehensive System. *Journal of Personality Assessment, 78*, 104–129.

Moore, C. L. (2001). Racial and ethnic members of under-represented groups with hearing loss and VR services: Explaining the disparity in closure success rate. *Journal of Applied Rehabilitation Counseling, 32*, 15–23.

Moore, C. L., Feist-Price, S., & Alston, R. J. (2002). VR services for persons with severe/profound mental retardation: Does race matter? *Rehabilitation Counseling Bulletin, 45*, 162–167.

Moore, C. L., Giesen, J. M., & Cavenaugh, B. S. (2005). Latino VR access rates by disability type and proportions in the general population with disabilities. *Journal of Applied Rehabilitation Counseling, 36*, 25–32.

Neisser, U., Boodoo, G., Bouchard, T. J., Boykin, A. W., Brody, N., Ceci, S. J. et al., (1996). Intelligence: Knowns and unknowns. *American Psychologist, 51*, 77–101.

Novy, D. M., Stanley, M. A., Averill, P., & Daza, P. (2001). Psychometric comparability of English- and Spanish-language measures of anxiety and related affective symptoms. *Psychological Assessment, 13*, 347–355.

Okazaki, S. (1997). Sources of ethnic differences between Asian American and White American college students on measures of depression and social anxiety. *Journal of Abnormal Psychology, 106*, 52–60.

Okazaki, S., & Sue, S. (2000). Implications of test revisions for assessment with Asian Americans. *Psychological Assessment, 12*, 272–280.

Pace, T. M., Robbins, R. R., Choney, S. K., Hill, J. S., Lacey, K., & Blair, G. (2006). A cultural-contextual perspective on the validity of the MMPI-2 with American Indians. *Cultural Diversity and Ethnic Minority Psychology, 12*, 320–333.

Padilla, A. M. (1995). Issues in culturally appropriate assessment. In L. A. Suzuki, J. G. Ponterotto, & P. J. Meller (Eds.) *Handbook of multicultural assessment: Clinical, psychological, and educational applications,* (2nd ed., pp. 5–27). San Francisco: Jossey-Bass.

Ritzler, B. (2001). Multicultural usage of the Rorschach. In L. A. Suzuki, J. G. Ponterotto, & P. J. Meller (Eds.), *Handbook of multicultural assessment: Clinical, psychological, and educational applications,* 22, 237–252. San Francisco: Jossey-Bass.

Robin, R. W., Greene, R. L., Albaugh, B., Caldwell, A., & Goldman, D. (2003). Use of the MMPI-2 in American Indians: I. Comparability of the MMPI-2 between two tribes and with the MMPI-2 normative group. *Psychological Assessment, 15,* 351–359.

Rushton, J. P., & Jensen, A. R. (2005). Thirty years of research on race differences in cognitive ability. *Psychology, Public Policy, and Law, 11,* 235–294.

Ryan, J. J., Dai, X., & Paolo, A. M. (1995). Verbal-Performance IQ discrepancies on the mainland Chinese version of the Wechsler Adult Intelligence Scale (WAIS-RC). *Journal of Psychoeducational Assessment, 13,* 365–371.

Samuda, R. J. (1998). *Psychological testing of American minorities: Issues and consequences* (2nd ed.). Thousand Oaks, CA: Sage.

Sears, D. O. (1986). College sophomores in the laboratory: Influences of a narrow data base on social psychology's view of human nature. *Journal of Personality and Social Psychology, 51,* 515–530.

Shiota, N. K., Krauss, S. S., & Clark, L. A. (1996). Adaptation and validation of the Japanese MMPI-2. In J. N. Butcher (Ed.), *International adaptations of the MMPI-2: A handbook of research and applications* (pp. 67–87). Minneapolis, MN: University of Minnesota Press.

Sternberg, R. J., & Grigorenko, E. L. (2001). Unified psychology. *American Psychologist, 56,* 1069–1079.

Stevens, M. J., Kwan, K. L., & Graybill, D. (1993). Comparison of MMPI-2 scores of foreign Chinese and Caucasian-American students. *Journal of Clinical Psychology, 49,* 23–27.

Sue, D. W., Arredondo, P., & McDavis, R. J. (1992). Multicultural competencies and standards: A call to the profession. *Journal of Multicultural Counseling and Development, 20,* 64–89.

Thomas, D. F., Rosenthal, D. A., Banks, M. E., & Schroeder, M. (2002). *Diversity in vocational rehabilitation: People, practice, and outcomes.* Community-based rehabilitation: Research for improving employment outcome conference. 2002 State-of-the-science conference proceedings. Retrieved March 25, 2008, from *http://www.tamas.gov.il/NR/rdonlyres/32BD2068-AF73-4381-BACF-914CAECA8309/0/Diversity.pdf*

Thomason, T. C. (1999). *Psychological and vocational assessment of Native Americans.* Flagstaff, AZ: American Indian Rehabilitation Research and Training Center.

Timbrook, R. E. & Graham, J. R. (1994). Ethnic differences on the MMPI-2. *Psychological Assessment, 6,* 212–217.

Tsai, D. C, & Pike, P. L. (2000). Effects of acculturation on the MMPI-2 scores of Asian American students. *Journal of Personality Assessment, 74,* 216–230.

Tulsky, D. & Zhu, J. (1997). *WAIS-III/WMS-III Technical Manual.* San Antonio: Psychological Corporation.

U. S. Census Bureau. (2001). *Census 2000 shows America's diversity.* Retrieved March 25, 2008, from *http://www.census.gov/Press-Release/www/2001/cb01cn61.html*

Wechsler, D. (1968). *Manual para la Escala de Inteligencia Wechsler para Adultos.* New York: Psychological Corporation.

Wechsler, D., Chen, Y. H., & Chen, X. Y. (2002). *WAIS-III Chinese version technical manual.* San Antonio, TX: Psychological Corporation.

Wiebe, J. S., & Penley, J. A. (2005). A psychometric comparison of the Beck Depression Inventory-II in English and Spanish. *Psychological Assessment, 17,* 481–485.

Whitworth, R. H., & McBlaine, D. D. (1993). Comparison of the MMPI and MMPI-2 administered to Anglo- and Hispanic-American university students. *Journal of Personality Assessment, 61,* 19–27.

Whitworth, R. H., & Unterbrink, C. (1994). Comparison of MMPI-2 clinical and content scales administered to Hispanic and Anglo-Americans. *Hispanic Journal of Behavioral Sciences, 16,* 255–264.

Wilson, K. B. (2000). Predicting vocational rehabilitation acceptance based on race, education, work status, and source of support at application. *Rehabilitation Counseling Bulletin, 43,* 97–105.

Yao, S., Chen, H., & Tam, W. C. (2007). Replication of factor structure of Wechsler Adult Intelligence Scale-III Chinese version in Chinese mainland non-clinical and schizophrenia samples. *Psychiatry and Clinical Neurosciences, 61,* 379–384.

Yeung, A., Howarth, S., Chan, R., Sonawalla, S., Nierenberg, A. A., & Fava, M. (2002). Use of the Chinese version of the Beck Depression Inventory for screening depression in primary care. *Journal of Nervous and Mental Disease, 190,* 94–99.

Zea, M. C., García, J. G., Belgrave, F. Z., & Quezada, T. (1997). Socioeconomic and cultural factors in the rehabilitation of Latinos with disabilities. In J. G. Garcia, & M. C. Zea (Eds.). *Psychological interventions and research with Latino populations,* (pp. 217–234). Needham Heights, MA: Allyn & Bacon.

Zheng, Y., Wei, L., Lianggue, G., Guochen, Z., & Chenggue, W. (1988). Applicability of the Chinese Beck Depression Inventory. *Comprehensive Psychiatry, 29,* 484–489.

CHAPTER 5

Access to Vocational Rehabilitation Services for Black Latinos with Disabilities: Colorism in the 21st Century

Keith B. Wilson, PhD, CRC, NCC, ABDA, LPC; and
Julissa Senices, PhD

INTRODUCTION

With the influx of Latinos in many of the major cities across the U.S., cultural competency is vital (Quiñones-Mayo, Wilson, & McGuire, 2000). The U.S. Census Bureau projects that non-White people will become a numerical majority by the year 2050; however, according to some private polls, this demographic shift will occur by the year 2030 (Sue, 1996). Therefore, it is likely that future human service workers, counselors, and educators will be serving a much larger number of clients from racially and ethnically diverse backgrounds (Sue, Arrendondo, & McDavis, 1992; Wilson, 2002).

The U.S. Census Bureau (2001b) reported that the Latino population has become the largest ethnic minority group in the U.S. For example, in 1980, Latinos made up 6.4% of the total population and in 2000, the Latino population grew to approximately 14.% (U.S. Census Bureau, 2001b).

It has been substantiated for several years that access to Vocational Rehabilitation (VR) services is more difficult for Black Latinos and African Americans than for White people in the U.S. (Wilson, Harley, McCormick, Jolivette, & Jackson 2001; Wilson & Senices, 2005). The difficulties in access to the VR system are underscored by changing demographics. For example, between 1980 and 1990, the White population increased only 7.7%, while the African American population increased by 15.8% (Rogers, Conoley, Ponterotto, & Wiese, 1992). While the demographic trends are gradually changing to reflect more diversity in the U.S., White people, who work in the human services, for example, must change how they relate to groups who are different from them. This is one of the challenges of the 21st century.

Despite the fact that the Latino population is the largest ethnic minority population in the U.S., very little research has been conducted on the Latino population relative to VR acceptance and eligibility (Wilson, 2005; Wilson & Senices, 2005). More
striking is the lack of research in the disability literature dividing the Latino population into racial categories based on how Latinos racially self-identify. Obviously,
Latinos with disabilities are deserving of more attention in the human services literature because of their sheer numbers in many parts of the U.S. and in the VR system.
Thus, the distinctive contribution of this chapter is to examine past investigations
focused on people with disabilities and the discrepant outcomes between people
with disabilities who classify racially as White, including White Latinos, and those
who classify racially as Black, including African Americans and Black Latinos.

Definition of Terms

Colorism

The key characteristic of colorism is distinguishing people with lighter skin col-
ors/hues from darker skin colors/hues. The darker skin-toned individuals are considered to be less desirable. This notion of colorism seems to stem back hundreds of
years when slaves with lighter skin colors/hues were favored by the slave master
(Carr, 1997). One may also use the word phenotype when referring to colorism in the
most general sense. Phenotype is defined as the physical characteristic of a person or
organism, such as skin color/hue or eye shape. While we recognize that there may
be negative perceptions within a group based on the color/hue of a person, this
chapter focuses on the relationship between skin colors/hues across some racial and
ethnic groups and VR outcomes.

Race and Ethnicity

While the word "race" may have appeared in writings centuries ago, the term continues to be misused. There is an obvious overlap in the meaning of the terms race
and ethnicity. The Rehabilitation Services Administration (RSA, 1995), a part of the
U.S. Department of Education, the U.S. Census Bureau, and several authors, such as
Wilson and Senices (2005), define race and ethnicity in two separate ways. According
to Sue et al. (1992), one of the two definitions of race is based on a constellation of
biological and physical traits. The race definition by Sue et al. implies that race could
be viewed as the outward appearance of a person. Because most people view race as
color and/or outward physical appearance (i.e., phenotype), the authors are inclined
to support this view of race in this chapter. Carter (1995) prefers to use the word race
instead of ethnicity because the experiences that people of color have in the U.S. are
superseded by the color of their skin. Many other authors support Carter's assertion

(Bennett, 1995; Devine & Elliott, 1995; Hacker, 1995; Schulman et al., 1999; Wilson, 2005). As with Carter and other research teams (e.g., Wilson & Senices, 2005), we believe that one's skin color is a principal characteristic in determining the intensity of discrimination in the U.S. Why? Because skin color is overt. Thus, in this chapter, race and colorism will be used synonymously.

On the other hand, ethnicity deals with shared culture, values, beliefs, foci of control, language, and the spirituality of a particular group of individuals (Banks, 1991; Dana, 1998). Ethnicity also tends to be land-based. The term ethnicity is more comprehensive and also includes both race and culture of origin (Phinney, 1996). "Although an ethnic minority group shares a common culture [e.g., behavior patterns, values, symbols], a historic tradition, and a sense of peoplehood, it also has unique physical and/or cultural characteristics that enable individuals who belong to other ethnic groups to identify its members easily, often for discrimination purposes" (Banks, p. 64; Hacker, 1995).

Hispanic or Latino

Just as it is important to distinguish between the terms race and ethnicity, it is important to differentiate the terms Hispanic and Latino. "Hispanics constitute an ethnic group rather than a racial category, and their members may classify themselves as White, Black, or some other race" (Rawlings & Saluter, 1994, p. xii), including being of mixed races (U.S. Census Bureau, 2001a). This illustrates that Hispanics and other groups can select more than one race to self-classify. "Currently, there appears to be a divided opinion regarding preference for the terms 'Hispanic' and 'Latino'" (Smart & Smart, 1996, p. 174). People in academia are steadily phasing out the Hispanic label and substituting Latino in its place (Gonzalez, 1995). The term Latino includes individuals of diverse Latino-based national origins including those from Mexico, the countries of Central America (i.e., Guatemala, Honduras, Costa Rica, El Salvador, Nicaragua, and Panama), the Spanish-speaking countries of South America (i.e., Colombia, Venezuela, Peru, Chile, Ecuador, Uruguay, Paraguay, Argentina), the Spanish-speaking countries of the Caribbean (i.e., Cuba, the Dominican Republic), and the United States territorial island of Puerto Rico (Casas & Pytluk, 1995). We have decided to use Latino rather than Hispanic because the term Hispanic emphasizes Spain, the period of conquest, and the Spanish language. The term Latino reflects a group's self-definition, and is inclusive of the wide range of cultures, ethnic backgrounds, languages, and races found among the 20-plus nations that comprise the Latino population of Central and South America, including the Caribbean islands (Quiñones-Mayo et al., 2000). As one would expect, Latinos exemplify a rainbow of skin colors and diverse physical attributes. We will retain the word "Hispanic" when quoting the work of other researchers.

It is increasingly clear that when forced to choose between classifying themselves racially as either Black or White, Latinos are likely to classify as White (U.S. Census Bureau, 2001a; Wilson & Senices). In the 1990 U.S. Census general population data, approximately half, or 52%, of Latinos identified as White (U.S. Census Bureau, 1990). Using a national database from the RSA which holds data on people with disabilities in the U.S., Wilson and Senices reported that 92% of all Latinos tended to select White as their race. While there was no way of knowing whether Latinos or other racial groups in the aforementioned references phenotypically looked White, cursory evidence suggest that most Latinos may look more White than Black. Until recently, the racial classification system in the U.S. did not include an option for "mixed race" that would allow Latinos, as well as other groups, to classify themselves according to the gradations in the color of the skin.

VOCATIONAL REHABILITATION OUTCOMES

Outcomes for African Americans

Colorism exists and has extremely negative consequences for people with disabilities in the U.S. Atkins and Wright (1980) were the first research team to empirically analyze VR acceptance by race (African Americans vis-à-vis White people). They found that African Americans were accepted proportionately less for VR services than their White counterparts with disabilities. Herbert and Martinez (1992) provided similar findings to those of Atkins and Wright; particularly, that African Americans were more likely to be determined ineligible for VR services and less likely to be successfully rehabilitated than White clients with disabilities. Taken together, these studies show that African Americans with disabilities tend to have problems accessing VR services when compared to their White counterparts.

These individual studies laid the foundation for another decade of research showing that people of color with disabilities tended to have different VR experiences than White people with disabilities in the U.S. One year after the Herbert and Martinez (1992) investigation, Dziekan and Okocha (1993) examined the accessibility of rehabilitation services among African Americans, Latinos, Native Americans, Asian Americans, and White people with disabilities for the years 1985 through 1989. Dziekan and Okocha's findings were consistent with those reported earlier by Atkins and Wright (1980) and Herbert and Martinez (1992), showing that White people were accepted for VR services at a higher rate than African American and others from non-White racial/ethnic backgrounds, considered both individually and collectively, in each of the five years of the study. In addition, in 2000 and 2002, Wilson's results provided further empirical support that African Americans are less likely to be accepted for VR services than White people—congruent with previous research findings regarding race, ethnicity, and VR acceptance (e.g., Atkins & Wright; Bowe, 1992; Feist-Price, 1995; Herbert & Martinez). Finally, Capella (2002) commented "that differences based on race do still exist for some [multiethnic and racial] groups in terms of acceptance rates and employment outcomes" (p. 150).

In contrast to the aforementioned studies, Wheaton (1995) concluded that "the proportions of Whites and African Americans found eligible for VR services are not significantly different statistically" (p. 228). Peterson (1996) and Wilson (1999) also found no statistical differences between African American and White consumers in VR acceptance rates. The contrasting findings may be due to different methodologies and samples used. For example, Wilson (1999) did not use a random sample. However, Peterson used a proportional sampling procedure. Although these few studies did not find a statistically significant difference in VR acceptance based on race, several other studies noted did have statistically significant findings that African Americans and others who are not White do not achieve the same acceptance status within the VR system.

This body of research suggests that preferential treatment of White people with disabilities may be due to skin color at either the conscious or unconscious level. It is evident that groups of people with disabilities with a darker skin color/hue like African Americans, tended to be accepted less for VR services than clients with a lighter skin color/hue.

Outcomes for Latinos

To clarify outcomes based on skin color and investigate the effects of colorism on people with disabilities, several researchers have conducted studies on Latino VR acceptance specifying skin color/hue as a predictor variable. For example, Herbert and Martinez (1992) divided people who classified as Latino into two racial groups, Black and White. The authors reported that Black Latinos tended to be accepted less for VR services than White people and White Latinos. Furthermore, Herbert and Martinez reported that not only did Black Latinos have problems gaining access to VR services, but once they gained access to VR services, they were less likely to find a job when compared to White Latinos with disabilities.

The following year, Dziekan and Okocha (1993) also reported findings relative to Latinos with disabilities in the VR system. The authors found that Latinos with disabilities are less likely to be accepted for VR services when compared to White people with disabilities. White people with disabilities in their study tended to be accepted for VR services more than any other racial and/or ethnic groups. However, it was not clear whether the Latinos sampled in the Dziekan and Okocha study were Black, White, or a combination of both Black and White Latinos. While the first two studies investigating Latinos with disabilities laid the foundation for colorism research in VR, external validity was one major weakness of the Dziekan and Okocha study due to use of state samples rather than national samples. It is clear that White Latinos with disabilities (Wilson, 2005; Wilson & Senices, 2005) and Latinos in the general population (Rosenbaum, 1996), enjoy similar benefits as White people in the U.S. Furthermore, evidence unmistakably suggests that when several demographic variables are controlled, one's skin color is a salient feature for being discriminated against in the U.S. The following studies by Wilson and his colleagues employed a sampling frame that allowed for more external validity by using a national sample.

In a national study in 2005 looking at the VR acceptance rates of Latinos and non-Latinos with disabilities, Wilson and Senices reported that White Latinos tended to be accepted for VR services more than non-Latinos (e.g., African Americans, Native Americans, etc.). Thus, the outcomes of Latinos were equal to those of White Latinos in the Wilson and Senices study. In another study, Wilson (2005) also reported that the majority of Latinos in the VR system tended to classify themselves racially as White. Again, there is a strong colorism association in the Wilson (2005) study. The VR outcomes of Black Latinos and White Latinos are similar to those of African Americans with disabilities and White people with disabilities (Wilson, 1999; Wilson, 2002). It is apparent that Latinos have the flexibility to classify themselves as White which is not afforded to other groups who are marginalized. As we will see later in this chapter, there are some noted benefits to being able to classify yourself racially as White in the U.S. While classifying oneself based on color is common, Latinos who classify themselves as Black have similar outcomes to African Americans not only in the VR system, but in other areas as well, such as education, housing, health, and employment (Institute of Medicine, 2003). Thus, the results of investigations by Wilson and his colleagues suggest that skin color plays an important part in the selection process of the VR system and that the VR system is nothing more than a microcosm of the general society in which we reside.

In summary, VR results for both Black Latinos and White Latinos with disabilities are similar to results comparing African Americans and White people with disabilities in the U.S. Although these studies are limited because Latinos are forced to choose between White and Black racial classifications that do not fully account for the variation in color within the Latino populations, the consistent theme in these studies is that those Latinos who classify racially as Black have greater difficulty accessing human services for people with disabilities than those who classify racially as White. Empirical evidence based on prior outcome studies investigating African Americans/Black Latinos and White Americans/White Latinos with disabilities has lead to additional evidence to support the claim that lighter skinned people with disabilities have preferential treatment when compared to darker skinned people with disabilities in the U.S. VR system.

COLORISM: A BRIEF HISTORICAL PERSPECTIVE

It is vital to give a historical account and background of the effects of colorism in the U.S. (Wilson, 2005; Wilson & Senices, 2005). During colonialism, the time period in which Europeans were conquering the Americas, a social hierarchy was established with Europeans designating Whites as superior and people of other races as inferior (Lancaster, 1999). Furthermore, the influence of skin color became loaded with connotations, implying that it is "natural" for White people to be accorded higher status over non-White people (Lancaster; Loewen, 1995). Throughout history, discrimination based on skin color has been a serious problem for people who did not have white skin.

European colonists assigned individuals born in European countries with the highest prestige. In the hierarchal structure, individuals born in America with European heritage had the next highest markers of privilege, followed by a large intermediate group such as individuals with mixed heritage. Finally, those with pure Native and/or African lineage were at the bottom of the social order. In time, the two White populations (those born in European countries and those born in America with European heritage) fused, developing a social hierarchy based on skin color (Montalvo, 1991). While there are numerous reasons why one's skin color served as either a disadvantage or advantage in the past (Wilson, Edwards, Alston, Harley, & Doughty, 2001), it is clear from American history that people of color are still at the bottom of the social, political, and economic hierarchy (Chideya, 1995). Undoubtedly, skin color is not the problem; it is what skin color represents for citizens on the North American continent. For example, in many of the old western movies, the good guy would wear a white outfit, and the bad guy would wear the black or dark outfit. Thus, the color of the outfit represented good (white) and evil (black or dark). The same parallel is adduced about skin color in many parts of the world.

As with the VR literature in the U.S., most of the literature on skin color has revolved around the African American community. As a result, prior research has clarified how Blackness has become a marker for discrimination and has highlighted the lack of material gain and privilege for African Americans in the U.S. (Hughes & Hertel, 1990; Jones, 1966; Lee, 1999). Therefore, given the importance of research on

Latinos in adding evidence of the adverse effects of colorism on people with disabilities, it seems important to highlight the influence of colorism in Latin America as well.

Colorism Influences Outside of the United States: Latinos

Skin color variability has had a direct impact on most Latino families within Latin American and Caribbean communities, with those at the lighter end of the continuum having access to more opportunities (Falicov, 1998). The numerous color gradations in the Latin communities create a challenge for racially mixed individuals to classify themselves in a color-coded hierarchy. Racially mixed individuals may have light skin and therefore develop a "White" identity, which is associated with more opportunities and privilege.

Caribbean societies have been shown to function under a multiracial stratification system that uses color gradations, ranging from White to Brown to Black, in association with class status and nationality, to maintain a social hierarchy. For example, both the Dominican Republic and Puerto Rico consist of racially mixed individuals, yet they blur the distinctions between Creoles, Whites, light Coloreds, and Mulattos, thereby creating the impression of, and functioning as, a predominantly White population (Itzigsohn & Dore-Cabral, 2000). Moreover, both countries emphasize "progressive whitening," which encourages individuals to establish their identity on the basis of color, or more specifically, as White (Duany, 1998). As observed in both Dominican Republic and Puerto Rican societies, within-group colorism results from the need to socially classify as White. These societies also give a broader perspective on the overall social structures within Latino countries (Falicov, 1998; Montalvo, 1991) that can be generalized to the U.S. While the continent of North America has a historical context of colorism, the Caribbean and other Latin American countries have similar manifestations of colorism discrimination as well. We assert that colorism is a global concern that does not have geographic boundaries.

It is the worth that we, as a society, attach to the color/hue of being Black or White that has been beneficial for White Latinos and White people and detrimental for Black Latinos and African Americans in the U.S. While one may not be able to readily identify a person who is Latino, a Latino who is Black can be immediately distinguished by the pigmentation of his or her skin color, and thus, be more readily targeted for discrimination because of the color/hue of their skin. The same illustration can be used for other groups, such as females, with certain phenotypical outward markers in our society. In most cases, because there are certain physical features that females share, people in our society who are sexist can readily target women because of general physical markers of what females may look or should look like, generally. The more identifiable a person is based on their skin color/hue, the more discrimination they are likely to encounter based on how people perceive that particular skin color. Although acknowledging that many variables including race, language proficiency, socioeconomic status, and gender, cause people to be discriminated against is painful and unfortunate, historically skin color, or race, has been the most divisive and even life threatening when compared to other characteristics (Smith, 2006).

LIMITATIONS OF RESEARCH ON COLORISM

The Able-bodied Population

Outside of the disability literature, prior studies focusing on skin color have used subjective measures, such as the researcher assuming the race or ethnicity of the participant. This was considered to be a limitation of some studies researching colorism. The literature on skin color has suffered because researchers are skeptical of the validity of studies that only use subjective measures. In certain studies (Arce, Murguia, & Frisbie, 1987), indicators of colorism were based on subjective interviewer ratings since the raters had no points of reference. It is unclear whether interviewers systematically assigned participants to a color category, which suggests possible interviewer bias, increasing the likelihood that the measure of skin color is unreliable. Objective measures of skin color, such as equipment or machines to record melanin, are costly, limiting their use in the skin color literature. In addition, prior studies have neglected to explore the influence of gender differences in the skin color literature. Men and women are socialized differently, which makes the influence of gender identity on skin color significant and worthy of future research consideration.

Vocational Rehabilitation and People with Disabilities

In the studies involving Latinos with disabilities in the VR system reviewed within this chapter, there was no way in which the researcher could validate whether White Latinos were indeed White Latinos (i.e., Latinos with light or white skin tone and/or White European American features). Many of the studies investigating Latinos with disabilities in the VR system used a secondary source to retrieve the data for analysis. When using many secondary data sources, the actual participants in the study are not observed by the researcher. More specifically, only the numbers with associated values are seen in the database. Although Wilson and Senices (2005) reported they had no way of knowing whether Latinos in the VR system could visibly pass as White or White Latino based on their skin color, the results from the Rodriquez and Cordero-Guzman (1992) investigation reported that Puerto Ricans are prone to identify as White, if they think people from the U.S., for example, would view them as White. The Rodriquez and Cordero-Guzman study supports the notion that people who classify themselves as White Latino may indeed have the same phenotypical European features as White people.

As reported, several investigations relied on a secondary data analysis or archival data. Thus, no cause and effect can be assumed. For example, classifying racially as White Latino or Black Latino does not cause one to be accepted into VR services in the U.S. Likewise, being non-Latino (Black or White) does not cause one to be rejected for the same VR services. However, our investigations (Wilson, 2005; Wilson & Senices, 2005) found a significant correlation between race/ethnicity and VR acceptance in the U.S. It is also important to note that the research findings mentioned in all of the VR studies that highlighted racial discrepancies were statistically significant, indicating a positive correlation between VR acceptance and the skin colors/hues of the participants.

Lastly, external validity is also limited to the races and ethnicities that were used in the colorism investigations. The VR studies can only be generalized to the populations used in the sampling procedure. While there is a strong case to be made for generalizing the results of the VR studies because they used a national sampling frame, caution must be stressed when looking to generalize beyond the groups used in the studies. On the other hand, there is evidence that able-bodied African Americans and Black Latinos with disabilities are likely to receive more overt discrimination as a result of being darker than their White Latino counterparts in the U.S. and other parts of the world. Thus, the case for being able to reasonably generalize to other populations not included in these investigations is tenable.

It is also obvious that other variables like limited English proficiency, thick accents, education, and socioeconomic status (SES) may have contributed to individuals not having access to general goods and services in the human services. For example, it is common knowledge that people who present well verbally may be perceived as more assimilated than people who tend to use jargon that is related to urban vernacular. Hence, one possibility is that gatekeepers of human service organizations may be prejudiced toward people with lower levels of education and SES.

There is always a concern with committing a type I error with large samples. Consequently, there may have been sensitivity, or over-fitting, between the number of variables in some of the investigations and the large sample size (Wilson, 2002). This sensitivity is also known as the additive effect of sample size. As the sample size increases, the probability of finding statistical significance also increases. Although many of the studies with large sample sizes use techniques to decrease the additive effect, such as sampling the same number of participants from each group studied, results must be interpreted with caution.

THE STRENGTHS OF RESEARCH ON COLORISM

The most obvious benefit of conducting research on colorism is to focus attention on the discrimination experienced by different groups in the U.S. We view exposure to research on colorism as a way to increase the knowledge base of another salient variable of discrimination that is experienced by a significant part of the racially marginalized population in the U.S. As a result, research on colorism may allow for people to openly communicate and dialogue about the degrees to which perceptions differ among certain groups. The fact of the matter is that people are discriminated against based on their skin color. Thus, becoming knowledgeable about the effects of colorism can potentially mobilize people who are White to facilitate social justice for people of color.

While some studies may have sample size limitations, the sample sizes of most of the VR outcome research regarding African Americans, Black Latinos, and White Latinos with disabilities is a major strength. For example, the study by Wilson and Senices (2005) used a national database with a subsample of 34,563 Latinos and 157,131 non-Latinos and no missing values (Wilson, 2002) to gather the needed information for their investigations. A study regarding able-bodied individuals by Hughes and Hertel (1990) used the National Survey to gather data for their sampling frame as well. Both samples in the aforementioned studies represented several hundred cases, increasing the statistical power to detect a statistical difference. In the aforementioned studies, the results can only be generalized to people in the databases and/or sample frame.

IMPLICATIONS FOR FUTURE RESEARCH

Although there is an obvious lack of research regarding colorism among people with disabilities in the U.S., in future studies researchers may want to use more objective measures of skin color in appraising colorism discrimination. Using more objective measures will continue to ensure that researchers are measuring what they aim to measure. Additionally, future studies should incorporate multiple measures of skin color. This way, it may be possible to cross-validate research findings with other assessments that measure the same or similar variables related to skin color. As stated before in this chapter, some prior studies using subjective measures of skin color have been deemed unreliable. For example, if using self-reports, it seems important to cross-validate self-reports with other criteria, such as an objective measure of skin color. While the results of many studies on colorism are relatively consistent, the use of multiple measures may continue to increase the likelihood of consistency among future outcomes regarding colorism.

Finally, it seems important for future studies to be sensitive to language, gender, and SES differences. Prior studies investigating skin color have neglected the influence of gender (Arce et al., 1987; Relethford, Stern, Gaskill, & Hazuda, 1983; Vasquez, Garcia-Vasquez, Bauman, & Sierra, 1997). Yet, gender identity allows for variability in the socialization process. Males have more of a tendency to adopt the norms, values, and beliefs of the dominant culture than females (Denton & Massey, 1993), which may possibly be due to their higher level of involvement with the American culture. For example, Latino men are expected to be the primary breadwinners and therefore spend more time away from home. Thus, Latino women place a higher priority on the home, which allows for more involvement with their ethnic culture. Adding gender to the equation on phenotypes will enhance what we know about the relationship between other variables and colorism in the U.S.

IMPLICATIONS FOR PRACTICE

Historically, the U.S. has placed a higher value on people who are White than on people who are not. Thus, many forms of discrimination are manifested in a lack of respect and dislike for people who are African American and Black Latino, whether they have disabilities or are able-bodied (Thomas & Sillen, 1972). Based on prior research (Denton & Massey, 1989; Rodriquez & Cordero-Guzman, 1992), people have different experiences based on the color of their skin. Because there is also a lack of research looking at colorism relative to people with disabilities in the U.S., research on colorism could be used to: (a) increase the visibility of an often isolated group of individuals (i.e., Blacks, Latinos) with disabilities, and (b) increase discussions about skin color discrimination relative to people who are African American and/or Black Latino with disabilities. More studies will enable researchers to plan for interventions that may facilitate the success of people of color through many of the human service systems in the U.S.

Whitney-Thomas, Timmons, Gilmore, and Thomas (1999) reported that the majority of VR administrators tend to be White people. Ninety-two percent of administrators and 93% of counselors were identified as White, while 6% of administrators and 5% of the counselors were identified as Black, and 4% of both administrators and counselors were identified as Hispanic. Since Black Latinos with disabilities tend to experience similar kinds of discrimination as African Americans with disabilities, the VR system could consider mandating cross-cultural training for VR counselors and administrators. These trainings could reduce discriminatory practices and improve outcomes for people with disabilities who are Black Latinos. To influence VR counselors, human services workers, and their consumers in a positive way, the trainings need to be extensive, ongoing, and system-wide. While we recognize that cross-cultural training is not a panacea, it could be a start to building cultural competence among gatekeepers in the human services.

CONCLUSION

The information presented in this chapter reviews empirical evidence of a significant relationship between skin colors/hues and services received for African Americans and Latinos with and without disabilities. As validated by several authors (e.g., Chideya, 1995; Rosenbaum, 1996), White Latinos enjoy similar privileges as White people in the U.S. There is also evidence that African Americans are consistently being denied access to VR services (Wilson, 1999; Wilson, 2005; Wilson & Senices, 2005). As we observed, there is a significant association between skin color and VR access. Would the "color," Black or White, of certain Latinos facilitate VR acceptance in the U.S.? Evidence suggests a resounding yes! The investigations by Wilson and Senices and Herbert and Martinez (1992), for example, indicate that White Latinos with disabilities are more likely to be accepted for VR services when compared to Black Latinos with disabilities. It is unmistakable that both Black Latinos and White Latinos with disabilities have different experiences in the VR system, just as African Americans and White people tend to have diverse experiences in the general U.S. population.

To lend further support to the colorism discrimination assertion, Rosenbaum (1996) empirically compared both White Latinos and Black Latinos and controlled for a host of independent variables in his investigation (e.g., socioeconomic status and place of residence). He concluded that White Latinos have privileges similar to those enjoyed by White people in the U.S., based on skin color.

REFERENCES

Arce, C. H., Murgia, E., & Frisbie, W. P. (1987). Phenotype and life chances among Chicanos. *Hispanic Journal of Behavioral Sciences, 9*, 19–22.

Atkins, B. J., & Wright, G. N. (1980). Three views: Vocational rehabilitation of Blacks: The statement. *Journal of Rehabilitation, 46*(2), 40, 42–46.

Banks, J. (1991). *Teaching strategies for ethnic studies*. Needham Heights, MA: Allyn & Bacon.

Bennett, C. (1995). *Comprehensive multicultural education: Theory and practice* (3rd ed.). Needham Heights, MA: Allyn & Bacon.

Bowe, F. (1992). *Adults with disabilities: A portrait*. Washington, DC: President's Committee on Employment of People with Disabilities, U.S. Department of Labor.

Capella, M. E. (2002). Inequities in the VR system: Do they still exist? *Rehabilitation Counseling Bulletin, 45*, 143–153.

Carr, L. (1997). "Color Blind" Racism. Thousand Oaks, CA: Sage.

Carter, R. T. (1995). *The influence of race and racial identity in psychotherapy: Toward a racially inclusive model.* New York: John Wiley.

Casas, J. M., & Pytluk, S. D. (1995). Hispanic identity development: Implications for research and practice. In J. G. Ponterotto & J. M. Casas (Eds.), *Handbook of multicultural counseling* (pp. 155–180). Thousand Oaks, CA: Sage.

Chideya, F. (1995). *Don't believe the hype: Fighting cultural misinformation about African Americans.* New York: Penguin Group.

Dana, R. H. (1998). *Understanding cultural identity in intervention and assessment. (Multicultural aspects of counseling series. Volume 9.)* Thousand Oaks, CA: Sage.

Denton, A., & Massey, D. (1993). *American apartheid: Segregation and the making of the underclass.* Cambridge, MA: Harvard University Press.

Denton, N., & Massey, D. S. (1989). Racial identity among Caribbean Hispanics: The effect of double minority status on residential segregation. *American Sociological Review, 54,* 790–808.

Devine, P. G., & Elliot, A. J. (1995). Are racial stereotypes really fading? The Princeton trilogy revisited. *Personality and Social Psychology Bulletin, 21,* 1139–1150.

Duany, J. (1998). Reconstructing racial identity. *Latin American Perspectives, 25*(3), 147–172.

Dziekan, K. I., & Okocha, A. G. (1993). Accessibility of rehabilitation services: Comparison by racial-ethnic status. *Rehabilitation Counseling Bulletin, 36,* 183–189.

Falicov, C. J. (1998). *Latino families in therapy.* New York: Guilford Press.

Feist-Price, S. (1995). African Americans with disabilities and equity in vocational rehabilitation services: One state's review. *Rehabilitation Counseling Bulletin, 39,* 119–129.

Gonzalez, J. (1995). *Roll down your windows: Stories of a forgotten America.* London: Verso Press.

Hacker, A. (1995). *Two nations: Black and White, separate, hostile, unequal.* New York: Macmillan.

Herbert, J. T., & Martinez, M. Y. (1992). Client ethnicity and vocational rehabilitation case service outcome. *Journal of Job Placement, 8,* 10–16.

Hughes, M., & Hertel, B. R. (1990). The significance of color remains: A study of life chances, mate selection, and ethnic consciousness among Black Americans. *Social Forces, 68,* 1105–1120.

Institute of Medicine (2003). *Unequal treatment: Confronting racial and ethnic disparities in health care.* Washington, DC: National Academies Press.

Itzigsohn, J., & Dore-Cabral, C. (2000). Competing identities? Race, ethnicity, and panethnicity among Dominicans in the U.S. *Sociological Forum, 15*(2), 225–247.

Jones, B. F. (1966). James Baldwin: The struggle for identity. *British Journal of Sociology, 17,* 107–121.

Lancaster, R. (1999). Skin color, race, and racism in Nicaragua. *Ethnologies, 30,* 339–353.

Lee, W. (1999). One whiteness veils three uglinesses: From border crossing to a womanist interrogation of gendered colorism. In T. K. Nakayama & J. N. Martin (Eds.), *Whiteness: The communication of social identity,* (pp. 27–41). Thousand Oaks, CA: Sage.

Loewen, J. W. (1995). *Lies my teacher told me.* New York: Touchstone.

Montalvo, F. F. (1991). Phenotyping, acculturation, and biracial assimilation of Mexican-Americans. In M. Sotomayor (Ed.), *Empowering Hispanic families* (pp. 97–120). Milwaukee, WI: Family Service America.

Peterson, G. E. (1996). *An analysis of participation, progress, and outcome of individuals from diverse racial and ethnic backgrounds in the public vocational rehabilitation program in Nevada.* Unpublished doctoral dissertation, University of Northern Colorado.

Phinney, J. S. (1996). When we talk about American ethnic groups, what do we mean? *American Psychologist, 51*, 918–927.

Quiñones-Mayo, Y., Wilson, K. B., & McGuire, M. V. (2000). Vocational rehabilitation and cultural competency for Latino populations: Considerations for rehabilitation counselors. *Journal of Applied Rehabilitation Counseling, 31*, 19–26.

Rawlings, S. W., & Saluter, A. F. (1994). Household and family characteristics: U.S. Bureau of the Census, Current Population Reports, Series P20-483. USGPO, Washington, DC.

Rehabilitation Services Administration. (2004). *Reporting manual for the RSA 911 case service report.* Washington, DC: Author.

Relethford, J. H., Stern, M. P., Gaskill, S. P., & Hazuda, H. P. (1983). Social class, admixture, and skin color variation in Mexican-Americans and Anglo-Americans in San Antonio, Texas. *American Journal of Physical Anthropology, 61*, 97–102.

Rodriquez, C. E., & Cordero-Guzman, H. (1992). Placing race in context. *Ethnic and Racial Studies, 15*, 523–542.

Rogers, M., Conoley, J., Ponterotto, J., & Wiese, M. (1992). Multicultural training in school psychology: A national survey. *School Psychology Review, 21*, 603–616.

Rosenbaum, E. (1996). The influence of race on Hispanic housing choices: New York City, 1978–1987. *Urban Affairs Review, 32*(2), 217–243.

Schulman, K. A., Berlin, J. A., Harless, W., Kerner, J. F., Sistrunk, S., Gersh, B., et al. (1999). The effect of race and sex on physicians' recommendations for cardiac catheterization. *The New England Journal of Medicine, 34*(8) 618–628.

Smart, J. & Smart, D. (1996). Hispanic Americans: Topics of interests to rehabilitation counselors. *Rehabilitation Education, 10*(2, 3), 171–184.

Smith, T. W. (2006). *Taking America's pulse III: Intergroup relations in contemporary America.* National Opinion Research Center, University of Chicago. New York: National Council for Community and Justice.

Sue, D. W. (1996). ACES endorsement of the multicultural counseling competencies: Do we have the courage. *Spectrum, 57*(1), 9–10.

Sue, D. W., Arrendondo, P., & McDavis, R. J. (1992). Multicultural competencies/standards: A pressing need. *Journal of Counseling and Development, 70*, 477–486.

Thomas, A., & Sillen, S. (1972). *Racism and psychiatry.* New York: Carol Publishing Group.

U.S. Census Bureau (1990). *1990 U.S. Census with race and ethnicity with Hispanic origin.* U.S. Department of Commerce, Bureau of the Census, Washington, DC.

U.S. Census Bureau (2001a). *Overview of race and Hispanic origin: Census 2000 brief.* Retrieved January 27, 2007, from *http://www.census.gov/prod/2001pubs/cenbr01-1.pdf*

U.S. Census Bureau (2001b). *Residential segregation of Hispanics or Latinos: 1980 to 2000. Census 2000 brief.* Retrieved November 27, 2002 from *http://www.census.gov/hhes/www/housing/resseg/ch6.html.*

Vasquez, L. A., Garcia-Vasquez, E., Bauman, S. A., & Sierra, A. S. (1997). Skin color, acculturation, and community interest among Mexican American students: A research note. *Hispanic Journal of Behavioral Sciences, 19*, 377–386.

Wheaton, J. E. (1995). Vocational rehabilitation acceptance rate for European Americans and African Americans: Another look. *Rehabilitation Counseling Bulletin, 38*, 224–231.

Whitney-Thomas, J., Timmons, J. C., Gilmore, D. S., & Thomas, D. M. (1999). Expanding access: Changes in vocational rehabilitation practice since the 1992 Rehabilitation Act Amendments. *Rehabilitation Counseling Bulletin, 43*, 30–40.

Wilson, K. B. (1999). Vocational rehabilitation acceptance: A tale of two races in a large Midwestern state. *Journal of Applied Rehabilitation Counseling 30*, 25–31.

Wilson, K. B. (2000). Predicting vocational rehabilitation acceptance based on race, education, work status, and source of support at application. *Rehabilitation Counseling Bulletin, 43*, 97–105.

Wilson, K. B. (2002). The exploration of vocational rehabilitation acceptance and ethnicity: A national investigation. *Rehabilitation Counseling Bulletin, 45*, 168–176.

Wilson, K. B. (2005). Vocational rehabilitation closure statues in the U.S.: Generalizing to the Hispanic ethnicity. *Journal of Applied Rehabilitation Counseling, 36*(2), 4–11.

Wilson, K. B., Edwards, D. W., Alston, R. J., Harley, D. A., & Doughty, J. D. (2001). Vocational rehabilitation and the dilemma of race in rural communities: The debate continues [Electronic version]. *Journal of Rural Community Psychology, 2*, 55–81.

Wilson, K. B., Harley, D. A., McCormick, K., Jolivette, K., & Jackson. R. (2001). A literature review of vocational rehabilitation acceptance and explaining bias in the rehabilitation process. *Journal of Rehabilitation, 32*, 24–35.

Wilson, K. B., & Senices, J. (2005). Exploring the vocational rehabilitation acceptance rates of Hispanics and non-Hispanics in the United States. *Journal of Counseling and Development 83*(1), 86–96.

CHAPTER 6

Challenges to Providing Culturally Competent Care in Medical Rehabilitation to African Americans

Felicia Hill-Briggs, PhD, ABPP;
Kennesha Kelly, BA.; and
Charisse Ewing, MA

INTRODUCTION

The physical medicine and rehabilitation setting, historically developed for persons with primary physical disabilities, continues to serve individuals needing medical treatment and physical, occupational, speech, cognitive, and behavioral treatments for improving functional independence in mobility and activities of daily living. Since medical inpatient and outpatient rehabilitation settings treat individuals with a range of chronic diseases (e.g., multiple sclerosis, diabetes, HIV/AIDS); acute medical events (e.g., heart attack, stroke, organ transplantation); and traumatic injuries (e.g., acquired brain injury, spinal cord injury), people of multiethnic backgrounds, who have an elevated risk for adverse health events, comprise a significant proportion of this rehabilitation population nationally. The presence of individuals from different cultures within inpatient rehabilitation settings necessitates attention to methods for providing care that are culturally appropriate and effective.

African Americans, in particular, experience disparities in disease, injury, and disability (U.S. Department of Health and Human Services [DHHS], 2005; Centers for Disease Control and Prevention [CDC], 2005). The 2000 Census reported that the prevalence of disability is highest among persons reporting Black or African American race (24.3%), as compared to non-Hispanic Whites (18.3%) (U.S. Census Bureau, 2000). Additionally, a higher prevalence of disability among African Americans is found across age groups. Among children (ages 5–15 years), the rate of disability was 7.0% for African Americans, as compared to 5.6% for Whites. Among African American working-aged adults (ages 16–64 years), 26.4% were disabled, as compared to 16.8% of Whites. Finally, among older adults (ages 65 and older), the rate of disability was 52.8% in African Americans versus 40.6% in Whites (U.S. Census Bureau).

Moreover, African Americans experience a higher incidence of many chronic diseases that lead to impairments and disability (DHHS, 2005). African Americans, as compared with their White counterparts, have a higher incidence of HIV/AIDS and certain cancers (e.g., lung, prostate, pancreatic, rectal) (CDC, 2005). African American men and women are 50% more likely to have a stroke, and survivors are at greater risk for long-term complications and disability when compared to non-Hispanic Whites (CDC, 2005). In the case of diabetes, African Americans are twice as likely to develop diabetes as non-Hispanic Whites. Once they have diabetes, African Americans have a 50% higher prevalence of retinopathy (eye disease that can result in blindness), a 30% higher likelihood of receiving a lower limb amputation, and an almost 60% higher likelihood of developing end-stage kidney disease (National Institute of Diabetes and Digestive and Kidney Diseases [NIDDK], 2005).

These racial and ethnic disparities in disease and disability increase the rehabilitation utilization needs of African Americans. African Americans experience poorer quality of healthcare and medical outcomes in the context of general medical care (Institute of Medicine [IOM], 2003), and there is evidence that such disparities exist in rehabilitation care as well (Bhandari, Kushel, Price, & Schillinger, 2005; Gregory, LaViest, & Simpson, 2006; Haider et al., 2007; Krause, Broderick, Saladin, & Broyles, 2006). Therefore, it is critical that the field of rehabilitation develop evidence-based practices to ensure quality and effectiveness of rehabilitation treatments for African American and underserved patients.

This chapter addresses issues that apply to the physical medicine and rehabilitation care of African Americans, but especially to rehabilitation psychology practice in this setting. On the rehabilitation treatment team, rehabilitation psychologists and neuropsychologists attend to the psychological and cognitive assessment and intervention needs of patients to facilitate optimal physical, psychological, and social functioning (Wegener et al., 2007). In this regard, this chapter addresses four topics. First, from the broader mental health literature, challenges of diagnostic accuracy, appropriateness, and effectiveness of treatments with African Americans are discussed. Second, considerations regarding how to provide culturally proficient psychological care to African Americans in medical rehabilitation are presented. Third, three different examples of promising research directions, which can be modeled in the rehabilitation setting, are presented to examine approaches to conducting research leading to more effective assessment and intervention with African Americans. Finally, a research agenda to further examine disparities and develop an evidence base for effective practices to deliver care to African Americans in medical rehabilitation settings is proposed.

ISSUES OF DIAGNOSTIC ACCURACY, TREATMENT APPROPRIATENESS, AND TREATMENT EFFECTIVENESS: AFRICAN AMERICANS AND MENTAL HEALTH

Rehabilitation psychology care for African Americans is impacted by the status of psychological and mental health care for African Americans in general. In 2001, the Department of Health and Human Services issued a Surgeon General's report on mental health, with a supplement addressing issues of diagnosis, utilization, and treatment of people of multiethnic backgrounds (DHHS, 2001). According to this report, African Americans remain at risk for inadequate psychological care. Key findings from the report, which have implications for rehabilitation, are presented here.

Diagnostic Accuracy

Diagnostic accuracy is one factor contributing to the risk of inadequate care among African Americans. African Americans are more frequently misdiagnosed by mental health professionals as having a severe mental illness. For example, anger may be mislabeled as emotional dyscontrol, a poor relationship with a practitioner may be mislabeled as probable personality disorder, and depression may be misdiagnosed as schizophrenia or other psychotic symptomatology (DHHS, 2001). Psychological assessment standards of care recommend consideration of cultural and demographic factors when interpreting diagnostic tests as one means of improving diagnostic accuracy (American Educational Research Association, 1999). Additional needs include examination of differential symptom presentations among persons of differing cultures and testing validity of commonly used diagnostic instruments.

Utilization and Race Concordance

Utilization is another factor impacting receipt of care. Fifty percent of African Americans discontinue psychological services after the initial session (DHHS, 2001). Many African Americans prefer, and report having greater trust in, a same-race practitioner (Cooper et al., 2003). However, there are not enough African American practitioners in institutions and facilities serving large numbers of multiethnic patients to meet this preference. To reduce health disparities, it has been recommended that institutions should ensure diversity in their professional medical workforce so that the race/ethnicity of their patient populations are represented (IOM, 2003). However, the small number of African American healthcare professionals, particularly in the field of rehabilitation medicine, make patient-practitioner race concordance challenging to achieve as a short-term goal.

Evidence-Based Psychological Treatments

There are several challenges to providing evidence-based care with African Americans. First, although evidence-based psychological treatments do exist (DHHS, 1999), African Americans have not been systematically included in the research development and testing of most of these psychological treatments. As a result, it is not known whether standardized treatments and treatment-as-usual are equally effective when administered to African Americans. It is also unclear whether in the natural practice setting clinicians diagnose problems correctly and make appropriate treatment recommendations for effective forms of psychological treatment for African Americans (Chambless & Ollendick, 2001; DHHS, 2001).

Evidence-Based Medication Treatments

The Surgeon General's report (DHHS, 2001) documented disparities in the receipt of treatments deemed efficacious for African Americans compared to Whites. For example, data suggest that African Americans on antidepressants may be less likely than Whites on antidepressants to be prescribed selective serotonin reuptake inhibitors (SSRI's), which have fewer negative side effects than older classes of antidepressant medications. Moreover, medications may have differential effects in African Americans. More African Americans than Whites metabolize antidepressants and antipsychotic medications slowly and demonstrate higher rates and severity of symptoms of medication hypersensitivity. As a result, when treated with doses commonly used for Whites, African Americans may exhibit higher sensitivity to psychotropic medications, as manifested in a faster and higher rate of response and more severe side effects, including delirium. In addition, despite a potential for hypersensitivity, African Americans are at risk for receiving medication overdosing. Clinicians working in inpatient services tend to prescribe both more and higher doses of oral and injectable antipsychotic medications to African Americans than to Whites. African Americans are also more likely to receive neuroleptics than are Whites, even for nonpsychotic symptoms (DHHS, 2001).

Mechanisms contributing to these challenges and disparities in the mental health care of African Americans are complex, and solutions are multifaceted. Although there is not a body of literature to date examining psychological and mental health care for African Americans during rehabilitation, it is likely that factors contributing to the risk of misdiagnosis and inadequacy of treatment approaches can impact mental health care in the rehabilitation setting. Research is needed to examine causal pathways and to test diagnostic and intervention tools.

However, in the absence of a body of research to date, recommendations have been proposed to assist healthcare professionals in improving cultural proficiency of care.

CONSIDERATIONS AND RECOMMENDATIONS FOR CULTURALLY PROFICIENT CARE

General Psychological Care with African Americans

In response to the need for recommendations for culturally appropriate and proficient psychological care for people of multiethnic backgrounds, *Psychological Treatment of Ethnic Minority Populations* was compiled by members of the Council of National Psychological Associations for the Advancement of Ethnic Minority Interests (2003) (representing The Asian American Psychological Association, The Association of Black Psychologists, The National Latina/o Psychological Association, and The Society of Indian Psychologists). The document was designed to present expert opinion regarding appropriateness of theory and practice of psychological treatment, with recommendations to empower consumers and to inform professionals and funders. Key information and recommendations regarding treatment of persons of African decent, as presented by Myers, Young, Obasi, and Speight (2003), is presented here.

Among the knowledge and skills recommended for professionals are: awareness of clients' thresholds of psychological distress and tolerance, natural support systems and healing modalities, variability in symptomatology and presentation, and treatment effects. Communication skills, including understanding of the nuances of verbal and nonverbal communication, are emphasized as well. To ensure that the care provided is culturally appropriate and acceptable to clients of African descent, professionals are encouraged to gain awareness of such factors as cultural values, beliefs, worldviews, and acculturation, which may influence the client's perspective. Table 6-1 lists some aspects of an "Africentric" viewpoint that may be considered.

Culturally proficient care, in this model, relies on a holistic approach to treatment. For persons of African descent who uphold traditional values, mental health is viewed as an inseparable relationship between an individual's social, psychological, physical, and spiritual well-being. Therefore, the role of the mental health professional is to engage in holistic and integrative analyses to identify the target of intervention to restore balance into the holistic system and develop better measures for understanding how culture affects the manifestation of behavior disorders. Clinicians

Table 6-1 Historical "Africentric" Views of Health and Illness

• There is a purpose for illness and disease; chance is unrecognized.

• The challenges caused by illness or disease serve a greater good.

• Getting to the cause of illness or disease is more important than resolving symptoms; it is worthwhile to tolerate discomfort to gain understanding.

• Natural remedies are preferable to artificially manufactured compounds.

• To hear or see things unheard or unseen by others does not mean one is crazy; one may be gifted, chosen.

• For a treatment to be effective, it must reintegrate the identified patient into family, community, and/or other systems.

• Health is difficult to achieve and sustain in a society or majority culture that is toxic.

Adapted from The Council of National Psychological Associations for the Advancement of Ethnic Minority Interests. (2003). *Psychological Treatment of Ethnic Minority Populations.* Washington, DC: Association of Black Psychologists.

must also be able to effectively communicate cross-culturally in order to increase their capacity to identify the aspects of psychospiritual and sociocultural practices that can be used to reinstate harmony necessary for maintaining good mental health (Myers et al., 2003).

The strength of this holistic approach to African American mental health care is that it offers insight into ways of rethinking health behaviors as adaptations to vulnerability, disenfranchisement, lack of socioeconomic resources, and oppression as opposed to biased assumptions based on race and fragmented attempts to define Black culture. However, further research is needed to understand the pathways by which distinct health behaviors and cultural norms have emerged within populations of African descent. This analysis has the capacity to provide a foundation for more effective evidence-based research initiatives.

Rehabilitation Care with African Americans

There is a "rehabilitation culture" implicit in the rehabilitation mission, goals, and organizational structure. This culture includes an emphasis on commonly accepted objectives including increasing the individual's functional independence, encouraging acceptance of and adaptation to functional limitations, and emphasizing the setting of *realistic goals*

(Lane, 2007). Clients may generally receive individual therapies to work on skill-building. Families and other social networks may be integrated into the rehabilitation process only as deemed necessary from the standpoint of the need for functional assistance. Based on this rehabilitation culture, the rehabilitation setting may be perceived as within the cultural norms of the patient (culturally congruent) or as different from, or in conflict with, the patient's cultural experiences and values (culturally incongruent).

Belgrave and Jarama (2000), using an Africentric worldview framework, highlighted examples of factors that may be relevant for integration into rehabilitation treatment: (a) the importance of an extended family network in adaptation following disability, not only in an assistance role but as an integrated social system; (b) the use of a communal and group orientation in preserving status following disability and in-treatment modality, perhaps more than one-on-one interactions with therapists; (c) understanding the role of spirituality and *negativity to positivity* in coping, allowing for a wider range of what may be accepted as realistic goals, as goals are not based only on medical advances; and (d) understanding harmony in perception of disability and integration of all aspects of self in treatment.

Combining insights from the United States Surgeon General's report, and aspects of an Africentric worldview, several general recommendations can be proposed for improving cultural proficiency in rehabilitation care with African Americans. These are presented in Table 6-2.

These recommendations are reasonably deduced from existing literature exploring cultural incongruence and inadequate quality of care experienced by African Americans. However, each warrants research to develop an evidence base and to investigate whether these aspects of cultural proficiency do in fact result in an improved rehabilitation experience and improved health outcomes among African Americans.

TOWARD A NEW BEGINNING: CULTURAL COMPETENCE IN RESEARCH AND EVIDENCE-BASED PRACTICE

A Model for Evidence-Based Rehabilitation Practice Incorporating Cultural Competence Factors

Gathering and examining evidence about how well treatments work is deemed important in helping clinicians make the best treatment decisions regarding the care for individuals, and such processes form the basis of evidence-based medicine (Sackett & Rosenberg, 1995). As discussed, many common psychological and behavioral practices in rehabilitation currently lack adequate evidence of effectiveness. They assume validity of assessments and interventions across settings (nonrehabilitation, rehabilitation)

Table 6-2 General Recommendations for Culturally Competent Rehabilitation Psychology Care for African Americans

• Maximize provision of care (not just assessment) during the initial contact.

• Ask patient's preference regarding treatment modality (e.g. individual, couple, family, or group) as opposed to assuming an individual modality.

• Listen carefully to the patient's expressed perspectives and worldview and recognize that the worldview may differ from your own.

• Be careful not to mislabel hope, a firm belief in healing powers/potential, or a positive view of the meaning of disability as denial or lack of insight.

• Be aware of medication hypersensitivity and overdosing. Be cautious with recommendations for psychotropic medications, with standard dosing, and with dosage increases.

• Be aware of increased risk of delirium with psychotropic medications (and resulting behavioral symptom worsening) due to combination of multiple comorbidities and medication hypersensitivity.

• Understand the potential for psychological misdiagnosis based on different symptom presentations as well as sociodemographic influences on psychological diagnostic tests.

• Be aware that we currently lack evidence that commonly used psychological treatments found efficacious with Whites are as effective with African Americans.

• Use clinical judgment and keen observation to help guide use and adaptation of psychological treatments.

and persons (all races/ethnicities), and they have been guided primarily by clinical experience and expert opinion, without follow-up testing for effectiveness using systematic research methods within rehabilitation. For determination of best treatment practices, therefore, parallel processes are needed: (a) the development of proven effective rehabilitation practices (evidence-based practice), and (b) the demonstration that these behavioral practices are effective in improving healthcare and outcomes for persons from differing cultural and racial/ethnic groups (cultural competence).

In an evidence-based practice model, in order to make the best treatment decisions, the clinician's expertise and the individual's own values are used in addition to the best research evidence regarding the treatment's effectiveness (Spring, 2007). When considering treatment decision-making for people of multiethnic backgrounds with disabilities, key cultural competence factors must also be considered, including: (a) evidence of treatment effectiveness specifically with racial/ethnic and disability subgroups, (b) preferences for treatment based on the individual's own cultural values and priorities, (c) the clinician's experience and expertise, including cultural competence both with the racial and ethnic population and with persons with disabilities, and (d) an additional factor of treatment accessibility to the individual with functional impairment or disability. Such a model is presented in Figure 6-1. The state-of-the-science in this area of combined evidence for treatment effectiveness and cultural competence remains formative, and in order to achieve the joint goals of evidence-based practice and culturally competent care, clear research

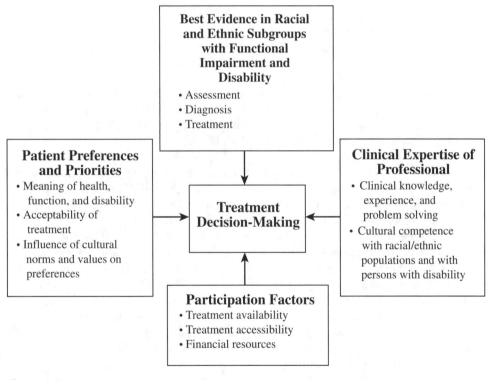

Figure 6-1
Evidence-Based Practice Model

directions and funding for systematic programs of research, translation, and dissemination are needed. There are, however, emerging opportunities and examples upon which to build.

Examples of Current Evidence-Building Research with Implications for Culturally Competent Rehabilitation Practice

Programs of research that will provide data for establishing evidence-based and effective care are growing. Three examples of such research directions, which have implications for rehabilitation care with African Americans, have been selected for discussion here.

Multicenter Databases on Processes of Rehabilitation Care and Outcomes: Model Systems

Racial and ethnic disparities in rehabilitation care and outcomes have not received systematic investigation, as data on clinical variables, psychosocial and functional measures, processes of care, and outcomes have not previously been available from national, representative samples of rehabilitation patients from different geographic and racial and ethnic groups. The Traumatic Brain Injury Model Systems (TBIMS), Model Spinal Cord Injury Systems (MSCIS), and Burn Model Systems (BMS) programs provide an example of research methods for gathering such data. The model systems research programs are multicenter studies funded by the National Institute on Disability and Rehabilitation Research (NIDRR). The primary goals of the TBIMS, MSCIS, and BMS are to longitudinally examine delivery of rehabilitation services, course of recovery, and outcomes of patients with TBI, SCI, and burn injury, respectively.

Establishment of the model systems longitudinal databases will help to meet the need for rigorous, systematic rehabilitation research, conducted with research protocols that have been standardized across centers, and data storage and dissemination mechanisms that allow for efficiency. Benefits of the TBIMS, MSCIS, and BMS include the following: (a) access to extensive sociodemographic, medical, functional, cognitive, and psychosocial data in order to examine associations and predictors among risks and outcomes; (b) opportunities to conduct evidence-based rehabilitation outcomes research and determination of *best practices*; and (c) collection of data from multiple centers, representing different geographic regions, leading to reduced bias in sampling, larger sample sizes, and representativeness. These characteristics allow for future systematic investigation of similarities and differences, within and between racial and ethnic groups, with regard to risk factors and rehabilitation utilization, care, and outcomes.

Neuropsychological Test Use, Interpretation, and Normative Data

Cognitive testing, using neuropsychological measures and/or mental status screening tests, is a common practice for the purposes of assessment, diagnosis, and treatment planning within rehabilitation settings treating patients with neurological and psychiatric disorders or impairments (Wegener et al., 2007). However, the accuracy of clinical interpretations and diagnoses derived from the use of normative data has not been demonstrated for people of multiethnic backgrounds. Manly and colleagues (e.g., Manly, Miller et al., 1998; Manly, Jacobs, Touradji, Small, & Stern, 2002; Manly, Byrd, & Touradji, 2004) have undertaken a series of studies to address the problem of potential bias in standardized neuropsychological test scoring and interpretation when used with people of multiethnic backgrounds and underserved populations. This research has highlighted: (a) the need for availability of test validation and normative data research with people of multiethnic backgrounds, an issue with implications for test diagnostic accuracy, and (b) methods for systematically examining causes for patterns of score discrepancies between people of multiethnic backgrounds and Whites on cognitive tests.

The aim of the research program is to improve the diagnostic accuracy specifically of neuropsychological tests used to detect cognitive impairments and Alzheimer's disease among African American and Hispanic elders. The studies clarify the independent influences of language, acculturation, educational experiences, racial socialization, and socioeconomic status on cognitive test performance. Several studies to date have addressed the issue of poor specificity among multiethnic populations by investigating the cultural and educational determinants of individual variation in neuropsychological test performance (Manly, Jacobs et al., 1998; Byrd, Sanchez, & Manly, 2005; Manly et al., 2002). These studies have identified aspects of cultural and educational experiences that can be explicitly measured and have related these variables to test performance both in cross-sectional and longitudinal designs.

Manly (2005) has also investigated the advantages and disadvantages of establishing separate norms for African Americans, and she has proposed an alternate approach that deconstructs race and education to help clarify the independent influences of race, culture, quality of education, literacy level, and socioeconomic status on cognition and neuropsychological test performance. Continued research examining discrepancies in test performance with African Americans emphasizes the importance of using culturally appropriate norms when evaluating ethnically diverse elderly for dementia. This line of research facilitated the publication of demographic-corrected normative data for the Wechsler Adult Intelligence Scale III (WAIS-III; Heaton, Miller, Taylor, & Grant, 2004; Heaton, Taylor, & Manly, 2001).

Development of Evidence-Based Interventions with African Americans with Functional Impairment and Disability

Recommendations to improve health disparities have included a call for conducting more research designed to intervene upon processes of care that may improve health and functioning of health disparate populations (Beach et al., 2004). In the case of behavioral and psychological intervention research in the context of health and disease, research is needed that leads to an evidence base regarding intervention effectiveness for specific diseases. Diabetes, for example, is a disease with racial/ethnic disparities that is commonly encountered in the medical rehabilitation setting because it influences a higher incidence of heart attack, stroke, lower extremity amputation, retinopathy and blindness, and end-stage renal disease (NIDDK, 2005). However, despite the association of diabetes with disability and health disparities, standard diabetes behavioral and educational programs to improve the ability to perform self-care have not been systematically designed to meet the needs of persons with disabilities (American Association of Diabetes Educators, 2002; Williams, 2002), or the combined cultural competence needs of race/ethnicity and disability.

Project DECIDE (Decision-Making Education for Choices In Diabetes Everyday) is a pilot program of research designed to: (a) develop culturally competent diabetes education for African Americans with poorly-controlled type 2 diabetes and the challenges of diabetes complications, functional limitations, and disability; and (b) pilot a randomized controlled trial to determine effectiveness of this adapted education versus brief traditional education, on outcomes of disease knowledge, problem-solving skills for independent self-care, and clinical outcomes of blood sugar, blood pressure, and cholesterol control, which contribute to excess diabetes-related complications and disability.

Six methodological steps are described here as an example of designing, implementing, and testing an intervention specifically to meet goals of both evidence-based practice and cultural competence in multiethnic populations with functional impairment and disability. First, the study sample was intentionally inclusive to ensure that the research would be generalizable. Therefore, there were no *exclusion criteria* based on prior treatment nonresponsiveness, presence of diabetes complications, or presence of physical, visual, and/or cognitive disability. Second, qualitative and quantitative research was conducted to inform intervention needs and priorities within the urban, African American population of interest. This identified key areas needed for intervention, including socioeconomic and family problems adversely impacting diabetes self-care (Hill-Briggs, Gary, Hill, Bone, & Brancati, 2002), specific difficulties adhering to treatments (Hill-Briggs, Cooper, Brancati, & Cooper, 2003; Hill-Briggs et al., 2005), and lower literacy impacting understanding and use of educational materials (Hill-Briggs, Renosky et al., 2007; Hill-Briggs & Smith, 2008). Third, instruments to assess behavioral aspects of diabetes self-care in the context of managing barriers were developed and validated within an urban AfricanAmerican sample (Hill-Briggs, Yeh et al., 2007). Fourth, a behavioral and educational intervention was designed to meet standards for diabetes self-management education (Mensing et al., 2006), but adapted using guidelines to meet disability accessibility needs (American Association of Diabetes Educators, 2002; Williams, 1999), and non-diabetes specific guidelines for development and presentation of print information for lower literacy (e.g. reading grade levels, sentence length, layout, typography) (CDC, 1999; Doak, Doak, & Root, 1996; National Cancer Institute, 1994). Moreover, the accessible education module was designed in a format for ease of use for persons with diabetes during an inpatient or outpatient rehabilitation program. Fifth, a randomized controlled trial design was utilized to test evidence of effectiveness as compared to traditional diabetes education. Sixth, in addition to medical and clinical outcomes, key outcomes included evaluation of accessibility and acceptability of treatment by the participants themselves. Effectiveness studies to date have demonstrated that the education is accessible, acceptable, and effective in increasing skills for self-care in persons with visual impairment, physical impairment, cognitive impairment, and low literacy (Hill-Briggs, Renosky et al, 2007; Hill-Briggs, Lazo, Renosky, & Ewing, 2008). In sum, within the example of Project DECIDE, it is demonstrated that evidence-based research investigating effectiveness of culturally competent interventions within subgroups with health disparities and disability is feasible.

IMPLICATIONS FOR RESEARCH: SETTING FORTH A RESEARCH AGENDA

Within medical rehabilitation specifically, there are several research needs with regard to understanding and ensuring provision of optimal care for African Americans. A general research agenda can be proposed to examine disparities and develop an evidence base for effective rehabilitation care (see Table 6-3). This agenda includes research to examine rehabilitation medical and mental health/behavioral outcomes (short and long term) among African American populations; health services research to examine African Americans' access to, and utilization of, acute and postacute rehabilitation programs and services, particularly those that address mental health, psychosocial, and cognitive needs; and clinical research to develop and test treatments and interventions aimed at improving medical rehabilitation care and

Table 6-3 A Proposed Research Agenda

1. Determine nature and extent of racial and ethnic disparities in medical rehabilitation quality of care and outcomes.

   a. When population-based studies and intervention studies are conducted, ensure samples are of a sufficient size to conduct subgroup analyses for racial and ethnic minority groups.

   b. Address the particular need for research examining mental health, psychosocial, and cognitive outcomes in medical rehabilitation populations.

   c. Examine cultural and behavioral factors as mediators of quality of care and outcomes.

2. For areas of disparity, examine causal models and generate testable hypotheses.

3. Conduct clinical research to improve the specificity and diagnostic accuracy of assessments.

   a. Test the validity of diagnostic tests and measures.

   b. Develop and test psychometric properties of new assessment instruments, as needed, using the population(s) of interest.

4. Design interventions that are accessible, relevant, and appropriate for the selected population.

   a. Explore intervention models and hypotheses using qualitative and quantitative research methods with the population of interest.

   b. Design interventions and materials to meet the characteristics of the population of interest.

   c. Design and test outcomes related to interventions that incorporate "Africentric" or other cultural worldviews in rehabilitation treatment planning, conduct of care, and training of health professionals.

5. Conduct both efficacy and effectiveness studies with the population of interest to ensure that therapeutic and educational interventions are acceptable, accessible, and effective.

outcomes, and improving secondary and tertiary prevention among African Americans.

Translating the specific research objectives in Table 6-3 into effective programs and policy will be accomplished best through a progression of intervention studies, beginning with randomized controlled trials to test treatment efficacy in racial/ethnic subgroups with disabilities, followed by multicenter trials for projects demonstrating efficacy in pilot studies, and finally, effectiveness trials that target translation and program evaluation and dissemination research. This course of research will provide the data needed for systematic reviews with evidence grading, meta-analyses, and evidence reports that fulfill the key objectives of evidence in medical care (Clancy, Slutsky, & Patton, 2004). These objectives include: (a) to know whether current healthcare practices are effective or not *with multiethnic people with disabilities*, (b) to improve the quality of healthcare and consistent delivery of high quality healthcare *to multiethnic people with disabilities*, and (c) for impact on policy, as evidence from systematic reviews, meta-analyses, and evidence reports is used for informing and developing coverage/reimbursement decisions, quality measures/outcome standards, educational materials and tools, guidelines, and further research agendas.

CONCLUSION

Challenges faced in working with African American populations in medical rehabilitation include provision of culturally appropriate diagnostic procedures, ensuring culturally congruent or acceptable practices, and employing evidence-based practices. Recommendations for culturally proficient psychological care with persons of African descent have been put forth by professional organizations. These recommendations highlight areas of practitioner awareness, knowledge, and skills to increase acceptability and applicability of psychology services.

However, systematic research involving African Americans is essential for the field of rehabilitation. Evidence is lacking to demonstrate that many standard psychological treatments are as effective with African Americans, and to date very little is known about whether incorporating aspects of culturally proficient care leads to improved outcomes. There are promising areas of current research involving African Americans that will, in the future, provide an evidence base for care. These lines of research, combined with a comprehensive, systematic proposed research agenda, will facilitate clinical practice and policy standards for ensuring optimal care and, hopefully, reduced disparities in clinical and functional outcomes for African Americans entering medical rehabilitation systems of care.

REFERENCES

American Association of Diabetes Educators. (2002). Diabetes education for people with disabilities. *Diabetes Educator, 28*, 916–921.

American Educational Research Association. (1999). *Standards for educational and psychological testing*. Washington, DC: American Educational Research Association, American Psychological Association, and National Council on Measurement in Education.

Beach, M. C., Cooper L. A., Robinson, K. A., Price, E. G., Gary, T. L., Jenckes, M. W., et al. (2004). *Strategies for improving minority healthcare quality: Evidence report/technology assessment No. 90.* (AHRQ Publication No. 04-E008-02). Rockville, MD: Agency for Healthcare Research and Quality.

Belgrave, F. Z. & Jarama, S. L. (2000). Culture and the disability and rehabilitation experience: An African American example. In R. G. Frank & T. R. Elliot (Eds.), *Handbook of Rehabilitation Psychology* (pp. 585–600). Washington, DC: American Psychological Association.

Bhandari, V. K., Kushel, M., Price, L., & Schillinger, D. (2005). Racial disparities in outcomes of inpatient stroke rehabilitation. *Archives of Physical Medicine and Rehabilitation, 86*(11), 2081–2086.

Byrd, D. A., Sanchez, D., & Manly, J. J. (2005). Neuropsychological test performance among Caribbean-born and U.S.-born African American elderly: The role of age, education and reading level. *Journal of Clinical and Experimental Neuropsychology, 27*, 1056–1069.

Centers for Disease Control and Prevention. (1999). *Scientific and technical information simply put* (2nd ed.). Atlanta, GA: Office of Communication, Centers for Disease Control and Prevention.

Centers for Disease Control and Prevention. (2005). Health disparities experienced by Black or African Americans—United States. *Morbidity and Mortality Weekly Report, 54*(1), 1–32.

Chambless, D. L., & Ollendick, T. H. (2001). Empirically supported psychological interventions: controversies and evidence. *Annual Review of Psychology, 52*, 685–716.

Clancy, C., Slutsky, J., & Patton, L. (2004). Evidence-Based Health Care 2004: AHRQ moves research to translation and implementation. *Health Services Research, 39*(5), xv–xxiii.

Cooper, L. A., Roter, D. L., Johnson, R. L., Ford, D. E., Steinwachs, D. M., & Powe, N. R. (2003). Patient-centered communication, ratings of care, and concordance of patient and physician race. *Annals of Internal Medicine, 139*(11), 907–915.

Council of National Psychological Associations for the Advancement of Ethnic Minority Interests. (2003). *Psychological treatment of ethnic minority populations*. Washington, DC: Association of Black Psychologists.

Doak, C. C., Doak, L. G., & Root, J. H. (1996). *Teaching patients with low literacy skills*. (2nd ed.). Philadelphia: J.B. Lippincott.

Gregory, P. C., LaVeist, T. A., & Simpson, C. (2006). Racial disparities in access to cardiac rehabilitation. *American Journal of Physical Medicine & Rehabilitation, 85*(9), 705–710.

Haider A. H., Efron, D. T., Haut, E. R., Dirusso, S. M., Sullivan, T., & Cornwell, E. E. III. (2007). Black children experience worse clinical and functional outcomes after traumatic brain injury: An analysis of the national pediatric trauma registry. *Journal of Trauma, 62*(5), 1259–1263.

Heaton, R. K., Miller, S. W., Taylor, M. J. & Grant, I. (2004). *Revised comprehensive norms for an expanded Halstead-Reitan battery: Demographically adjusted neuropsychological norms for African American and Caucasian adults*, Professional Manual. Odessa, FL: Psychological Assessment Resources, Inc.

Heaton, R. K., Taylor, M., & Manly, J. (2001). Demographic effects and demographically corrected norms with the WAIS-III and WMS-III. In D. Tulsky, R. K. Heaton, G. J. Chelune, I. Ivnik, R. A. Bornstein, A. Prifitera, et al. (Eds.), *Clinical interpretations of the WAIS-II and WMS-III* (pp. 181–210). San Diego, CA: Academic Press.

Hill-Briggs, F., Cooper, D. C., Brancati, F. L., & Cooper, L. A. (2003). A qualitative study of problem solving and diabetes control in type 2 diabetes self-management. *Diabetes Educator, 29,* 1018–1028.

Hill-Briggs, F., Gary, T. L., Bone, L. R., Hill, M. N., Levine, D. M., & Brancati F. L. (2005). Medication adherence and diabetes control in urban African Americans with type 2 diabetes. *Health Psychology, 24,* 349–357.

Hill-Briggs, F., Gary, T. L., Hill, M. N., Bone, L. R., & Brancati, F. L. (2002). Health-related quality of life in urban African Americans with type 2 diabetes. *Journal of General Internal Medicine, 17,* 412–419.

Hill-Briggs, F., Lazo, M., Renosky, R., & Ewing, C. (2008). Effectiveness of a diabetes and cardiovascular disease education module in an African-American, pilot sample with type 2 diabetes and physical, visual, and cognitive impairment. *Rehabilitation Psychology, 53,* 1–8.

Hill-Briggs, F., Renosky, R., Gemmell, L., Lazo, M., Peyrot, M., & Brancati, F. L. (2007). Effectiveness of literacy-adapted diabetes and CVD education module for high CVD risk, urban African Americans with type 2 diabetes. *Annals of Behavioral Medicine, 33*(1), 93.

Hill-Briggs, F., & Smith, A. S. (2008). Evaluation of diabetes and cardiovascular disease print patient education materials for use with low-health literate populations. *Diabetes Care, 31*(4), 667–671.

Hill-Briggs, F., Yeh, H. C., Gary, T. L., Batts-Turner, M., D'Zurilla, T., & Brancati, F. L. (2007). Diabetes problem-solving scale (DPSS) development in an adult, African-American sample. *Diabetes Educator, 33,* 291–299.

Institute of Medicine (2003). Unequal treatment: Confronting racial and ethnic disparities in health care. Washington, DC: National Academies Press.

Krause, J. S., Broderick, L. E., Saladin, L. K., & Broyles, J. (2006). Racial disparities in health outcomes after spinal cord injury: Mediating effects of education and income. *Journal of Spinal Cord Medicine, 29*(1), 17–25.

Lane, A. E. (2007). Achieving functional independence. In R.L. Braddom (Ed.), *Physical Medicine and Rehabilitation* (3rd ed., pp. 581–596). London: Elsevier.

Manly, J. J. (2005). Advantages and disadvantages of separate norms for African Americans. *The Clinical Neuropsychologist, 19,* 270–275.

Manly, J. J., Byrd, D. A., & Touradji, P. (2004). Acculturation, reading level, and neuropsychological test performance among African American elders. *Applied Neuropsychology, 11,* 37–46.

Manly, J. J., Jacobs, D. M., Sano, M., Bell, K., Merchant, C. A., Small, S. A., et al. (1998). Cognitive test performance among nondemented elderly African Americans and Whites. *Neurology, 50,* 1238–1245.

Manly, J. J., Jacobs, D. M., Touradji, P., Small, S. A., & Stern, Y. (2002). Reading level attenuates differences in neuropsychological test performance between African American and White elders. *Journal of the International Neuropsychological Society, 8*, 341–348.

Manly, J. J., Miller, S. W., Heaton, R. K., Byrd, D., Reilly, J., Velasquez, R. J., et al. (1998). The effect of African-American acculturation on neuropsychological test performance in normal and HIV-positive individuals. *Journal of International Neuropsychological Society, 4*, 291–302.

Mensing, C., Boucher, J., Cypress, M., Weinger, K., Mulcahy, K., Barta, P., et al. (2006). National standards for diabetes self-management education. *Diabetes Care, 29*(Suppl. 1), 78–85.

Myers, L. J., Young, A., Obasi, E., & Speight, S. L. (2003). Recommendations for the psychological treatment of persons of African descent. In *Psychological Treatment of Ethnic Minority Populations*. Council of National Psychological Associations for the Advancement of Ethnic Minority Interests. (pp. 13–18). Washington, DC: Association of Black Psychologists.

National Cancer Institute. (1994). *Clear and simple: Developing effective print materials for low-literate readers*. Bethesda, MD: U.S. Department of Health and Human Services.

National Institute of Diabetes and Digestive and Kidney Diseases. (2005). *National diabetes statistics fact sheet*. Bethesda, MD: U.S. Department of Health and Human Services.

Sackett, D. L., & Rosenberg, W. M. (1995). The need for evidence-based medicine. *Journal of the Royal Society of Medicine, 88*(11), 620–624.

Spring, B. (2007). Evidence-based practice in clinical psychology: What it is, why it matters; what you need to know. *Journal of Clinical Psychology, 63*(7), 611–631.

U.S. Census Bureau. (2000). *Disability status: 2000*. Retrieved May 1, 2007, from *http://www.census.gov*.

U.S. Department of Health and Human Services. (1999). *Mental health: A report of the Surgeon General*. Rockville, MD: Author.

U.S. Department of Health and Human Services. (2001). *Mental health: Culture, race, and ethnicity—A supplement to mental health: A report of the Surgeon General*. Rockville, MD: Author.

U.S. Department of Health and Human Services. (2005). *National healthcare disparities report*. (AHRQ Publication No. 06-0017). Rockville, MD: Author.

Wegener, S. T., Kortte, K. B., Hill-Briggs, F., Johnson-Greene, D., Palmer, S., & Solario, C. (2007). Rehabilitation psychology. In R.L. Braddom (Ed.), *Physical Medicine and Rehabilitation* (3rd ed., pp. 63–92). London: Elsevier.

Williams, A. S. (1999). Accessible diabetes education materials in low-vision format. *Diabetes Educator, 25*, 695–715.

Williams, A. S. (2002). A focus group study of accessibility and related psychosocial issues in diabetes education for people with visual impairment. *Diabetes Educator, 28*, 999–1008.

CHAPTER 7

Cultural Diversity and How It May Differ for Programs and Providers Serving People with Psychiatric Disabilities

Judith A. Cook, PhD;
Lisa A. Razzano, PhD; and
Jessica A. Jonikas, MA

INTRODUCTION

When he first started experiencing symptoms as a young [Hawaiian] man, he went to his Auntie and asked for help. His Auntie heard him out and then told him not to worry, because in a week he would receive the help he needed. Oishi was relieved and eagerly waited for the promised cure only to be presented, after a week, with a cucumber. Etched on the cucumber were characters in Japanese. His Auntie explained to him that he was supposed to rub the cucumber over his head and he would get better. "You can imagine my disappointment," says Oishi, when he retells the story. "I had been waiting a week and I thought I would get better and all I got was this cucumber. But I knew that I had serious problems and I knew that I needed some kind of real medicine." Oishi ended up "rebelling" by seeking western medical attention for his mental health problems. He credits this medical attention with allowing him to be the capable consumer advocate he is today (Heim & Kaapana 2001, p. 4.6).

Fieldwork was carried out in a Mahanubhav healing temple in Maharashtra (in western India on the coast). Women's responsibility for the health and well-being of the family is given a novel and literal interpretation in this setting. Women come as care givers accompanying a mentally ill family member. But although they arrive as care givers and, indeed, continue to fulfill that function,

they become afflicted by trance soon after their arrival. Women see this trans-
formation into patienthood as resulting from their devotion to their families.
Indeed, they pray that the illness be transferred from their sons, husband or
daughters to themselves. It is thought that regular trance will channel the force
of the earlier affliction away from the original patient. Thus women cultivate
trance as a sacrificial device to ensure the health and well-being of the rest of the
family (Skultans, 1987, p. 661).

Striking disparities characterize what we know about the mental health of members of diverse racial and ethnic groups as well as the care they receive for mental illness. Compared to White people, members of multicultural groups have less access to psychiatric services, are less likely to receive care when needed, and their care is more likely to be of inferior quality and efficacy (U.S. Department of Health & Human Services [DHHS], 2001).

In this chapter, we argue that many aspects of mental illness and the service system designed to treat it in the U.S. present unique challenges to organizations and providers aiming to deliver culturally competent services. The nature of mental illness and its disabling potential are both culturally diverse phenomena that may differ from other types of conditions and impairments often associated with disability. In what follows, we define cultural competence in the field of mental health and discuss six ways in which specific features of mental illness and its sociocultural context create challenges for mental health and rehabilitation agencies working across diverse cultures with people who have psychiatric disabilities. We describe the research supporting our assertions as well as gaps in our knowledge that also illustrate our points. We argue that unless the fields of mental health and rehabilitation begin to address some of these issues specifically and concretely, attempts to assess and promote cultural competence will miss the mark. As a result, the recovery of people with psychiatric disabilities will continue to lag behind that of individuals with other types of disabilities and medical conditions.

CULTURAL COMPETENCE IN MENTAL HEALTH

In this analysis, mental illness is defined as a disorder meeting criteria outlined in the *Diagnostic and Statistical Manual of Mental Disorders* or DSM (American Psychiatric Association [APA], 2000a). Disability is defined as a limitation in the performance of one or more age—and culturally-appropriate adult social roles resulting from an interaction between functional limitations and impairments related to individuals' health status and features of their cultural, social, natural, and built environments (Gross & Hahn, 2004). In this *new paradigm* framework (DeJong & O'Day, 1991), disability does not lie within the person but in the interface between individuals' characteristics (such as their functional status or personal or social qualities), and the features of the environments in which they operate. Psychiatric disability is defined as the co-occurrence of a mental illness and related level of disability. Rehabilitation is defined as recovery-oriented services and supports designed to restore an individual's role functioning, pursuit of daily activities, and goal attainment to optimal levels (Cook, 2003).

As defined by the DHHS in *Mental Health: Culture, Race, and Ethnicity: A Supplement to Mental Health: A Report to the Surgeon General* (2001), cultural competence starts with acknowledgement of features of individuals' cultures and a set of related clinical skills, professional knowledge, and organizational policies necessary for effective treatments. The notion of cultural competence in delivery of mental health services has as its foundation the belief that services tailored toward recipients' individual cultures will enhance access, engagement, treatment completion, and positive outcomes. Sue (1998) argues that the notion of cultural competence indicates a major shift in ethnic and race relations, placing responsibility for *competent* care on primarily White organizations and providers (Peterson et al., 1996). While many models of cultural competence exist, few have been empirically validated, and there is little information regarding the key components of cultural competence, whether these influence clinical outcomes, and the nature of such influences (Koss-Chioino & Vargas, 1999; Sue & Sue, 1999; Szapocznik et al., 1997). One feature common across models of cultural competence, noted by the Surgeon General's Report, is placing responsibility for competence on the provider, organization, and service delivery system rather than on the individual patient, client, or consumer (DHHS). In this chapter, we argue that this responsibility in the fields of mental health and rehabilitation has some unique features that are distinct from those of other disciplines of medicine and related areas of disability. These features are described and the research supporting our contentions is summarized in the following sections. Listed in Table 7-1 are the six focal areas most unique to those with mental health disorders included in this discussion.

Cultural Variation in Views of Mental Illness

The first uniquely challenging aspect of cultural competence in working with individuals who have psychiatric disabilities is the *cultural variation in definitions of mental illness, its causes, and manifestations.* Some cultures do not draw as fine a distinction between mental health and illness as do Western cultures. As noted in the Surgeon General's report (DHHS, 2001), racial and ethnic groups have widely varying perceptions of mental illness. These variations in views related to mental illness affect not only the understanding of psychiatric distress and its meaning among diverse groups, but also whether they are likely to seek professional help or treatment for a condition or experience that is perceived as troubling. An example is the culture-bound syndrome, defined clinically as a recurrent pattern of aberrant behavior and

Table 7-1 Aspects of Cultural Diversity Relevant to Psychiatric Disabilities

1. Cultural variations in definitions of mental illness, its causes, and manifestations	• In some cultures, unusual behaviors are attributed to "spirit possession" rather than biological illnesses.
2. Cultural diversity in help-seeking behavior for mental health difficulties	• Seeking help outside of the traditional family unit is considered taboo or shameful.
3. Cultural variations in use of language and verbal communication	• Gender can restrict emotional expression in certain cultures such that women do not discuss health issues with male providers.
4. Cultural attitudes toward use of western psychotropic medications	• Individuals from diverse groups express concerns over "mind control" as a result of using psychiatric medications.
5. Lack of cultural diversity in the mental health workforce	• While the U.S. Census Bureau demonstrates increased numbers of diverse citizens, there are relatively few providers who are members of these racial and ethnic groups.
6. Use of indigenous healers for mental health problems	• Shamans, faith healers, and other types of traditional healers creates a more culturally competent approach to mental health treatment.

troubling experience, limited to specific societies or culture areas and represented by localized, folk diagnostic categories (APA, 2000a). One example is the condition known as *ataque de nervios*, primarily reported by Latinas from the Caribbean, with symptoms including uncontrollable shouting, attacks of crying, trembling, palpitations, and verbal or physical aggression (Lewis-Fernández, 1994). Dissociative experiences, seizure-like or fainting experiences, and suicidal gestures are prominent in some attacks. People may experience amnesia for what occurred during the attack. Ataque de nervios has symptoms in common with affective and anxiety disorders, with which it can co-occur. However, it is not formally recognized as a type of mental illness by American psychiatry or included in the widely used DSM-IV (Oquendo, 1995).

Another culture-bound syndrome known as *amok* occurs in Malaysia, Philippines, Thailand, and Laos, when the victim, known as a *pengamok*, suddenly withdraws from family and friends, and then bursts into a murderous rage, attacking the people around him with whatever weapon is available. He does not stop until he is over-powered or killed; if the former, he falls into a sleep or stupor, often awakening with no knowledge of his violent acts (APA, 2000a). A third example is *ufufunyane*, a culture-bound syndrome found mainly among young women in Zulu-speaking and Xhosa-speaking communities of southern Africa, and in Kenya where it is called *saka*. This condition is characterized by shouting, sobbing, paralysis, convulsions, night-mares with sexual themes, and trance or loss of consciousness. It is attributed locally to spirit possession, witchcraft, or magical potions administered by rejected lovers or enemies (APA, 2000a). Yet another syndrome, known as *pibloktoq* and sometimes called arctic hysteria, is restricted mainly to Eskimo communities of North America and Greenland, characterized by a period of fatigue, social withdrawal, confusion, and irritability. This can continue for only a few hours or for days, leading up to an abrupt episode of dissociation that usually lasts only minutes, during which the afflicted person may strip or tear off clothes, roll in the snow, run about in a frenzied state, shout obscenities, destroy property, engage in other violent, dangerous, or anti-social forms of behavior, before lapsing into convulsions and losing consciousness, followed typically by complete amnesia for the dissociative episode (APA, 2000a).

Given the diversity of what is considered a culture-bound syndrome versus a mental illness as defined by Western medicine, some cultures look upon a psy-chiatric diagnosis with skepticism and suspicion, making it more challenging for mental health programs to be culturally sensitive. Another challenge is that some of these syndromes are not considered to be abnormal by members of the individual's culture. For example, ataque de nervios has a prevalence of 13.8% in Puerto Rico and is considered "normal" by many Latinos, yet studies show that it is often associated with mood and anxiety disorders (Guarnaccia, Canino, Rubio-Stipec, & Bravo, 1993) and with more formal diagnoses of panic disorder and dissociative disorders (Lewis-Fernández et al., 2002). On the other hand, evidence from some studies supports the argument that culture-bound syndromes have physical causes. For example, early research reported by Wallace and Ackerman (1960) commonly found that the causes of pibloktoq (arctic hysteria) among the Eskimo populations studied were linked with poor nutrition, principally a lack of calcium. In contrast, Dick (1995) later reviewed the complete literature on pibloktoq to show how the accounts of "running wild" among polar Inuit arose from a situation of sexual exploitation and abuse by arctic explorers.

Working from a perspective of cultural psychiatry, Kirmayer and Jarvis (1998) argue that many of what psychiatry considers to be culture-bound syndromes are not really syndromes at all. In their formulation, the folk term for each "syndrome" refers to an illness attribution or explanation rather than a demarcated cluster of interrelated symptoms and behaviors that characterize a psychiatric diagnosis. While psychiatric nosology (or diagnostic formulation) has as its foundation individual psychopathology, many culture-bound syndromes represent *idioms of distress* or culturally defined expressions of bodily discomfort, social conflict, or personal malaise that are locally understood (Kirmayer & Jarvis, p.185). Thus, they may occur with or without the coexistence of any clinical disorder and are better studied using ethnopsychological theories of emotion and social relations than exclusively through individual psychopathology. Additionally, culture-bound syndromes that reflect elements of dissociation or have been theorized to result from exploitation (such as pibloktoq) might best be approached using trauma-informed mental health treatment (Elliot, Bjelajac, Fallor, Markoff, & Reed, 2005). This type of treatment was developed in response to the high rates of self-reported abuse among people using public mental health and substance abuse services (Goodman, Rosenberg, Mueser, & Drake, 1997). The approach specifically addresses the conscious and unconscious effects that trauma and posttraumatic stress disorder have on people's emotional well-being.

This wide cultural diversity in understanding of the nature and causes of mental illness places unique demands on United States mental health providers and agencies seeking to provide culturally competent services. Providers must walk a fine line between educating people with these conditions and their families about psychiatric disorders and effective treatments, versus imposing what may be construed as a culturally insensitive Western conceptualization of mental health and illness. They also must be alert to manifestations of what appear to be psychiatric disorders but may instead be culture-bound syndromes caused by social dislocation, culture clash, and racial oppression. This ambiguity between diagnosis of psychiatric disability compared to cultural mental health manifestations calls for great caution and care in interpreting and understanding what clients believe and understand when attempting to engage and treat racially and ethnically diverse populations.

Cultural Diversity in Help-Seeking Behavior for Mental Health Difficulties

The second aspect of cultural diversity that is especially relevant to psychiatric disability is the fact that *different cultures have different likelihoods of help-seeking for mental illness* and these may influence ways in which programs and providers handle engagement and the forging of effective therapeutic relationships. While Western culture distinguishes between mind and body, many Asian cultures do not (Lin, 1996). The Confucian, collectivist tradition discourages emotional display as a sign of personal weakness or a sign of familial or social disharmony. Another factor for some Asians experiencing mental health problems is a strong sense of stigma owing to the belief that mental illness reflects negatively on one's ancestry (Ho, 1984). Taken together, these are thought to contribute to the denial of the experience of emotions and the tendency of many Asians to express psychological distress through the body in the form of somatic (i.e., physical) complaints (Chun, Enomoto, & Sue, 1996; Gaw, 1993). A complementary argument is that this somatization is influenced by *display rules* that, in turn, influence what symptoms are shown, to whom, and where they are manifested. Similarly, data from large national studies indicate that African Americans' voluntary mental health treatment-seeking is related to an idiom of distress in which somatization-like symptoms are related to a greater likelihood of seeking services. Research on African Americans' attitudes toward help-seeking for mental health problems has found that many African Americans endorse the belief that life is difficult for people with black skin and that they should display strength in the face of personal problems rather than seek professional assistance (Jackson, 2006). Recent studies have also found that African Americans hold the belief that formal mental health treatment is only appropriate for those who are severely mentally ill, while less serious problems should be dealt with within the individual's family (Snowden, 2001). This belief may be related to the fact that the dominant experience for many African Americans with mental illness was involuntary commitment to a psychiatric inpatient setting that was perceived as punitive and restrictive (Snowden & Cheung, 1990). Finally, Latinos who seek help for mental health difficulties often use multiple providers in different service sectors. One epidemiologic survey of Californians of Mexican origin found that they were more likely to use medical doctors, counselors, ministers/priests, and chiropractors than mental health specialists (Vega, Kolody, & Aguilar-Gaxiola, 2001). Other research suggests that many Latino communities have promoted the notion that mental health problems, including severe mental illness, should be dealt with using natural support systems in the family and community rather than professional care (Cox & Monk, 1993; Vega & Lopez, 2001).

Wide variations in how different cultures view help-seeking for mental health problems presents unique challenges in mental health and rehabilitation. Since different groups have different likelihoods of seeking professional help for mental illness, this variation places responsibility for assertive outreach to diverse communities on mental health agencies and providers. It also influences how providers manage the process of engaging people with mental illness into treatment and how they build therapeutic relationships that respect specific cultural boundaries defining the roles and responsibilities of the helper and the recipient of help.

Cultural Variations in Use of Language and Verbal Communication

There are distinct issues that arise in mental health as a result of *cultural differences in verbal communication and preferred language*, depending on the help-seekers' levels of acculturation. Of particular significance is the fact that mental health treatment and rehabilitation are often heavily focused on language and verbal communication, which may be unfamiliar or uncomfortable across cultures. For example, values associated with Western psychotherapeutic formulations emphasize open and intimate communication, along with verbal exploration of personal problems and intrapsychic conflicts. This type of intimate conversation with care providers is atypical in many non-Western cultures, and thus, may cause disorientation or distress among diverse individuals (especially those with no or lower acculturation to Western cultures) when they receive mental health services in the United States. For example, it has been shown that Asian Americans, who often are raised to be private and circumspect, are uncomfortable with the emphasis on verbalizing intense emotions in psychotherapy (Leong & Lau, 2001). Moreover, cross-cultural communication conflicts can be compounded by gender and age dynamics, such as among traditional cultures where men might find it impossible to discuss intimate feelings and suffering with female providers, or where elders would be loath to unburden worries to younger clinicians. Additionally, some cultural groups may discourage the sharing of personal problems outside of the family due to beliefs that the family best solves its own problems (Alvidrez, 1999). Restoring the health of the distressed individual may be considered the work of the entire family unit (Al-Krenawi & Graham, 2000). Moreover, a diagnosis of mental illness could compromise the family's honor or reputation due to the stigma that surrounds it (Heim & Kaapana, 2001).

The emphasis on directive communication and factual information about problems and their solutions typical in Western-oriented mental health settings leads to communication conflicts across cultures as well. A direct approach may be disconcerting to cultural groups that rely on metaphors to express strong feelings and emotions. For example, terms such as *anxiety* and *depression* do not exist in the Alaska Native or the Native American lexicons. Certainly, Native people describe intense emotional, spiritual, or grieving states, but they do not typically use Western medical terminology to do so. As one example, among the Hopi Indians, the term *Qo vis ti* or turning one's face to the wall, can include symptoms of depression—such as despondency and suicidal ideation—but this emotional state would not be recognized as "depression" by tribal members (Manson, Shore, & Bloom, 1985). Similarly, Arabic individuals may express symptoms of depression as having a *dark life* or express fearfulness by using the phrase *my heart fell down* (Al-Krenawi & Graham, 2000), while in Latvia people in distress are told to *bury [their] suffering under a stone and step over it singing* (Kirmayer, 2001). This metaphorical use of language to describe emotional duress is largely unfamiliar to, and sometimes rejected by, Western clinicians (Al-Krenawi, 1999). Such metaphors of negative affect can lead to misunderstandings between them and the diverse people they serve, along with other serious problems such as the under- or misdiagnosis of psychiatric disorders.

Yet another communication conflict can arise in mental health and rehabilitation settings that tend to emphasize independence, self-direction, and personal growth during discussions of treatment and service planning. Among the many cultures that emphasize the needs of the collective over the needs of any one individual (Triandis, Bontempo, & Villareal, 1988), this individualistic approach may be confusing or even distressing. For example, in the Arab culture, suggestions that the family be less involved or less protective of their ill relative may be viewed as tantamount to asking them to neglect or abandon the person in need (Al-Krenawi & Graham, 2000). Similarly, family members of the African American and Latino cultures may find suggestions that the person with a psychiatric disability should be more independent and live outside of the family home challenging conceptions of what it means to be a family and the positive caretaking that families provide would lead them to care for the family member in need within the family home (Guarnaccia & Parra, 1996).

Lack of linguistic competence also presents a significant barrier for diverse individuals served in mental health and psychiatric rehabilitation programs. As implied above, effective communication is critical to developing an effective therapeutic alliance. Additionally, within Western health care settings, people seeking services are expected to understand psychiatric vocabulary or jargon, ask appropriate questions, provide detailed information about their symptoms and current medications, and comprehend often complex treatment instructions (Parker, 2000). For people with limited English proficiency (or low literacy), these tasks are difficult to impossible. Yet, most community-based programs have both a dearth of providers who can speak the languages represented among their target neighborhoods and program/treatment materials written in those languages (and at lower reading levels).

A lack of language capacity is doubly concerning for people who have recently migrated to the United States. Without access to professional interpreters, the families may be forced to rely on their children or other relatives as interpreters (Gilbert, 2005), including when seeing a physician about their mental health problems. The need to use minors as interpreters has the potential to greatly inhibit effective communication for the adults who do not want their children exposed to private information, the physicians who are speaking to the adults through minors, and the children who are functioning in an adult role for which they are ill-prepared (Singleton, 2002).

As a result of differing cultural backgrounds, many providers may misunderstand clients' perspectives, leading to miscommunication in therapeutic settings and resulting in poor client outcomes for people with mental illnesses. Therapeutic communication relies on specialized cultural knowledge and appropriate styles of discourse, yet many clinicians lack exposure to these skills. Thus, many of those who could benefit from mental health services exit the treatment process prematurely. Therefore, cross-cultural communication skills and linguistic sensitivity assume greatly enhanced importance for people with psychiatric disabilities undergoing mental health treatment. While communication between providers and recipients is critical in all aspects of healthcare, it is paramount in the treatment of mental disorders, since these disorders influence the individual's thoughts, moods, and integrative aspects of behavior (DHHS, 2001).

Cultural Attitudes toward Use of Western Psychotropic Medications

The fourth feature of mental disorders with important cross-cultural implications is the fact that *different cultures have different attitudes toward, and acceptance of, psychotropic medications.* Some cultures strongly resist taking medication for mental health problems. In one study, African Americans and Latinos were less likely to view medications as acceptable treatment for depression compared to White people (Cooper et al., 2003). In another study, African Americans expressed concerns about whether medication treatment is effective, the side effects they would experience, and the potential for addiction to the medications themselves (Cooper-Patrick et al., 1997). In one of the few studies to examine the influence of ethnicity on treatment preferences among patients with anxiety disorders, Hazlett-Stevens et al. (2002) reported that both African American and Asian patients were less likely to consider taking medication to control panic episodes than White patients. Some cultures may see medication as a way to control them or harm them.

> *Related to attitudinal variations, there are also studies demonstrating that certain psychotropic medications are metabolized differently among different ethnic populations. According to Lin, Anderson, and Poland, (1997), compared to White patients, African Americans and Asians metabolize pharmacological treatment for depression and psychosis more slowly. Clinicians who are unaware of these differences may unintentionally prescribe doses that are too high or too low for racial and ethnic minority patients when using guidelines standardized on White people. These metabolic differences may then result in greater medication side effects or patient nonadherence (Lin & Cheung, 1999). The fact that most clinical trials of new pharmaceuticals do not include adequate numbers of diverse racial and ethnic group members compounds this problem (DHHS, 2001).*
>
> *Because psychopharmacology now constitutes one of the major evidence-based treatment modalities for some forms of major mental illnesses such as depression, bipolar disorder, and schizophrenia (APA, 1994, 1997, 2000b), the uneasy relationship between diverse racial and ethnic groups and psychotropic medications is problematic. Equally problematic is the lack of inclusion of mem-*

bers of diverse racial and ethnic groups in randomized clinical trials of medication efficacy. Until specific information is available about the impact of pharmacologic interventions for diverse groups, the mental health field is unable to make a strong rebuttal case for the skepticism and fear with which some culturally diverse groups view this treatment modality.

Lack of Cultural Diversity in the Mental Health Workforce

The fifth important influence on cultural competence in the mental health field is the *lower representation of multicultural groups in its service provider population*. For example, in the United States, most mental health providers are White. Manderscheid and Henderson (1998) report that among diverse ethnic and racial groups, certain communities have even fewer providers indigenous to their culture. One example is the number of psychiatrists of color in the treatment community. According to Manderscheid and Henderson's report, there are approximately 1.5 Native American/Alaska Native psychiatrists per 100,000 Native American/Alaska Natives in this country, and only 2.0 Latino psychiatrists per 100,000 Latinos. Given the substantial increase in Latinos in the general population and the fact that they now represent a larger proportion of the American population than African Americans (U.S. Census Bureau, 2001), the lack of Latino providers will continue to have negative effects on mental health services and recovery within that community.

Studies examining clinician-client matching indicate that when providers and clients are from different ethnic groups, there is an increased potential for therapists to overlook symptoms clients consider important (Hunt, 1995). These providers also are less likely to have a comprehensive understanding of the fears, needs, and treatment concerns of individuals with mental illnesses (Porter, 1997). The lack of a culturally diverse workforce is certainly not restricted to the fields of mental health and psychiatric rehabilitation, since this is a problem shared in all of the human services. However, the inability to engage in provider-client cultural matching is particularly acute in its impact for individuals with psychiatric disabilities given the many other ways in which mental health is culturally constructed and the strong use of culturally grounded communication in assessing and treating mental illness.

The Use of Indigenous Healers for Mental Health Problems

A sixth aspect of cultural competence in the field of mental health relates to the documented *high frequency of use of indigenous healers for mental health problems* in diverse racial and ethnic populations. Several studies of Alaska Natives and Native Americans find that they are more likely to use alternative therapies than White people. In one study of clients at a rural New Mexico Indian Health Service clinic (Kim

& Kwok, 1998), 62% of Navajos reported use of Native healers while 39% said they used them routinely. Diverse racial and ethnic group members are also more likely than Whites to use culturally traditional healers in conjunction with more traditional providers (DHHS, 2001). A study of urban Wisconsin individuals representing 30 tribal affiliations found that 38% reported concurrent use of a Native healer and a traditional mental health clinician (Marbella, Harris, Diehr, Ignace, & Ignace, 1998). Another study of mental health service use among veterans in two Native American tribes found that concurrent use of traditional and alternative healers was common for both physical and psychiatric problems (Gurley et al., 2001). Among African Americans, spiritual counselors and ministers often take on the roles played by more traditional mental health therapists and counselors (Snowden, 2001).

> As the preceding points out, there is a need to develop and test models so the fields of psychiatry, psychology, social work, nursing, and counseling can work effectively with indigenous healing communities and alternative therapies. Traditional healing practices and spirituality are important aspects of the lives of most members of racial and ethnic minority groups. The failure to incorporate these forces in the treatment process can be construed as a waste of valuable resources and natural supports.

IMPLICATIONS FOR PRACTICE

In this chapter, we have sought to illuminate special issues that arise when treating and supporting multicultural individuals with mental health difficulties. There are many points of contact within mental health systems where providers and diverse people come into conflict due to differing worldviews and multiple group memberships. A comprehensive look at specific strategies to improve cultural competency at all system levels is beyond the scope of this chapter. For additional information regarding multisystem level strategies to promote competence, see Chapter 14. However, renowned cultural expert Sue (1998) offers three key skills that can help service providers and their clients become cognizant of the six cultural variations we describe, and thus begin to interact in more culturally-attuned, recovery-oriented ways.

First, Sue (1998) describes the importance of *culture-specific expertise*. Culturally competent providers become experts in the issues we describe in this chapter, as well as other important features and beliefs of the cultures represented in their targeted service areas. They explore their own worldviews and how these meld with or diverge from other perspectives. They are willing to learn more about cultural alternatives to traditional treatments, and to use these alternatives in complementary ways with other services and supports.

Secondly, Sue (1998) describes the value of what he calls *scientific mindedness* within the clinical or rehabilitation alliance. Providers use scientific mindedness when they avoid making assumptions about what an individual is experiencing, and instead, form hypotheses. Then they test these hypotheses with the individual (and his/her family when relevant) for accuracy and, based on the findings, act upon them accordingly. In this way, providers do not respond to people based on prejudgments or commonly held Western beliefs that do not apply across diverse cultures. For example, consider an initial appointment between a White psychiatrist and a Japanese woman. On the surface the physician may prejudge that the woman is depressed, due to her seemingly low affect, unwillingness to speak much, and inability to make eye contact. However, a psychiatrist in this situation using scientific mindedness would also consider an alternate hypothesis—that perhaps the woman is showing deference to an authority figure as is expected in her culture. She would wait to decide until she learns more about how the woman describes what has brought her to treatment and from speaking with her family (with her permission) about her mood and behaviors when at home. Sue (1998) suggests that scientifically minded providers ask themselves a series of questions in working with diverse individuals:

1. How proficient is this person with the English language (assuming the provider is not bi- or multilingual)? Will there be communication difficulties, either from limited English skills or a lack of similar world views?
2. How acculturated is this person to Western society and views?
3. How familiar is this person with Western mental health services and approaches?
4. What does this person think of me? How can we best work together to assess strengths and problems, and to form a plan?

A final key skill involves what Sue (1998) calls "dynamic sizing," or the ability to know when to generalize group experiences to the individual and when to see experiences as unique to that individual. As Jones (1997) notes, major conflicts arise when providers (or anyone) wittingly or unwittingly form stereotypes about others based on their group memberships. To illustrate, a social worker may see that he is scheduled to meet with a Latina for the first time. As such, he may consciously or unconsciously form stereotypes about this woman, thinking that she would have strong family/kin attachments, would not use a medical framework to understand her problems, and would be hesitant to use psychotropic medications. Instead, a social worker using dynamic sizing would keep in mind the things he has learned about Latin culture and how they may influence his client. However, this social worker would not assume that those group experiences generalize to this person until they meet and get to know one another. When using dynamic sizing, Sue (1998) offers these questions for providers to consider in thinking about the group and the individual within that group:

1. What are my stereotypes, biases, or impressions about this person's culture?
2. What can I learn about the parts of her culture that this person embraces or rejects?

Although by and large not evidence-based, consensus of many experts across cultures provides guidance about what it takes to be a culturally competent mental health organization. As described by several authors (Goode, Jones, & Mason, 2002), competent organizations and their personnel have the capacity to value diversity, conduct provider and organizational self-assessment, manage the dynamics of difference, acquire and institutionalize cultural knowledge, and adapt to the diversity and cultural contexts of the individuals and communities served. Competent organizations generally establish a Diversity Committee with direct access to the executive director and an earmarked budget to oversee development, implementation, and benchmarking of diversity activities. They recruit, mentor, and promote diverse individuals at all levels of staffing, and they ensure an agency environment that is welcoming and representative of various cultures through artwork, magazines, and the food served (Chow et al., 2008). Such organizations also hire people who speak the languages represented in their surrounding communities, or engage interpreters, to ensure adequate linguistic capacity (Brach & Fraserirector, 2000). Successful clinical and educational programs have also used such strategies as employing a "cultural consultation team" to improve diagnostic assessment and treatment for diverse individuals (Kirmayer, Groleau, Guzder, Blake, & Jarvis, 2003), collaborating with cultural leaders such as ministers to improve public education about mental health and mental illness (National Alliance on Mental Illness, n.d.), and hiring Native American *Medicine People* to function as paid consultant educators, interpreters, and referral sources for traditional native services/supports (National Technical Assistance Center for State Mental Health Planning, 2000). With dedication, patience, and perseverance, strategies to engage and support individuals across the many cultural groups living in the U.S. can be as varied, unique, and strengths-oriented as the people themselves.

IMPLICATIONS FOR FUTURE RESEARCH

Calls for cultural competence in mental health have been put forth for more than 25 years, with a growing recognition that theories and models developed within a Euro-American context are likely to have limited applicability across ethnically, racially, and culturally diverse groups in the U.S. (Sue, 2001). In response, various government offices and professional associations have created clinical and treatment guidelines to develop, implement, and evaluate culturally competent behavioral health services. The Office of Minority Health Web site (*http://www.omhrc.gov*) and the document titled *Guidelines on Multicultural Education, Training, Research, Practice, and Organizational Change for Psychologists* from the APA (2002) are examples.

In spite of these promising trends, however, few rigorous studies have been conducted regarding the effectiveness of evidence-based mental health interventions across and within specific cultural groups (DHHS, 2001). Randomized controlled trials are needed that include sizeable multicultural samples to shed light on the effectiveness of established medications and interventions across cultures. Culture-specific treatments that could maximize positive mental health outcomes for these individuals also merit careful examination. Along these lines, there is a great need for rigorous research on effective public education and rehabilitation programs that sensitively (and differentially by culture) respond to the issues previously identified in this chapter. These include but are not limited to cultural variations in the explanations for emotional distress and mental health problems, cross-cultural communication conflicts, and lack of a diverse provider workforce.

Additionally, there are cultural competency organizational assessments available to the public (Vancouver Ethnocultural Advisory Committee of the Ministry for Children and Families, n.d.). Nonetheless, there has been virtually no rigorous research on how culturally and linguistically competent policies, procedures, and services impact organizations, the people they serve, and their surrounding communities (Goode, Dunne, & Bronheim, 2006).

Of particular importance in our field is the need for epidemiological studies to address the incidence and prevalence of mental illness among our country's various racial, ethnic, and cultural groups. To this end, several large efforts were funded and will continue to yield important information in the coming years (DHHS, 2001), such as the National Latino and Asian American Study (Center for Multicultural Mental Health Research, n.d.) and the American Indian Services Utilization, Psychiatric Epidemiology, Risk and Protective Factors Project (American Indian and Alaska Native Programs [AIANP], n.d.). More large-scale studies of this nature are necessary to accurately determine the extent and impact of mental illness among the many diverse groups living in the United States.

Goode and her colleagues (2006) cogently summarize future directions for cultural and linguistic competence research, which apply to the fields of mental health and rehabilitation as well. Specifically, they note that 21st century research will include:

Use of validated and shared definitions of cultural and linguistic competence; refined population definitions to include cultural variables other than race, ethnicity, or language; use of designs that test the specific effects of cultural and linguistic competence; implementation of longitudinal and large sample studies to investigate ultimate [mental] health outcomes; and use of methods and measures that examine the relationship among organizational policies, structures, and practices, quality and effectiveness of care, and outcomes and well-being (p. viii).

Additionally, there is a need for more participatory action research (Whyte, 1991) that would involve multicultural individuals in the design, implementation, and interpretation of findings about the emotional resiliency and mental health challenges faced specifically within their communities. A study conducted by Kelly et al. (2004) to understand collaborative models for leadership development within one African American community serves as a useful example. Finally, members of diverse cultures have a critical role to play as advocates and shapers of public policy given the current federal emphasis on "transformation" of the mental health service system to one that further promotes prevention, recovery, and resiliency, as well as being driven by consumers and their families (New Freedom Commission on Mental Health, 2003).

CONCLUSION

While much that has been argued in the foregoing analysis is also true for other medical conditions and disability groups, there is also ample evidence for the contention that working with individuals who experience disabling mental health problems poses particular challenges to the establishment and maintenance of culturally competent treatments and services. The formidable barriers that individuals with mental illness face in today's world are heightened by the fact that the United States treatment system has failed to understand and address many of these issues. Although some progress has been made within the academic community, until these barriers are better understood and clinical skills and training are comprehensively altered, the mental health workforce will have a limited ability to maximize rehabilitation and recovery outcomes among culturally diverse individuals.

REFERENCES

Al-Krenawi, A. (1999). Explanations of mental health symptoms by the Bedouin-Arab of the Negev. *International Journal of Social Psychiatry, 45*(1), 56–64.

Al-Krenawi, A. & Graham, J. R. (2000). Culturally sensitive social work practice with Arab clients in mental health settings. *Health & Social Work, 25*(1), 9–22.

Alvidrez, J. (1999). Ethnic variations in mental health attitudes and service use among low-income African American, Latina, and European American young women. *Community Mental Health Journal, 35*(6), 515–530.

American Indian and Alaska Native Programs. (n.d.). *American Indian service utilization, psychiatric epidemiology, risk and protective factors project (AI-SUPERPFP)*. Retrieved October 23, 2008, from http://aianp.uchsc.edu/ncaianmhr/research/superpfp.htm

American Psychiatric Association. (1994). Practice guidelines for treatment of patients with bipolar disorder. *American Journal of Psychiatry, 151*(Suppl. 12), 1–36.

American Psychiatric Association. (1997). Practice guidelines for treatment of patients with schizophrenia. *American Journal of Psychiatry, 154*(Suppl. 4), 1–63.

American Psychiatric Association. (2000a). *Diagnostic and statistical manual of mental disorders* (4th ed. text revision). Washington, DC: Author.

American Psychiatric Association. (2000b). Practice guidelines for treatment of patients with depression. *American Journal of Psychiatry, 157*(Suppl. 4), 1–45.

American Psychological Association. (2002, August). *Guidelines on multicultural education, training, research, practice, and organizational change for psychologists*. Retrieved October 26, 2008, from http://www.apa.org/pi/multiculturalguidelines/homepage.html

Brach, C., & Fraserirector, I. (2000). Can cultural competency reduce racial and ethnic disparities? A review and conceptual model. *Medical Care Research and Review, 57*(1), 181–217.

Center for Multicultural Mental Health Research. (n.d.). *National Latino and Asian American study*. Retrieved October 23, 2008, from http://www.multiculturalmentalhealth.org/nlaas.asp#aims

Chow, C. M., Ostrow, L., Cave, C., Camacho-Gonsalves, T., Leff, S. H., Jonikas, J. A., et al. (2008). *A guide to cultural competence in community mental health: A six-module web-based course*. Chicago: University of Illinois at Chicago National Research and Training Center on Psychiatric Disability.

Chun, C. A., Enomoto, K., & Sue, S. (1996). Health care issues among Asian Americans: Implications of somatization. In P. M. Kato & T. Mann (Eds.), *Handbook of diversity in health psychology*. New York: Plenum.

Cook, J. A. (2003). Depression, disability, and rehabilitation services for women. *Psychology of Women Quarterly, 27*, 121–129.

Cooper, L. A., Gonzales, J. J., Gallo, J. J., Rost, K. M., Meredith, L. S., Rubenstein, L. V., et al. (2003). The acceptability of treatment for depression among African-American, Hispanic, and White primary care patients. *Meds Care, 41*, 479–489.

Cooper-Patrick, L., Powe, N. R., Jenckes, M. W., Gonzales, J. J., Levine, D. M., & Ford, D. E. (1997). Identification of patient attitudes and preferences regarding treatment for depression. *Journal of General Internal Medicine, 12*, 431–438.

Cox, M. C., & Monk, A. (1993). Hispanic culture and family care of Alzheimer's patients. *Health and Social Work, 18*, 92–100.

DeJong, G., & O'Day, B. (1991). *Materials prepared for the NIDRR Long Range Plan 1999–2003*. Washington, DC: U.S. Department of Education, Office of Special Education and Rehabilitative Services, National Institute on Disability and Rehabilitation Research.

Dick, L. (1995). 'Pibloktoq' (Arctic hysteria): A construction of European-Inuit relations? *Arctic Anthropology, 32*, 1–42.

Elliott, D. E., Bjelajac, P., Fallor, R. D., Markoff, L. S., & Reed, B. G. (2005). Trauma-informed or trauma-denied: Principles and implementation of trauma-informed services for women. *Journal of Community Psychology, 33*(4), 461–477.

Gaw, A. C. (1993). Psychiatric care of Chinese Americans. In A. C. Gaw (Ed.), *Culture, ethnicity and mental illness* (pp. 245–280). Washington, DC: American Psychiatry Press.

Gilbert, M. J. (2005). The case against using family, friends, and minors as interpreters in health and mental health care settings. In *Process of inquiry—Communicating in a multicultural environment.* From the Curricula Enhancement Module Series. Washington, DC: National Center for Cultural Competence, Georgetown University Center for Child and Human Development.

Goode, T., Jones, W., & Mason, J. (2002). *A guide to planning and implementing cultural competence organization self-assessment.* Washington, DC: National Center for Cultural Competence, Georgetown University Child Development Center.

Goode, T. D., Dunne, M. C., & Bronheim, S. M. (2006). *The evidence base for cultural and linguistic competency in health care.* New York: The Commonwealth Fund.

Goodman, L. A., Rosenberg, S. D., Mueser, K. T., & Drake, R. E. (1997). Physical and sexual history in women with serious mental illness: Prevalence, correlates, treatment, and future research directions. *Schizophrenia Bulletin, 23*(4), 685–696.

Gross, B. H., & Hahn, H. (2004). Developing issues in the classification of mental and physical disability. *Journal of Disability Policy Studies, 15*, 341–350.

Guarnaccia, P. J., Canino, G., Rubio-Stipec, M., & Bravo, M. (1993). The prevalence of ataques de nervios in the Puerto Rico Disaster Study. *Journal of Nervous and Mental Disease, 181*, 157–165.

Guarnaccia, P. J., & Parra, P. (1996). Ethnicity, social status, and families' experiences of caring for a mentally ill family member. *Community Mental Health Journal, 32*(3), 243–260.

Gurley, D., Novins, D. K., Jones, M. C., Beals, J., Shore, J. H., & Manson, S. M. (2001). Comparative use of biomedical services and traditional health options by American Indian veterans. *Psychiatric Services, 52*, 68–74.

Hazlett-Stevens, H., Craske, M. G., Roy-Byrne, P. P., Sherbourne, C. D., Stein, M. B., & Bystritsky A. (2002). Predictors of willingness to consider medication and psychosocial treatment for panic disorder in primary care patients. *General Hospital Psychiatry, 24*, 316–321.

Heim, P., & Kaapana, K. (2001). Oahu's "mixed plate" speakers bureau. In E. Alderton (Ed.), *A cultural competency toolkit: Ten grant sites share lessons learned* (pp. 4.1–4.8). Alexandria, VA: National Mental Health Association, National Consumer Supporter Technical Assistance Center.

Ho, M. K. (1984). Social group work with Asian Americans. *Social Casework, 57*(3), 195–201.

Hunt, G. J. (1995). Social and cultural aspects of health, illness, and treatment. In H. H. Goldman (Ed.), *Review of General Psychiatry* (4th ed., pp. 87–98). Norwalk, CT: Appleton & Lange.

Jackson, Y. (2006). *Encyclopedia of multicultural psychology.* Thousand Oaks, CA: Sage.

Jones, J. M. (1997). *Prejudice and racism.* San Francisco: McGraw-Hill.

Kelly, J. G., Azelton, L. S., Lardon, C., Mock, L. O., Tandon, S. D., & Thomas, M. (2004). On community leadership: Stories about collaboration in action research. *American Journal of Community Psychology, 33*(3/4), 205–216.

Kim, C., & Kwok, Y. S. (1998). Navajo use of native healers. *Archives of Internal Medicine, 158,* 2245–2249.

Kirmayer, L. J. (2001). Cultural variations in the clinical presentation of depression and anxiety: Implications for diagnosis and treatment. *Journal of Clinical Psychiatry, 62*(Suppl. 13), 22–28.

Kirmayer, L. J., Groleau, D., Guzder, J., Blake, C., & Jarvis, E. (2003). Cultural consultation: A model of mental health service for multicultural societies. *The Canadian Journal of Psychiatry, 48*(3), 145–153.

Kirmayer, L. J., & Jarvis, E., (1998). Cultural psychiatry: From museums of exotica to the global agora. *Current Opinion in Psychiatry, 11*(2), 183–189.

Koss-Chioino, J. D., & Vargas, L. A. (1999). *Working with Latino youth.* San Francisco: Jossey-Bass.

Leong, F. T. L., & Lau, A. S. (2001). Barriers to providing effective mental health services to Asian Americans. *Mental Health Services Research, 3*(4), 201–214.

Lewis-Fernández, R. (1994). Culture and dissociation: A comparison of ataque de nervios among Puerto Ricans and possession syndrome in India. In D. Spiegel (Ed.), *Dissociation: Culture, mind, and body* (pp. 123–167). Washington, DC: American Psychiatric Press.

Lewis-Fernández, R., Guarnaccia, P. J., Martinez, I. E., Martinez, I. E., Salman, E., Schmidt A., & Liebowitz, M. (2002). Comparative phenomenology of ataques de nervios, panic attacks, and panic disorder. *Culture, Medicine, and Psychiatry, 26,* 199–223.

Lin, K. M. (1996). Culture and DSM-IV: Asian-American perspectives. In H. Fabrega Jr. & D. Parron (Eds.), *Culture and psychiatric diagnosis* (pp. 35-38). Washington, DC: American Psychiatric Press.

Lin, K. M., Anderson, D., & Poland, R. E. (1997). Ethnic and cultural considerations in psychopharmacotherapy. In D. Dunner (Ed.), *Current psychiatric therapy II* (pp. 75–81). Philadelphia: WB Saunders.

Lin, K. M., & Cheung, F. (1999). Mental health issues for Asian Americans. *Psychiatric Services, 50,* 774–780.

Manderscheid, R. W., & Henderson, M. J. (Eds.). (1998). *Mental Health, United States, 1998.* Rockville, MD: Center for Mental Health Services.

Manson, S. M., Shore, J. H., & Bloom, J. D. (1985). The depressive experience in American Indian communities: A challenge for psychiatric theory and diagnosis. In A. Kleinman & B. Good (Eds.), *Culture and depression* (pp. 331–368). Berkeley: University of California Press.

Marbella, A. M., Harris, M. C., Diehr, S., Ignace, G., & Ignace, G. (1998). Use of Native American healers among Native American patients in an urban Native American health center. *Archives of Family Medicine, 7,* 182–185.

National Alliance on Mental Illness. (n.d.). African American faith-based initiative. Retrieved May 21, 2008, from *www.nami.org/Template.cfm?Section=Multicultural_Support1&Template=/ ContentManagement/ContentDisplay.cfm&ContentID=55931.*

National Technical Assistance Center for State Mental Health Planning. (2000). *Examples from the field: Programmatic efforts to improve cultural competence in mental health services.* Alexandria, VA: Author.

New Freedom Commission on Mental Health (2003). Achieving the promise: Transforming mental health care in America. Final report [DHHS Pub. No. SMA-03-3832]. Rockville, MD: Center for Mental Health Services, Substance Abuse and Mental Health Services Administration.

Oquendo, M. A. (1995). Differential diagnosis of ataque de nervios. *American Journal of Orthopsychiatry, 65*, 60–65.

Parker, R. (2000). Health literacy: A challenge for American patients and their health care providers. *Health Promotion International, 15*(4), 277–283.

Peterson, J. L., Coates, T. J., Catania, J. A., Hauk, W. W., Acree, M., Daigle, D., et al. (1996). Evaluation of an HIV risk reduction intervention among African-American homosexual and bisexual men. *AIDS, 10*(3), 319–325.

Porter, R. (1997). *The greatest benefit to mankind: A medical history of humanity from antiquity to the present*. London: Harper Collins.

Singleton, K. (2002). *Health literacy and adult English language learners*. Retrieved May 19, 2008, from Center for Adult English Language Acquisition Web site: *www.cal.org/caela/esl_resources/digests/healthlit.html/*.

Skultans, V. (1987). The management of mental illness among Maharashtrian families: A case study of a Mahanubhav healing temple. *Man, 22*(4), 661–679.

Snowden, L. R. (2001). Barriers to effective mental health services for African Americans. *Mental Health Services Research, 3*(4), 181–187.

Snowden, L. R., & Cheung, F. K. (1990). Use of inpatient mental health services by members of ethnic minority groups. *American Psychologist, 45*(3), 347–355.

Sue, D. W. (2001). Multidimensional facets of cultural competence. *The Counseling Psychologist, 29*, 790–821.

Sue, D. W., & Sue, S. (1999). *Counseling the culturally different: Theory and practice* (3rd ed.). New York: Wiley.

Sue, S. (1998). In search of cultural competence in psychotherapy and counseling. *American Psychologist, 53*, 440–448.

Szapocznik, J., Kurtines, W., Santisteban, D. A., Pantin, H., Scopetta, M., Mancilla, Y., et al. (1997). The evolution of structural ecosystemic theory for working with Latino families. In J. Garcia & M. C. Zea (Eds.), *Psychological interventions and research with Latino populations* (pp. 156–180). Boston: Allyn & Bacon.

Triandis, H. C., Bontempo, R., & Villareal, M. J. (1988). Individualism and collectivism: Cross-cultural perspectives on self-in group relationships. *Journal of Personality and Social Psychology, 54*(2), 323–338.

U.S. Census Bureau. (2001). *Overview of race and Hispanic origin. Census 2000 Brief.* Washington, DC: Author.

U.S. Department of Health and Human Services. (2001). *Mental health: Culture, race, and ethnicity: A supplement to mental health: A report of the Surgeon General.* Rockville, MD: U.S. Department of Health and Human Services, Substance Abuse and Mental Health Services Administration, Center for Mental Health Services.

Vancouver Ethnocultural Advisory Committee of the Ministry for Children and Families. (n.d.). *Cultural competency assessment tool.* Retrieved October 26, 2008, from http://www.llbc.leg.bc.ca/public/PubDocs/bcdocs/339295/assessment_tool.pdf

Vega, W.A., Kolody, B., & Aguilar-Gaxiola, S. (2001). Help seeking for mental health problems among Mexican Americans. *Journal of Immigrant Health, 3*(3), 133–140.

Vega, W. A., & Lopez, S. R. (2001). Priority issues in Latino mental health services research. *Mental Health Services Research, 3*(4), 189–200.

Wallace, A. F. C., & Ackerman, R. E. (1960). An interdisciplinary approach to mental disorder among the Polar Eskimos of northwest Greenland. *Anthropologica, 2*(2), 249–260.

Williams, A. S. (1999). Accessible diabetes education materials in low-vision format. *Diabetes Educator, 25,* 695–715.

Whyte, W. F. (Ed.). (1991). *Participatory Action Research.* Newbury Park, CA: Sage.

CHAPTER 8

Community Infrastructure and Employment Opportunities for Native Americans and Alaska Natives

Julie Clay, MPH;
Tom Seekins, PhD; and
Jeanie Castillo, MA

INTRODUCTION

About 52 million Americans, or 19% of the United States population, experience some level of disability due to impairments caused by injuries, chronic diseases, and other conditions (U.S. Census Bureau, 2006, May, para. 5). People with disabilities experience an extraordinarily high rate of unemployment. According to the National Council on Disability (2008, Exhibit 5.2), the average rate of employment for people with disabilities is only 38% as compared to 78% for working age adults without a disability.

Compared with other social/ethnic groups, unemployment and disability rates increase when discussing Native Americans and Alaska Natives living on tribal lands, which include federal and state reservations, Alaska Native villages, rancheros, and pueblos. The approximately 4.1 million Native Americans and Alaska Natives in the U.S. experience the highest rate of disability of any ethnic group population in the U.S. at 22% (National Council on Disability, 2003b, p. 5). Added to this high disability rate is a high rate of unemployment for the population as a whole. According to the 2000 United States Census, Native Americans and Alaska Natives had the highest rate of unemployment at 7.6% compared to 3.7% overall (U.S. Census Bureau, 2003, August, Table 2). These percentages increase considerably depending on the tribe (U.S. Census Bureau, 2003, December, Table 9). One reason for these high unemployment rates is the lack of infrastructure to support employment on Native American reservations and Alaskan Native villages, and this infrastructure is even more lacking for tribal members with disabilities (National Council on Disability, 2003a, General Barriers, para. 4).

In larger, urban communities, we take for granted the infrastructure needed to support employment for people with disabilities (Clarkson, 2007). Disability infrastructure includes those features of a community that facilitate a person with a disability participating in all aspects of the community. It includes employment, transportation, education and training, housing, health and public services, laws, as well as policies and procedures that facilitate participation of members with disabilities. Within urban communities, there are numerous programs and organizations that take different roles in building and maintaining disability infrastructure. For instance, vocational rehabilitation (VR), employment networks, and Centers for Independent Living (CILs) can focus on promoting employment opportunities for people with disabilities through training and placement (Fugelberg, 2005); other organizations generally take the lead role in maintaining community and economic development infrastructure. Entrepreneurs, private businesses, community organizations, and not-for-profit organizations are constantly developing new employment opportunities. Local government agencies coordinate efforts to facilitate transportation through roadways or public transit systems. State organizations and some local agencies develop strategic plans to both build infrastructure and accommodate people with disabilities.

This level of infrastructure is not nearly as established on tribal lands (Clarkson, 2007; Jojola, 2007). Tribal governments struggle to promote economic development and create employment opportunities on their tribal lands for able-bodied tribal members let alone those with disabilities (National Council on Disability, 2003a). There are a limited number of private, governmental, and nongovernmental organizations that can lead any part of community or economic development. Entrepreneurs, whether individual or organizational, often have a hard time securing capital to invest in new businesses that create employment opportunities in tribal lands (Clarkson).

Indeed, Native Americans and Alaska Natives rank at the bottom of virtually every social statistical indicator and average one of the highest rates of unemployment, the lowest level of educational achievement, the lowest per capita income, and the poorest housing and transportation in the nation (Clarkson, 2007). Many Native American and Alaska Native households lack even the most basic services as plumbing, electricity, and telephone service. For instance, 20% of Native American and Alaska Native homes on tribal lands do not have indoor plumbing or modern sewage disposal systems (Clarkson), 14% lack electricity, and 23% do not have telephones (Jojola, 2007). Transportation infrastructure is another important concern as tribal lands often lack an extensive network of passable roadways. Consider differences between the Navajo Nation and the state of West Virginia; although they are roughly the same size, only 2000 miles of roads are paved on the Navajo Nation compared to 18,000 miles of paved roads in West Virginia (Clarkson). Tribal governments are not only struggling to promote economic development and employment opportunities in their communities, but are also struggling to provide their tribal members with the basic services most U.S. citizens take for granted.

While direct job placement as a service is an important support, given the economic conditions on most tribal lands, working to build disability infrastructure is critical to promoting and sustaining employment for tribal members with disabilities. Such efforts require approval of the tribal government and close ties with the other efforts designed to promote tribal community and economic development (Scalpcane, 2005).

This chapter considers the approaches utilized to address the traditionally high rates of unemployment for people with disabilities and further explores the factors behind the high unemployment rates on tribal lands. The role of disability infrastructure in promoting employment for people with disabilities is explored and shown to be lacking in tribal communities compounding unemployment for Native Americans and Alaska Natives with disabilities. The Tribal Disability Actualization Process (TDAP) is introduced and described as one potential tool for addressing the lack of disability infrastructure. We present case studies of tribes that have used this model.

APPROACHES TO ADDRESS HIGH UNEMPLOYMENT RATES FOR PEOPLE WITH DISABILITIES

Several approaches to promote employment of people with disabilities have been developed depending upon different conceptualizations of disability. According to Hahn (1985), an early "definition of disability focuses on work disability . . . [where] emphasis . . . is placed primarily on changing or altering the individual as the primary solution to the problem [of unemployment]" (p. 33). More recent definitions focus on disability as a consequence of the interaction between the individual and his or her environment (World Health Organization [WHO], 1999).

This earlier definition of disability led to a strong presumption that discrepancies in employment had a relationship to the skills, education, and functional capacity of individuals with disabilities (Hahn, 1985). The VR system emerged to help remedy this presumed discrepancy. The goal of this system was to help individuals compensate for their disability by acquiring new skills and functional competencies (Wright, 1980). An additional goal was to build the capacity of individuals to adapt to what was viewed as a relatively stable environment.

Following the return of veterans from World War II, Korea, and Vietnam, many of whom had disabilities, discrimination against people with disabilities was identified as another factor contributing to unemployment (DeJong, 1979). This sociopolitical concept of disability led to the development and passage of several laws intended to prohibit discrimination and promote employment of people with disabilities. Arguably, the most significant of those laws was Section 504 of the Rehabilitation Act of 1973. This provision prohibited discrimination in employment on the basis of disability by entities receiving federal funds. It also articulated the importance of the physical environment as a source of barriers to participation and set the groundwork for the creation of standards for workplace accessibility.

In the later decades of the 20th century, several laws and policies focused on environmental barriers to participation in work (National Council on Disability, 2008, chap. 5). Chief among these is the Americans with Disabilities Act (ADA) of 1990 (West, 1993). Importantly, the 1990 ADA not only extended prohibition against discrimination in employment to the private sector, it also solidified standards of accessibility.

As assessments of the causes of high rates of unemployment among people with disabilities have changed and the approaches to addressing the problem have evolved, so have the programs to promote the employment of people with disabilities (National Council on Disability, n.d.). For many years, the national and state partnership that forms the VR system served as the primary program for providing direct employment supports to people with disabilities. More recently, additional programs have been added and existing ones reorganized. The 1998 Workforce Investment Act established a national workforce preparation and employment system, America's Workforce Network, to bring together organizations that help employers find qualified workers and help people manage their careers (Office of Disability Employment Policy, 2001, para. 2). In 1999, Congress created the Plan for Achieving Self-Support (PASS) as part of the Social Security Ticket-to-Work and Work Incentives Improvement Act. The PASS helps individuals with disabilities set aside resources in order to achieve a work goal (Social Security Administration, 2004). Most recently, the Ticket-to-Work program has removed some barriers to Social Security recipients with disabilities returning to work by providing beneficiaries more choice in obtaining employment services, VR services, or other support services (Social Security Online, n.d., para. 1). Programs such as these are integral to providing support for work goals for individuals with disabilities. These efforts are part of a long and evolving effort to rectify the low rate of employment of people with disabilities.

Despite the variety of programs that have been developed to address unemployment among people with disabilities, Native Americans and Alaska Natives are underserved by these programs (National Council on Disability, 2003b). Research data from the National Council on Disability found that "American Indians and Alaska Natives have the most disproportionate rate of disabilities and limited opportunity for access to culturally sensitive programs and services of all races" (National Council on Disability, 2003b, para. 3).

UNEMPLOYMENT AMONG NATIVE AMERICANS AND ALASKA NATIVES

In general, the rates of unemployment are very high among Native Americans and Alaska Natives living on tribal lands. Two groups with particularly high general unemployment rates are the Fort Peck Assiniboine and Sioux, at 56.5%, and the Alaskan Athabascan Native Village of Tanacross, at 68.2% (U.S. Census Bureau, 2003, December, Table 9). Many causal factors contribute to the poor employment situation on tribal lands and slow attempts to promote economic development. These factors include locations in economically disadvantaged areas, the inability of tribes to utilize land as an economic resource, poor educational opportunities on tribal lands, tribal mistrust of government programs due to years of discrimination and broken promises, and the struggle to maintain tribal sovereignty while working with state and federal governments (Clarkson, 2007; Cornell & Kalt, 2003; Jojola, 2007).

Location of Tribal Lands

Most tribal lands are not located in economically advantageous places. The system was set up by the U.S. government to isolate Native Americans and Alaska Natives; the land that was set aside was perceived to be some of the least desirable land then available (Locke, 2001). Today, this means that most tribal lands have poor access to transportation used for commerce such as highways and railroads (Cornell & Kalt, 2003). In addition, most tribal lands have limited natural resources for development. The geographical isolation also contributes to a lack of access to outside resources.

Inability to Use Land as an Economic Resource

The most valuable resource of many tribes, their land, can never be used to directly promote economic development. Because a tribe can never relinquish title to its tribal lands as they are held in trust by the federal government, it cannot use them as collateral for investment (Clarkson, 2007). This seriously limits tribal and Native entrepreneurs' access to capital for business and job creation.

Lack of Educational Opportunities on Tribal Lands

Education is a critical element of economic development (Cornell & Kalt, 2003). Unfortunately, the educational system available to most Native Americans and Alaska Natives has been notoriously poor. In 2000, 33.1% of the population living in Native American areas and 31.8% in Alaska Native villages had less than a high school diploma, compared to 19.6% of the total U.S. population (U.S. Census Bureau,

2006, February, Figure 13). One factor contributing to this disparity in education levels includes the fact that "local school systems depend on property taxes for their existence, and tribal lands are exempt from taxation" (National Indian Education Association [NIEA], 2003, State Governments section, para. 2). As a result, the education system available to most residents on tribal lands lacks financial resources (NIEA, 2005, No Child Left Behind: Achieving High Goals Requires Flexibility and Adequate Resources Section, para. 3). Furthermore, only 4% of the residents in Alaskan Native villages and 8.1% of those on Native American land have a Bachelor's degree or more, contrasted with 24.4% in the U.S. as a whole (U.S. Census Bureau, 2006, February, Figure 13). Consequently, these communities often lack the highly educated and skilled labor force that typically drives current-day economic development.

Tribal Mistrust of Government Programs

Native Americans and Alaska Natives in general have suffered from decades of discrimination (Deloria, 1999; Smith, 1999). Relationships with the broader business and government sectors have been seriously strained by centuries of exploitation, distrust, and mismanagement (American Indian Policy Center, 1998, Threats to Tribal Sovereignty are Nothing New section, para. 2; Deer, 1993; Goldberg-Ambrose, 1994). For example, explicit discrimination can easily be seen in the election arena. Native Americans were not recognized as U.S. citizens capable of voting until the Indian Citizenship Act of 1924, and even in the recent past, a Montana judge ruled, "official acts of discrimination. . . interfered with the rights of Indian citizens to register and vote" (Svingen, 1987, p. 275).

Struggle to Maintain Tribal Sovereignty

Tribal governments constitute sovereign nations but exist within the structure of the federal and state government. There are constant battles to protect the sovereignty of each tribe from encroachment by outside forces. Goldberg-Ambrose (1994) suggested that "the constantly endangered quality of tribal sovereignty suggests that any public expression that could jeopardize the legal hold of tribal sovereignty would be subject to criticism from organized Indian interests" (p. 1127). These battles drain precious energy and resources away from development efforts.

In addition to the numerous barriers to improving economic conditions for Native Americans and Alaska Natives living on tribal lands previously discussed, two additional factors affect employment opportunities for tribal members with disabilities. First, the network of employment services and other human service programs is less established on tribal lands, and the linkage with external resources is often tenuous. While Title I, Part C, Section 121 of the Rehabilitation Act Amendments of 1992 provides funding for VR services over a five year period for Native American tribes and Alaska Native communities, few programs are in existence today. As of 2007, only 77 tribal VR programs had been established among the more than 560 federally recognized tribes (Consortia of Administrators for Native American Rehabilitation, 2008). A second factor that affects employment opportunities for people with disabilities living on tribal lands is the lack of disability rights legislation. Because tribal governments are sovereign nations, they are not required to adopt the same disability rights legislation as the rest of the country. The ADA, for example, specifically excludes applications of its provisions to tribal governments. This exclusion means that the established laws that protect all Americans with disabilities do not apply on tribal lands (Dwyer, 1999; National Council on Disability, 1999). However, this does not exclude tribal governments from enacting similar legislation that both protects the rights of tribal members with disabilities while still maintaining the delicate balance of tribal sovereignty.

THE LINK BETWEEN DISABILITY INFRASTRUCTURE AND EMPLOYMENT

There are many views of community infrastructure and its relationship to employment. One is to view a community's economic vitality as a function of its natural, physical, financial, human, and social capital (e.g., Putnam, 2000). Natural and physical capital include such things as a community's location, available raw resources, shipping access, communications systems (e.g., phone and internet access), and its built environment. Financial capital involves the ease of access to funding for investment and development and the institutions (e.g., banks) that manage money and its investment (Emery, Wall, Bregendahl, Flora, & Schmitt, 2006, Table 2). Its human capital involves the number, energy, motivation, skills, and capacities of its residents. Finally, social capital involves the linkages between people and the degree of trust and commitment between community residents. It also includes the traditions and cultural norms of a community (Rainey, Robinson, Allen, & Christy, 2003). Whether these different forms of capital are high or low on tribal lands vary considerably due to the diversity across native communities. For instance, some tribal lands are rich in natural resources, thus high in natural capital, while others have fewer natural resources (Cornell & Kalt, 2003).

Disability infrastructure is built upon the existing resources of any community, and then extends them for people with disabilities. Similar to urban communities, disability infrastructure on tribal lands includes such items as: (a) education and training programs; (b) tribal laws, policies, and procedures; (c) transportation; (d) accessible public places; (e) medical and health services; (f) independent living and assistive technology services; and (g) other health and human services supports. Given the marginal status of general infrastructure on many tribal lands, building disability-related infrastructure poses great challenges. Some particular challenges to building adequate disability infrastructure on tribal lands include a lack of educational and training opportunities, tribal laws and policies that may not provide protections for tribal members with disabilities, lack of accessible public spaces and transportation, and limited independent living services.

Education and Training Opportunities

Native Americans and Alaska Natives with disabilities, until recently, received poor service and support from existing employment services. They are, of course, eligible for services from state job services and VR programs. Unfortunately, data have consistently shown that Native Americans and Alaska Natives with disabilities are seriously underserved by these programs (Ma, Coyle, Wares, & Cornell, 1999; National Council on Disability, 2003a, p. 37). In recognition of this problem, the Rehabilitation Services Administration developed a network of tribally run, culturally relevant employment programs under Section 121 of the Rehabilitation Act Amendments of 1998. These VR service programs for Native Americans and Alaska Natives with disabilities are operated by tribal governments. They mirror the general VR program but are located on tribal lands, are operated by tribal governments, and specifically serve tribal members. They contribute to building human capital by preparing counselors and by supporting education, training, and related services that can lead to employment both on and off tribal lands. However, as noted in a previous section, less than 15% of tribes have such programs leaving a significant number of Native Americans and Alaska Natives without direct access to culturally relevant training and employment services.

Tribal Law, Policies, and Procedures

For many people with disabilities, law, policies, and administrative procedures are in place to provide protection against discrimination in employment and other aspects of life. On tribal lands, however, many of these national and state civil rights laws, such as the ADA, simply do not apply due to issues of tribal sovereignty, and most tribal governments have not adopted similar disability legislation (Dwyer, 2000). Even though these laws do not apply, it does not mean that tribal leaders are insensitive to the needs and desires of their members with disabilities. Previous research has shown that tribal leaders are simply unfamiliar with the policy model for addressing issues of disability but are very interested in learning about it (Fowler & Dwyer, 1996, para. 3). This lack of knowledge, however, can have serious implications for employment of tribal members with disabilities. For example, one tribe had a specific policy stating that disability was a reason for termination of employment or not hiring an individual. When this issue was brought to the tribal council's attention by tribal disability advocates, the policy was immediately changed. More importantly, this change was voluntary given that there is no legal requirement for them to do so.

Another example comes from the Pine Ridge Oglala Lakota tribe who chose to adopt the ADA in response to a request of a tribal disability group. Similarly, the Confederated Salish and Kootenai Tribes created a tribally-mandated committee to develop and implement disability policies and passed a resolution that adopts the spirit of the ADA (Dwyer, 1999, Results section, para. 2). Such efforts set a tone for enhancing disability infrastructure.

Accessible Public Spaces

Most people take the architectural design infrastructure of public spaces for granted because they are designed for the typical person. People with disabilities, due to mobility and other impairments, cannot take for granted physical access to public spaces, or for that matter, to private homes (e.g. Maisel, 2007). For example, a building with even one step precludes a person who uses a typical wheelchair from entering independently. Therefore, many people with impairments cannot access training, employment services, or work.

The first national survey of tribal governments found that many tribal and Bureau of Indian Affairs facilities did not meet even basic access standards (Fowler, Dwyer, Brueckmann, & Seekins, 2000). For instance, the tribal government offices of one tribe lacked designated parking places in its parking area, the sidewalk was rimmed by curbs and gutters with no curb cuts, and the entrance to the building had stairs with no ramp. Such findings are of particular concern since tribal offices are a main source of both direct employment and civic participation information and opportunities.

Transportation

Transportation is a critical aspect of the community infrastructure that supports employment. For people with disabilities and those who serve them, the lack of accessible transportation is one of the most frequently cited problems in finding and maintaining employment (Brusin & Dwyer, 2002). On tribal lands, accessible transportation is often unavailable for a variety of reasons. First, because of the high levels of unemployment and poverty on tribal lands, owning a private vehicle is often out of reach for many families. Even when a family or individual owns a vehicle, it is often difficult to cover costs associated with operation and maintenance. Second, land-use patterns also exacerbate transportation problems. On some tribal lands, housing developments have been placed some distance from the major communities.

Having long distances to travel puts housing out of easy walking distance to business and employment sectors. At the same time, most tribal lands lack a public transit system (Brusin & Dwyer). In general, until recently, the federal government has not adequately supported rural transportation. Finally, legal problems experienced because of high rates of alcohol and drug use further complicate the transportation picture on or near tribal lands. Many otherwise capable drivers, who may own operating vehicles, have lost their driving privileges after being convicted of driving under the influence.

Independent Living Services

CILs are one disability model that has emerged over the past 30 years and has demonstrated its ability to build both community infrastructure and individual capacity for people with disabilities (Hanson & Temkin, 1999, para. 3). These programs provide information and referral, peer counseling, skill acquisition, and advocacy services. Many offer a range of other services, such as access to assistive technology (e.g., wheelchairs, assistive listening devices, etc.) that can improve the functional capacity of individuals. While most U.S. cities have a CIL, 40% of rural counties fall outside of a CIL's service area (Innes et al., 2000). Although some CILs offer services to those living on tribal lands, only a handful of CILs are operated by tribal programs. Moreover, the advocacy approach taken by these programs may conflict with tribal culture (Clay, 1992).

Tribal members with disabilities are faced with numerous challenges that hinder their success in finding employment, living independently, and participating fully in their communities. Some of the challenges outlined above include limited educational and training opportunities, tribal laws and policies that afford few protections for tribal members with disabilities, lack of accessible public spaces and transportation, and few independent living programs. Tribal governments, although interested in improving conditions for their constituents with disabilities, struggle to provide even the basic services, such as plumbing, electricity, telephone service, and passable roadways, for the reservation or village as a whole. Therefore, an approach to tribal development that addresses issues of disability but is directed by tribal members is needed.

IMPROVING CONDITIONS FOR PEOPLE WITH DISABILITIES ON TRIBAL LANDS

As already demonstrated, tribes and their members with disabilities living on tribal lands face a broad range of challenges. It is difficult to speak of tribal challenges, in general, since most tribal lands represent a tribe with a unique culture, while others are home to several tribes that may not be historically and culturally compatible since, in some cases, the U.S. government forced tribes that were historic enemies onto the same reservation (Goldberg-Ambrose, 1994). Tribal governments face many challenges as well, and often must address them in a context of scarce resources and multiple claims. Moreover, the structure of tribal governments varies significantly among different tribal lands. Because tribal members are so interconnected, any policy or allocation changes, no matter how small they may seem to an outsider, have the potential to seriously disrupt relationships. Thus, any changes to be made must be carefully weighed.

The complexity of the issues presented here makes it obvious that no one solution can be implemented that will result in increased employment opportunities or outcomes for tribal members with disabilities. Rather, tribes must be involved in the development of their own solutions that fit their particular circumstances, are respectful of tribal sovereignty, and are culturally relevant. Improving the infrastructure on tribal lands can promote and support the employment of Native Americans and Alaska Natives with disabilities, and such efforts can be greatly facilitated through technical assistance that is culturally sensitive and respectful of tribal sovereignty.

According to Cornell and Kalt (2003), two of the most important factors for successful economic development in tribal communities are true sovereignty and strong institutions. The first factor involves "genuine decision-making control over the running of tribal affairs and the use of tribal resources" (Cornell & Kalt, p. 15). Genuine control allows a tribe the opportunity to evaluate the problems, solutions, and consequences of each decision to best determine how well it suits the tribe's unique circumstances. The second key feature of effective and sustainable tribal economic development requires "capable institutions of self-governance" (Cornell & Kalt, p. 17), both formal and informal. Formal institutions entail the rules, laws, and constitutions that direct people's actions, whereas the informal institutions are the cultural standards that determine what is right and wrong. Thus, true and lasting change is only achievable when tribes have direct control over the decisions being made and both formal and informal institutions are in place to help shape what follows.

Internal and external pressures on tribal governments force them to focus on protecting sovereignty from encroachment by federal, state, and local governments, and private interests (EagleWoman, 2008). The tension of protecting sovereignty, combined with the close-knit nature of tribal communities, and the complex and time-consuming tribal deliberation process, requires concepts of disability and individual legal protections to be introduced in a contextually appropriate manner for tribal government and life. Tribal governments and members are wary of externally imposed solutions. In order to assure that tribal members and leaders mutually understand disability within the framework of their culture, government, and relationships, the process must be primarily internal.

Brown (1986) developed a decision-making process for tribes based on historical models. Dwyer et al (2000) modified her model to develop a culturally appropriate deliberation process, the Tribal Disability Actualization Process (TDAP), whereby tribal members become active participants in improving conditions and employment outcomes for members with disabilities.

The Tribal Disability Actualization Process (TDAP)

The TDAP was created as a model for flexible, culturally responsive, and respectful tribal deliberative process and involves four phases hinged on tribal community member participation and input (Dwyer et al., 2000). The phases involve identifying key tribal liaisons, gaining tribal government support and authorization, conducting a talking circle, and refining the goals and solutions from the talking circle to finalize recommendations.

Phase I

The first phase is to identify key leadership contacts (Dwyer et al., 2000). Local leadership, interest, and commitment are necessary to allow a tribe to address disability issues; therefore, a willing tribal contact is identified to serve as an advocate for the community. This individual acts as a liaison to the tribal government and is responsible for organizing and hosting the process. Tribal elders, tribal social service program directors or other respected members of the community make excellent contacts (Stromnes-Elias, 2007). Once a potential contact has been identified, a letter of introduction is sent explaining the purpose of the process and the intended outcomes (Stromnes-Elias). Introductions to potential contacts can also be facilitated by mutual acquaintances.

Phase II

The second phase of the TDAP seeks tribal government support and authorization (Dwyer et al., 2000). This phase is often attempted through a presentation to individual government leaders or governing bodies on the importance of disability issues. The goal of tribal authorization is to have the talking circle officially sanctioned by tribal lawmakers as a recognized body.

The tribal liaison plays a vital role in this phase of the process by helping to develop the best strategy for approaching the tribal government whether through a letter of introduction, written resolution or presentation to the government leaders (Stromnes-Elias, 2007). It is also an important point of etiquette for all nontribal individuals to make their presence known to government officials by visiting tribal government offices to introduce themselves to the appropriate officials and explain the reason for their visit to the community.

Phase III

The third phase of the TDAP is the talking circle, a method used to discuss and reach a consensus on important community issues (Fowler et al., 2000). The talking circle is based on a more traditional tribal decision-making process whereby group consensus is sought by patient deliberation and respectful discussion of different perspectives (American Indian Policy Center, 1997; Becker, Affonso, & Blue Horse Beard, 2006; Struthers, Hodge, Geishirt-Cantrell, & De Cora, 2003). According to Clay and Fugleberg (2005), "the circle arrangement emphasizes the connectedness of the participants, equal responsibility for leadership, and ownership of the solution by all participants in the circle" (p. 2). The structure and details of each talking circle may vary depending on the purpose and topic; however, most employ the use of a talking piece (e.g. stick, feather, stone) to determine who should speak. Only the one holding the talking piece is allowed to speak, which slows down the pace of the discussion and requires the other participants to actively listen to what is being said (Clay & Fugleberg).

The talking circle methodology has been adopted by the fields of health, social science, and education as a tool to discuss sensitive issues such as disability, race, justice, diabetes, cancer, violence, and even the environment (Becker et al., 2006; Greenwood, 2005; Struthers et al., 2003). In one particular study of Native American women, the talking circle was used to better understand the cultural meanings of cancer (Becker et al.). According to the researchers, "the Talking Circles application to focus group methodology provided culturally rich group discussions, because the circles bring forth conversations and stories about how a participant thinks and feels about negative topics such as cancer" (p. 29). Based on careful analysis of the conversations from the talking circles, numerous issues and cultural beliefs were brought to light that the researchers hope will provide public health professionals insight into the concerns and needs of Native American women dealing with cancer and cancer screenings.

To address issues of disability infrastructure, this self-directed model begins with tribal representatives arranging workshop logistics and inviting key tribal members as participants that may include tribal leaders, social services representatives, members with disabilities and their families, and local organizations. Essentially, the talking circle is a two-day workshop that has the goal of addressing issues of disability infrastructure. Two handbooks (Fowler, Brueckmann, & Dwyer, 1996; Fowler, Seekins et al., 1996) are provided to participants prior to the workshop to facilitate organization and familiarity with the process. Nontribal professionals attend initial meetings and subsequently work with the tribe to answer questions and provide technical assistance.

A talking circle begins with a discussion of individual and tribal beliefs, culture, and traditions related to disability (Fowler et al.). Next, the concerns of tribal members with disabilities are identified and discussed within this cultural and historical context. Since disability rights and rehabilitation language and terms used in tribal members' understanding of disability may be different, definitions are offered by nontribal professionals and then compared and contrasted with tribal beliefs.

Following the consideration of disability rights, rehabilitation vernacular, and community needs, the circle is encouraged to solidify as a group (Fowler et al., 2000). Leadership, advocacy, and systems-change training is provided, and education on disability issues continues. Existing state and local disability services are explored and new programs may be presented to address unique disability issues. These programs and services may include local CILs and state projects and agencies.

Next, the group explores solutions to the problems of disability infrastructure and policy. Current tribal administrative policies are reviewed by the group for omissions and instances of discrimination. Approaches to concerns are developed and discussed. The group suggests revisions to tribal law and works to draft adapted policies on accessibility, employment, transportation, and housing to protect the rights of Native Americans and Alaska Natives with disabilities living on tribal lands within self-directed tribal parameters.

Phase IV

The fourth phase of the TDAP refines the goals and solutions that have come out of the talking circle and finalizes recommendations (Dwyer et al., 2000). The group of tribal representatives then present their findings to the tribal government and continue to track the progress of their recommendations by observing tribal government actions and assisting with understanding and implementing the recommendations.

Impact of the TDAP

The TDAP was developed to be adaptable to the unique needs and characteristics of each tribe; for that reason, it cannot provide strict scientific control or quantifiable results as to its effectiveness. However, its effectiveness can still be judged based on the results of individual tribes in a case study approach. Looking at how the TDAP was implemented to address disability infrastructure on two different tribal lands, the Flathead Reservation in northwest Montana and the Pine Ridge Reservation in southwest South Dakota, provides some insight into how this process can be adapted to meet the distinct needs and considerations of different tribes (Dwyer et al., 2000). These case studies are based on the American Indian Disability Legislation

(AIDL) project which sought to help tribes address a lack of disability legislation and infrastructure by offering technical assistance and training on how to develop culturally appropriate disability legislation.

The Case of the Flathead Reservation in Montana

The Flathead Reservation in Montana is home to 4000 enrolled members of the Salish, Kalispell, Pend d'Oreilles, and Kootenai tribes. The TDAP model was employed by first making contact with the tribal VR project director who agreed to act as the tribal liaison. Next, AIDL staff members contacted the tribal vice-chairperson subsequently receiving authorization from the tribal government to hold the talking circle (Dwyer et al., 2000).

The tribal liaison took responsibility for identifying and contacting participants and coordinating the talking circle. Participants included representatives from tribal VR, facilities management, education, tribal health, the housing authority, the People's Cultural Center, and the Tribal Council.

During the talking circle, the group discussed the meaning of disability and shared their personal stories. They also discussed the importance of improving disability education and self-advocacy training and recognized the need for additional technical assistance in these areas. The group then went on to review tribal personnel policies discovering that disability could be used as a basis for not hiring an individual or even termination (Dwyer et al., 2000).

As a result of the activities and findings of the talking circle, the group developed a number of recommendations on improving access and addressing discrimination in hiring policies. Representatives of the group then took these recommendations to the Tribal Council for consideration.

Based on these recommendations, the actions taken by the Tribal Council produced the following outcomes: (a) a resolution was approved adopting the spirit of the ADA; (b) tribal hiring policies were amended to remove the discriminatory personnel policies; (c) the Tribal Complex Building was made accessible by bringing the ramp in front of the building up to code, and a crew was organized and trained to build ramps; and (d) the Tribal Council made plans to address accessibility issues with tribal housing (Dwyer et al., 2000).

The Case of The Pine Ridge Reservation in South Dakota

The Pine Ridge Reservation in southwest South Dakota is home to 23,000 Oglala Sioux. Members of a nonprofit Oglala Sioux disability advocacy group, the Quad Squad, contacted AIDL project staff requesting aid in addressing inadequate disability infrastructure on the reservation and agreed to act as tribal liaisons (Dwyer et al., 2000). Members of the Quad Squad first gained permission from the Tribal Council to hold a talking circle and then coordinated the event by identifying and contacting participants and hosting the talking circle. Participants in the workshop included representatives of the Quad Squad, the Oglala Lakota

continued

Tribal College, Indian Health Service, community health agencies, the tribe's Employment Rights Office, the Tribal Council, and family members of people with disabilities.

During the talking circle, the group recognized the need for increased awareness of disability issues and encouraged the Tribal Council to establish accessible parking and requested that government facility managers comply with Section 504 of the Rehabilitation Act. As a result of the group's recommendations, the Tribal Council passed the ADA in 1994 (Dwyer et al., 2000). A disability resources fair was also held to increase awareness of disability issues, and a tribal attorney was given the task of writing parking codes to address the lack of accessible parking. Unfortunately, there were some unforeseen consequences in implementing the ADA on the reservation, which included jurisdictional issues and difficulty in maintaining ADA training for Tribal Council staff due to regular changes in personnel. Additionally, although all recognized the importance of ensuring accessibility by addressing parking codes, tribal members agreed that basic needs, such as plumbing, electricity, heating, and telephone service, must take precedence, therefore, providing accessible parking could not be a top priority.

CONCLUSION

Because of the history of isolation of tribal lands, tribes often lack many of the resources needed to build, develop, and maintain economic and community infrastructure. While many outsiders view the recent emergence of casinos as the source of such financial capital, few tribal lands actually have casinos or significant income from them. There is a need for innovative solutions to overcome these barriers.

The Coeur d'Alene Tribe of Idaho provides a strong example of addressing community and economic development through innovative and diverse strategies (McNeel, 2007). The tribe has a comprehensive development plan to diversify its economic base which includes "strengthening resource management, improving infrastructure systems, developing an industrial park, expanding retail and wholesale enterprises, developing tourism, zoning development, and improving transportation" (Inland Northwest Economic Adjustment Strategy, 2001, Strategies section, para. 1). The Tribal Planning Department's mission seeks to empower the tribal community through sustainable economic and community development in the framework of traditional values, with attention given to public works, economic development, community development, and data collection and organization (Coeur d'Alene Tribe, 2006). For example, the tribe opened the Benewah Medical Center in 1990 and in subsequent years expanded the facility in order to serve more patients and offer more services including a Wellness Center. Through expansion of the medical center, the tribe has been able to create more employment opportunities for tribal members and better address the health concerns of its members (Inland Northwest Economic Adjustment Strategy).

Self-employment and business development is another strategy that tribes have successfully used to improve the employment outcomes of tribal members with disabilities. The Small Business Administration's 8(a) Business Development Program exists to award government procurement contracts to small businesses owned by minorities. The program introduces small businesses to many aspects of successful competition and then supports the businesses as they establish themselves. 8(a) businesses return revenues to a tribal budget in order to benefit all members of a tribal community (Reynolds, 2007).

In addition, several CILs have been established on tribal lands with the specific goal of providing vital, culturally appropriate services to Native Americans with disabilities. The ASSIST! to Independence program, located on the Navajo Reservation in Tuba City, Arizona, emphasizes "quality of life and community access. . . to cross-disability American Indian consumers. . . through the maximization of independence and improvement of functional skills" (National Council on Disability, 2003b, Section III, Assessing the Effectiveness of Strategies for Reducing Barriers to Provision of and Access to Appropriate Services section, para. 18). The ASSIST! program is a success story for Native American-operated, community-based programs to address the needs of tribal members living with disabilities. To fulfill its mission of improving quality of life and community access for Native Americans with disabilities, it collaborates with other organizations to provide the core services of advocacy, peer mentoring, skills training and information/referral, while also offering traditional healing, home modifications, environmental interventions, medical equipment, and transportation services (ASSIST! To Independence, n.d, para. 5; Blatchford, n.d., para. 5).

Despite these recent improvements, tribal governments and members still face a wide range of challenges in promoting integration and employment for people with disabilities. A major challenge involves building adequate community infrastructure that supports these goals. Tribal leaders and community members need to place a greater emphasis on infrastructure development over the long term, and the resources to achieve this goal need to come from diversified sources including federal, state, local, and tribal governments. As the case studies of the Flathead and Pine Ridge reservations demonstrate, improvements to the existing disability infrastructure can be implemented through a culturally appropriate tribal deliberation process that protects the tribe's sovereignty. The TDAP provides a means for self-directed change that is sensitive to the unique needs and circumstances of each tribe. However, the case studies also demonstrate that the changes can be slow and with unforeseen consequences. Sustainable economic and community development is an ongoing process that must continually be adapted to meet the changing needs of the community in question.

Unfortunately, research on issues of disability in Indian Country is sorely lacking. This means that directions and topics for future research in this area are many. One question of basic interest is what disability legislation and policy have tribal governments adopted: which tribes have such legislation and what have been the impacts of this legislation on the lives of tribal members with disabilities. It would also be interesting to look at tribes with successful economic and community development programs and whether or not they have been able to provide adequate infrastructure to support the full integration of tribal members with disabilities into the community.

REFERENCES

American Indian Policy Center. (1997). *Traditional American Indian leadership: A comparison with U.S. governance contents.* Retrieved May 14, 2008, from *http://www.americanindianpolicy center.org/research/tdlead.html*

American Indian Policy Center. (1998). *Threats to tribal sovereignty.* Retrieved May 15, 2008, from *http://www.airpi.org/research/sovthreat.html*

ASSIST! To Independence. (n.d.). *Competition regarding best CIL practices in rural outreach to emerging disability populations.* Retrieved May 1, 2008, from *http://www.assisttoindependence .org/bestpractices.html*

Becker, S., Affonso, D., & Blue Horse Beard, M. (2006). Talking circles: Northern Plains Tribes American Indian women's views of cancer as a health issue. *Public Health Nursing, 23*(1), 27–36.

Blatchford, M. (n.d.). *Round peg in a square hole: Independent living in Indian Country.* Retrieved May 1, 2008, from the ASSIST! To Independence Web site: *http://www.assisttoindependence .org/peg.html*

Brown, S. A. (1986, September). *The preventative and restorative aspects of cultural conflicts resolution through the native self-actualization model.* Paper presented at the Native American Rehabilitation National Research Symposium, Scottsdale, AZ.

Brusin, J., & Dwyer, K. (2002, December). *Tribal transportation: Barriers and solutions* (Brief No. 5). Retrieved May 8, 2008, from *http://rtc.ruralinstitute.umt.edu/Indian/Factsheets/transportation .htm*

Clarkson, G. (2007, May). *Capital and finance issues: Tribal enterprises.* Retrieved September 8, 2008, from *http://www.ncai.org/National_Native_American_Econo.228.0.html*

Clay, J. (1992). Native American independent living. *Rural Special Education Quarterly, 11,* 41–50.

Clay, J., & Fugleberg, A. (2005). *Talking Circles: A way for BPAO Benefits Specialists to build working relationships with Tribal communities and Native American SSA beneficiaries with disabilities.* (Issues Brief 1, Part 2, for the TANAC project). Retrieved October 9, 2008, from *http://www .nativeamericancwic.org/forms/issues_brief1_2005_2.rtf*

Coeur d'Alene Tribe. (2006). *Planning.* Retrieved June 15, 2007, from *http://www.cdatribe .com/planning.shtm*l

Consortia of Administrators for Native American Rehabilitation. (2008). *Vocational rehabilitation service projects for American Indians with disabilities.* Retrieved September 8, 2008, from *http://www.canar.org/map/stateAll.asp?sh=hide*

Cornell, S., & Kalt, J. P. (2003). Reloading the dice: Improving the chances for economic development on American Indian reservations. *Joint Occasional Papers on Native Affairs,* No. 2003-02. Retrieved September 8, 2008, from *http://www.jopna.net*

Deer, A. E. (1993). Statement of Ada Deer before the Senate Committee of Indian Affairs July 15, 1993. *Wicazo Sa Review, 9*(2), 105–108.

DeJong, G. (1979). Independent living: From social movement to analytic paradigm. *Archives of Physical Medicine and Rehabilitation, 60,* 435–446.

Deloria, V., Jr. (1999). Why Indians aren't celebrating the Bicentennial. In Deloria, B., Foehner, K., & Scinta, S. (Eds.), *Spirit and reason: The Vine Deloria, Jr., reader* (pp. 199–205). Golden, CO: Fulcrum.

Dwyer, K. (1999, January). *American Indian disability legislation research: Rural disability and rehabilitation research progress report #2.* Retrieved June 20, 2007, from *http://rtc.ruralinstitute.umt.edu/Indian/AIDLReProgressRpt.htm*

Dwyer, K., Fowler, L., Seekins, T., Locust, C., & Clay, J. (2000). Community development by American Indian Tribes: Five case studies of establishing policy for tribal members with disabilities. *Journal of the Community Development Society, 31*(2), 196–215.

EagleWoman, A. (2008). Tribal Values of Taxation within the Tribalist Economic Theory. *Indigenous Nations Journal, 6*(1). Retrieved October 10, 2008, from *http://papers.ssrn.com/sol3/papers.cfm?abstract_id=1020264*

Emery, M., Wall, M., Bregendahl, C., Flora, C., & Schmitt, B. (2006, April). Economic development in Indian Country: Redefining success. *Online Journal of Rural Research & Policy.* Retrieved July 22, 2008, from *http://www.ojrrp.org/issues/2006/04/0604Emery.pdf*

Fowler, L., Brueckmann, S., & Dwyer, K. (1996). *How to hold a successful focus group meeting.* Missoula: The University of Montana, Montana University Affiliated Rural Institute on Disabilities.

Fowler, L., & Dwyer, K. (1996). *AIDL survey results* (Factsheet). Retrieved July 17, 2008, from *http://rtc.ruralinstitute.umt.edu/Indian/Factsheets/AmILegSrv.htm*

Fowler, L., Dwyer, K., Brueckmann, S., & Seekins, T. (2000). *How to hold a successful talking circle.* (Rev. ed.). Missoula: The University of Montana Rural Institute, American Indian Disability Technical Assistance Center.

Fowler, L., Seekins, T., Guidry, J., Dwyer, K., Duffy, S., & Brueckmann, S. (1996). *American Indian Disability Legislation Project: A guide to developing disability policies on American Indian reservations.* Missoula: The University of Montana, Montana University Affiliated Rural Institute on Disabilities.

Fugelberg, A. (2005, September). *Independent living center employment programs: Important resources for American Indians and Alaska Natives with disabilities.* Retrieved October, 9, 2008, from Research and Training Center on Disability in Rural Communities Web site: *http://rtc.ruralinstitute.umt.edu/Indian/Factsheets/IL.htm*

Goldberg-Ambrose, C. (1994). Of Native Americans and tribal members: The impact of law on Indian group life. *Law & Society Review, 28*(5), 1123–1148.

Greenwood, J. (2005, October). *The circle process: A path for restorative dialogue.* Retrieved April 10, 2008, from the University of Minnesota's Center for Restorative Justice & Peacemaking Web site: *http://www.rjp.umn.edu/img/assets/13522/The_Circle_Process.pdf*

Hahn, H. (1985). A sociopolitical perspective. In R. Habeck (Ed.), *Proceedings from the Symposium: Economics and equity in the employment of people with disabilities: International policies and practices* (pp. 18–21). East Lansing: Michigan State University. (ERIC Document Reproduction Service No. ED261209)

Hanson, S., & Temkin, T. (1999). *RRTC-ILDP Issue Brief: Collaboration between publicly-funded rehabilitation programs and community-based independent living centers.* Retrieved May 1, 2008 from the World Institute on Disability Web site: *http://www.wid.org/publications/rrtc-ildp-issue-brief-collaboration-between-publicly-funded-rehabilitation-programs-and-community-based-independent-living-centers/*

Inland Northwest Economic Adjustment Strategy. (2001). *Coeur d'Alene Reservation, North Idaho: A case study.* Retrieved June 15, 2007, from *http://www.inlandnwregion.org/Phase1-2ID-CR.html*

Innes, B., Enders, A., Seekins, T., Merritt, D., Kirshenbaum, A., & Arnold, N. (2000). Assessing the geographic distribution of centers for independent living across urban and rural areas: Toward a policy of universal access. *Journal of Disability Policy Studies, 10*(2), 207–224.

Jojola, T. (2007, May). *Physical infrastructure and economic development.* Retrieved September 8, 2008, from *http://www.ncai.org/National_Native_American_Econo.228.0.html*

Locke, R. F. (2001). *The book of the Navajo.* Los Angeles: Mankind.

Ma, G. X., Coyle, C., Wares, D., & Cornell, D. (1999). Assessment of services to American Indians with disabilities. *Journal of Rehabilitation, 65*(3), 11–16.

Maisel, J. (2007). Toward inclusive housing and neighborhood design: A look at visitability. In J. Nasar & J. Evans-Crowley (Eds.), *Universal design and visitability: From accessibility to zoning* (pp. 31–43). Columbus: Ohio State University.

McNeel, J. (2007, April 24). Coeur d'Alene's economic success impacts neighboring communities. Indian Country Today. Retrieved July 18, 2008, from *http://www.indiancountry.com/content.cfm?id=1096414896*

National Council on Disability. (1999, December). *Lift every voice: Modernizing disability policies and programs to serve a diverse nation.* Retrieved June 20, 2007, from http://www.ncd.gov/newsroom/publications/1999/pdf/lift_report.pdf

National Council on Disability. (2003a, August 1). *People with disabilities on tribal lands: Education, health care, vocational rehabilitation, and independent living.* Retrieved May 25, 2007, from *http://www.ncd.gov/newsroom/publications/2003/tribal_lands.htm*

National Council on Disability. (2003b, August 1). *National Council on Disability says Native Americans with disabilities are underserved* (News Release, NCD #03-428). Retrieved July 25, 2008, from *http://www.ncd.gov/newsroom/news/2003/r03-428.htm*

National Council on Disability. (2008, April). *Keeping track: National disability status and program performance indicators.* Retrieved April 25, 2008, from *http://www.ncd.gov/newsroom/publications/2008/Indicators_Report.html*

National Council on Disability. (n.d.). *Achieving Independence: The Challenge for the 21st Century.* Retrieved May 13, 2008, from *http://www.ncd.gov/newsroom/publications/1996/achieving_1.htm*

National Indian Education Association. (2003). *History of Indian education.* Retrieved May 25, 2007, from *http://www.niea.org/history/educationhistory.php*

National Indian Education Association. (2005). *NIEA education issues—briefing papers: Tribal education departments.* Retrieved May 25, 2007, from *http://www.niea.org/issues/ NIEA_Education_BreifingPapers.pdf*

Office of Disability Employment Policy. (2001, July). *Workforce Investment Act of 1998: Its application to people with disabilities.* Retrieved May 25, 2007, from *http://www.dol.gov/odep/pubs/ ek01/act.htm*

Putnam, R. D. (2000). *Bowling alone: The collapse and revival of American community.* New York: Simon and Schuster.

Rainey, D., Robinson, K., Allen, I., & Christy, R. (2003, August). Essential forms of capital for sustainable community development. *American Journal of Agricultural Economics, 85*(3), 708–715.

[Section 504] Rehabilitation Act of 1973, 29 U.S.C. § 794

Rehabilitation Act Amendments of 1992, Pub. L. No. 102-569, § 121, 106 Stat. 4344 (1992).

Rehabilitation Act Amendments of 1998, Pub. L. No. 105-220, § 121, 112 Stat. 1092 (1998).

Reynolds, J. (2007). Native 8a Program: The other economic initiative success story. *Indian Country Today, 26*(51), A1, A4.

Scalpcane, H. (2005, September). *Tribal disability concerns report method: Respecting sovereignty and building capacity.* Retrieved October, 9, 2008, from Research and Training Center on Disability in Rural Communities Web site: *http://rtc.ruralinstitute.umt.edu/Indian/Factsheets/ concerns.htm*

Smith, L. (1999). *Decolonizing methodologies: Research and indigenous peoples.* London and New York: Zed Books.

Social Security Administration. (2004, February). Working while disabled. *A guide to plans for achieving self-support.* Retrieved June 20, 2007, from *http://www.ssa.gov/pubs/11017 .html#1*

Social Security Online. (n.d.). *About Ticket to Work.* Retrieved July 18, 2008, from *http://www .socialsecurity.gov/work/aboutticket.html*

Stromnes-Elias, K. (2007). *A field guide for community work incentives coordinators: How to improve services to Native American social security beneficiaries with disabilities in tribal and urban areas.* Retrieved June 10, 2008 from the University of Montana American Indian Disability Technical Assistance Center's Web site: *http://www.nativeamericancwic.org/issues_briefs .html*

Struthers, R., Hodge, F. S., Geishirt-Cantrell, B., & De Cora, L. (2003). Participant experiences of talking circles in Type 2 Diabetes in two Northern Plains American Indian tribes. *Qualitative Health Research, 13*(8), 1094–1115.

Svingen, O. J. (1987). Jim Crow, Indian style. *American Indian Quarterly, 11*(4), 275–286.

U.S. Census Bureau. (2003, August). *Employment Status: 2000.* Retrieved July 15, 2008, from *http://www.census.gov/prod/2003pubs/c2kbr-18.pdf*

U.S. Census Bureau. (2003, December). *Characteristics of American Indians and Alaska Natives by tribe and language: 2000.* Retrieved May 25, 2007, from *http://www.census.gov/prod/ cen2000/phc-5-pt1.pdf*

U.S. Census Bureau. (2006, February). *We the people: American Indians and Alaska Natives in the United States.* Retrieved June 15, 2007, from *http://www.census.gov/prod/2006pubs/ censr-28.pdf*

U.S. Census Bureau. (2006, May). *Americans with disabilities: 2002.* Retrieved May 25, 2007, from *http://www.census.gov/prod/2006pubs/p70-107.pdf*

West, J. (1993). The evolution of disability rights. In L. O. Gostin & H. A. Beyer (Eds.), *Implementing the Americans with Disabilities Act* (pp. 3–16). Baltimore: Paul H. Brookes.

World Health Organization. (1999). *International classification of functioning and disability: ICIDH-2* (Beta-2 draft, full version). Retrieved September 10, 2008, from *http://whqlibdoc .who.int/hq/1999/WHO_HSC_ACE_99.1.pdf*

Wright, G. N. (1980). *Total rehabilitation* (1st ed.). Boston: Little, Brown.

CHAPTER 9

Employment and Rehabilitation Issues for Racially and Ethnically Diverse Women with Disabilities

Diane L. Smith, PhD, OTR/L;
Reginald Alston, PhD

INTRODUCTION

Women with disabilities encounter dual discrimination with regard to employment (Burkhauser, Havemen, & Wolfe, 1990). They are much less likely to be employed than women without disabilities, and if employed, work in lower-paying, lower-skilled service and domestic jobs (Baldwin, Johnson, & Watson, 1993; Bowe, 1992; Johnson & Lambrinos, 1985; Randolph, 2004; Randolph & Andresen, 2004; Smith, 2007a; Smith, 2007b). Racially and ethnically diverse women with disabilities are subject to what has been termed "triple jeopardy" (Wright, 1988). This chapter presents information regarding employment issues of racially and ethnically diverse women with disabilities. Issues concerning women, racially and ethnically diverse persons with disabilities, and women with disabilities in general, are explored as we attempt to provide additional insight into this complex population. Unfortunately, there is minimal research and information regarding racially and ethnically diverse women with disabilities, particularly in the areas of employment and rehabilitation. In addition, we make suggestions for rehabilitation professionals with regard to how best to address some of the issues with this population in a culturally sensitive manner using supply-side (support for the employee) and demand-side (support for the employer) approaches.

THEORIES

The Intersection of Race/Ethnicity, Gender, and Disability

In order to better understand issues faced by racially and ethnically diverse women with disabilities, several theories have been postulated. While not exhaustive, the following represent some of the prevalent theories developed to explain the multiple issues affecting racially and ethnically diverse women with disabilities.

Minority Status Model

Women, persons with disabilities, and persons of color have all been viewed as minorities. Representation theories view the term *minority status* as referring to groups that share a history of being denied access to resources and privileges, such as economic opportunity, communicative self-representation, and preferred lifestyle (Foucault, 1986; Habermas, 1987; Wirth, 1945). Wirth expanded this concept by defining minorities as "a group of people, who, because of physical or cultural characteristics, are singled out from others in society in which they live for differential and unequal treatment, and who therefore regard themselves as objects of collective discrimination" (p. 347).

Although the term minority is often equated with numbers of racial or ethnic populations based on a census (e.g., 12.1% African American; 12.5% Latinos [U.S. Census Bureau, 2002]), from a representation theory perspective, numerical underrepresentation is not an intrinsic property of being a minority (Mpofu & Conyers, 2004). For instance, females comprise the larger proportion of people in most societies, yet are defined as minorities in many cases because of their economic and social oppression, defined as the first key characteristic of minority status (Solomon, 1995; Wilson, 1996).

Representation theory views restrictions on communicative self-representation as the second key characteristic of minority status (Habermas, 1984, 1987). Communicative self-representation is the right to self-identify or refer to the self in self-chosen or preferred terms (Gans, 1979; Habermas, 1984; Waters, 1996). By contrast, being subject to imposed restrictions on communicative self-representation indicates dependence and co-option into the worldview of another group.

A third characteristic by which representation theories characterize minority status is limitation in accessing a culturally preferred way of life (Foucault, 1986). The minority engendering effects are most likely to be experienced when a dominant culture overshadows or excludes alternative cultural expressions (Frosh, Phoenix, & Pattman, 2000; Lakoff & Johnson, 1980). Women, persons of color, and persons with disabilities have all experienced these characteristics as separate populations and as intersecting populations (racially and ethnically diverse women, women with disabilities, racially and ethnically diverse persons with disabilities, and racially and ethnically diverse women with disabilities).

Simultaneous Oppression

Stuart (1992) suggests that racism within disability is part of a process of simultaneous oppression defined as experiencing multiple types of oppression as a singular experience, which individuals of African descent experience daily in Western society. It is also an experience that divides persons with disabilities from their able-bodied peers. In fact, people from all races or cultures with a disability may be discriminated against within their own able-bodied community. Stuart identifies three areas that exemplify African Americans with disabilities' experiences as distinct forms of oppression. These are: (a) limited or no disability identity (the person is identified by others primarily as Black); (b) resource discrimination, (for example, inequitable access to financial opportunities); and (c) isolation within the African American community and family (often associated with limited resources and supports to promote the independence of the person with a disability). Stuart argues that although White people with disabilities also experience marginalization, they do so as accepted members of society. This opinion is not embraced by White scholars with disabilities.

Multiple Identities

Vernon (1999) argues that the concept of simultaneous oppression is too simplistic an analysis to capture the day-to-day experiences of those who possess negatively labeled multiple identities because it overlooks the importance of social class positioning. That is, not all people with disabilities (Morris, 1991) or individuals of African descent (Miles, 1989) are in the same social class position. The author argues that the reality of being a multiple "other" (Vernon, 1996c) results in shared alliances, as well as oppositional interests between different groups of others. Thus, people with disabilities who may also be racially and culturally diverse, women, gay men and lesbians, older people, or those from the working class, may experience oppression singularly, multiply, and simultaneously by other persons or entities depending on the context (Vernon, 1996a, 1996b).

In order to better understand the issues facing racially and ethnically diverse women with disabilities, issues facing women, women with disabilities, and racially and ethnically diverse persons with disabilities will first be described. Specific barriers to employment for each of these groups will be discussed. The final discussion will focus on the unique issues faced by racially and ethnically diverse women with disabilities, followed by mechanisms for intervention that can be implemented by rehabilitation professionals.

WOMEN

One of the most notable changes in the U.S. economy over the past decades has been the rapid rise in women's participation in the labor force. Between 1965 and 2000, the proportion of American women who work increased from 39% to 60% (U.S. Department of Labor, Bureau of Labor Statistics, 2001). Women now make up nearly half of the U.S. labor force at 46.5% of all workers (full-time and part-time combined). According to projections by the Bureau of Labor Statistics, women's share of the labor force will continue to increase to 48% by 2010 (Fullerton & Tossi, 2001).

Women and men are distributed differently across occupations. Female workers are most likely to be in technical, sales, and administrative support occupations (roughly 40% of all working women). Women's next most likely occupational group is managers and professionals (32.2%). About 17.4% of working women are in service occupations, and very small percentages work in skilled and unskilled blue collar jobs or in agricultural jobs. Men are more evenly spread across the six broad occupational categories. Their largest occupational group is managers and professionals (28.6%); followed by technical, sales, and administrative support occupations (at 19.7%); and operators, manufacturers, and laborers (at 19.4%; Fullerton & Tossi, 2001).

Even when women work in the highest paid occupations, such as managerial positions, they earn substantially less than men. An Institute for Women's Policy Research (IWPR) study in 1995 showed that women are unlikely to be among the top earners in managerial positions. The Fortune 500 list of CEOs for 2008 includes only 13 women or 2.6% of the total (Fortune, 2008, May 5). In addition, the top male CEO's salary for 2007 started at 350.7 million, while the top female CEO's salary started at 38.6 million that year, which was less than the 25th ranked male CEO in the Fortune 500 companies. Hamlin, Erkut, and Fields (1994) surveyed nine U.S. companies regarding development in managerial careers of women and minorities in the 1990s. A major finding of this survey is that there are still few racially and ethnically diverse or female managers in large U.S. companies. This was especially true at the top of the corporate hierarchy, where two out of nine companies surveyed did not have any racially and ethnically diverse or female officers. In the other seven companies, rarely more than 10% of the officers were female and/or racially and ethnically diverse. Furthermore, data from all nine companies clearly showed that the terms racially and ethnically diverse and women in management refer to racially and ethnically diverse men and White women. Racially and ethnically diverse women are scarce even in the lowest levels of management. It was also apparent that not only are there glass ceilings in managerial hierarchies beyond which few White women and racially and ethnically diverse men can be found, but there are also glass walls that keep women and racially and ethnically diverse managers out of some functional divisions and locked into others.

In the United States, women's wages continue to lag behind men's. In 2002, the median wages for women who worked full-time year-round were 76.1% of men's (Urban Institute, 2004). For racially and ethnically diverse women, the factors causing the gender wage gap are often compounded by specific racial- and ethnic-based inequities. Racial and ethnic discrimination continues to pose serious barriers to employment, promotion, and higher earnings for Latinas, African Americans, Asian Americans, and Native Americans in the United States (Blumrosen & Blumrosen, 2002). Industrial and occupational segregation can also be a source of racial and ethnic wage inequality. For instance, in 2002, nearly one-third of employees in the low-paying private households sector of the service industry were Latinas (Thomas-Breitfeld, 2003). Asian American women are also disproportionately represented in low-wage jobs such as garment work, high-tech contract assembly work (for example, Silicon Valley), and domestic work (Foo, 2003). For Native Americans, geographic isolation, reductions in state and federal public assistance, limited tribal economic development and employment opportunities, and inadequate investment in education and health services are also associated with lower wages (Vinje, 1996). Among Latinas, lower levels of educational attainment and English language ability both contribute to lower earnings (Thomas-Breitfeld; Trejo, 1997).

National data show that in 1999, the median annual earnings of African American women (in 2003 dollars) for full-time, year-round work were $27,600; those of Native American women were $25,500; and those of Latina women were $23,200, all substantially below that of White women, who earned $30,900. The earnings of Asian American women were the highest of all groups, at $33,100. These higher earnings, however, were also accompanied by higher poverty rates and disparities within the larger category of Asian American women (Caiazza, Shaw, & Werschkul, 2004). Figure 9-1 compares these median annual earnings.

WOMEN WITH DISABILITIES

According to the 2002 Survey of Income and Program Participation (Steinmetz, 2006), women have higher disability rates than men in all the major ethnic and racial groups (see Figure 9-2). Among females, African American and White women face the highest disability rates (20.5%), followed by Latina women at 15.2%. Among the female population, Asian/Pacific Islander females have the lowest disability rate at 11.5%. For those with severe disabilities, the gap between men and women narrows,

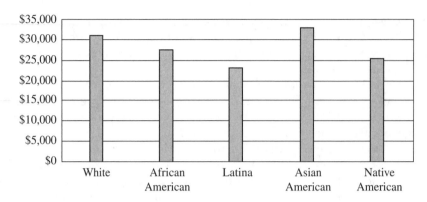

Figure 9-1 Median annual earnings of women in 2003

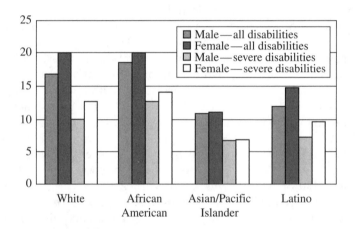

Figure 9-2 Percentage of adults with disabilities by race/ethnicity

however women still have higher disability rates. Disability rates for Native Americans were not included in this study.

Table 9-1 presents the employment rates for males and females with disabilities from the *2005 American Community Survey* (U.S. Census Bureau, 2005). In every disability category, females show a lower rate of employment than males. Randolph and Andresen (2004) also found that there was a significant difference in employment rates of women with and without disabilities compared to men with and without disabilities. Only in the case of those who identified themselves as "severely disabled" was there no greater risk of unemployment by gender. In adjusted models, these authors found that women with disabilities were approximately 1.4 times more

Table 9-1 Employment Rate by Disability and Gender

Disability Status	Employment Rate	
	Male	Female
No disability	80.8%	68.2%
Mental disability	31.1%	26.3%
Physical disability	33.4%	30.5%
Sensory disability	52.0%	40.7%
Any disability	41.1%	34.2%

Source: U.S. Census Bureau, 2005, American Community Survey.

at risk of being unemployed than men with disabilities. Women with disabilities also experience discrimination, both overt and unintentional, that produces lower pay and hinders opportunities for advancement. Earnings of women with disabilities with full-time jobs were only 65% of the earnings of men with disabilities employed full-time (Bowe, 1992).

Barriers to Employment for Women with Disabilities

Russo and Jansen (1988) claim that very little attention has been devoted to the disadvantaged employment status of women with disabilities. For example, compared to men, women with disabilities are less likely to receive quality training for competitive employment. The authors also indicate how the economy in general, and the specialized disability services in particular, restricts the employment opportunities and lives of women with disabilities. Burke (1999) notes that women with disabilities reported more negative work experiences than did nondisabled women, including higher levels of harassment, more hazards, greater demands, and more job insecurity.

According to the 2000 report, "Occupational Employment in Private Industry by Race/Ethnic, Group/Sex, and by Industry," completed by the U.S. Equal Employment Opportunity Commission (EEOC, 2000), women with and without disabilities have fewer jobs in the emerging computer industry and more often work in the lower-paying jobs as computer equipment operators than in the more lucrative jobs as computer programmers or scientists. Compared to men, more women with disabilities are employed in service occupations. In the category of managerial and professional occupations, women with disabilities are employed at higher rates and in greater numbers than men with disabilities. However, women with disabilities are represented in higher numbers primarily in traditionally female-dominated professions, including registered nurses and similar health professionals, elementary and secondary school teachers, and librarians (Jans & Stoddard, 1999).

Barriers to Employment for Racially and Ethnically Diverse Persons with Disabilities

Braddock and Bacheler (1994) reported that racial discrimination remains a major obstacle to the career advancement of racially and ethnically diverse employees, especially those with disabilities. White people with disabilities are almost twice as likely as African American or Latino persons with disabilities to receive an advancement opportunity through full-time employment. About 20% of applications to the state–federal Vocational Rehabilitation (VR) program were African American and 5% were Latino (U.S. General Accounting Office, 1993). This report also states that state agencies spend less for services received by racially and ethnically diverse groups than for services received by nonracially and ethnically diverse groups.

A report to the president and Congress by the National Council on Disability (1989), "The Education of Students with Disabilities: Where Do We Stand?" found that students with disabilities generally are at risk. Racially and ethnically diverse students with disabilities are particularly at risk of inadequate preparation for employment. As dysfunctional as conditions are for students generally, they are worse for students with disabilities and still worse for students with disabilities from racially and ethnically diverse backgrounds. The problems they face are further discussed in a subsequent report by the National Council on Disability (1993) entitled, "Serving the Nation's Students with Disabilities: Progress and Prospects."

Reports from the Rehabilitation Services Administration (RSA) database are sometimes contradictory. For instance, Wilson, Alston, Harley, and Mitchell (2002) found that compared to European Americans, African Americans were 2.12 times more likely to be accepted for VR services. However, in another study, Wilson (2002) found that European Americans are more likely to be accepted for VR services than are African Americans. Similarly, Capella (2002) found that acceptance rates favored European Americans over African Americans. Moore, Feist-Price, and Alston (2002) found that persons with severe/profound mental retardation who were of European American descent were significantly more likely to achieve closure success (i.e., employment) when compared to African Americans. Finally, Olney and Kennedy (2002) found that European American VR recipients had the highest rates of competitive employment, whereas African American VR recipients were placed in noncompetitive employment more often than other racial/ethnic groups.

RACIALLY AND ETHNICALLY DIVERSE WOMEN WITH DISABILITIES

According to Bowe (1990), 8.4% or about one in every 12 "working age" woman reports a working disability. Further examination of the data indicates that as of 1990, one in three (34%) African American or Latina women with disabilities were severely disabled, compared to three in ten in 1981. In addition, more than two-thirds of African American women with disabilities (69%) are categorized as severely disabled versus 51% of White women. African American women with disabilities comprise 20.4% of the working age population of women with work disabilities; although African American women are only 12.4% of all women ages 16–64. This is due to the fact that 13.8% of all African American women have work-related disabilities, as opposed to 7.7% of White women.

Disparities were also apparent for racial/ethnic status with regard to employment. Those who identified themselves as African American or as other ethnic groups had an increased risk for unemployment (Randolph & Andresen, 2004). Table 9-2 shows the prevalence of work limitation by race/ethnicity and gender (LaPlante & Carlson, 1996). Black non-Latino and Black Latino women show the highest rates of limited employment and inability to work.

Barriers to Employment for Racially and Ethnically Diverse Women with Disabilities

Similar to racially and ethnically diverse women who are not disabled, racially and ethnically diverse women with disabilities encounter work-role stereotypes such as the belief that women should seek employment in traditionally female occupations—like nurse, secretary, or childcare worker (Hollingsworth & Mastroberti, 1983). In addition, women with and without disabilities may be dealing with issues of role conflict and career aspiration. African American women experience greater difficulty with multiple role conflict as a result of group-specific factors such as a higher number of offspring, greater likelihood of single parent status, and greater work-environment stress (Richie, 1992; Staples, 1985; Sue & Sue, 1990). Thus, it can be argued that these factors heighten role conflict for African American women with disabilities (Alston & McCowan, 1994). For example, more children to care for can create greater feelings of inadequacy as a mother. The single parent status would compound the stress associated with daily care needs of children because of the absence of a spouse to assist in these responsibilities.

Barriers in the workplace such as combating negative stereotypes regarding gender, ethnicity, and disability status may amplify role conflict for African American

Table 9-2 Employment Status of Women with Disabilities by Race/Ethnicity

Characteristic	Limited in Amount or Kind of Work	Unable to Work	Total with Work Limitation
American Indian	6.5%	9.7%	16.1%
Asian/Pacific Islander	2.3%	3.8%	6.1%
Black non-Latino	3.9%	10.5%	14.4%
Black Latino	3.4%	13.3%	16.4%
White non-Latino	5.3%	6.1%	11.4%
White Latino	3.2%	5.8%	9.0%
Other/Unknown	3.0%	6.8%	9.7%

Source: LaPlante, P., Miller, S., & Miller, K., 1992.

women with disabilities (Richie, 1992). African American women in the workplace are faced with the challenge of dealing with the stereotypes related to race as well as gender. African American women with disabilities in the workplace are faced with the challenge of dealing with the stereotypes associated with disability as well as those of gender and race.

The career aspirations of women with disabilities may be adversely affected by the influence of perceptions about their limitations. Lower career aspiration is of particular concern for African American women with disabilities. The negative messages African American women receive on the basis of race and gender appear to lower their career aspirations and limit their career choices (Richie, 1992). Most adult African American women are employed in traditionally female occupations and 40% are employed in service jobs (Reid, 1984).

A key influence of career aspiration for any demographic group is the presence of role models and mentors. For example, an African American woman with a disability who aspires to be an engineer may find it difficult to identify a role model. Thus, she may abandon or redirect her career goals. Similarly, if an African American woman with a disability secures employment as a computer analyst, she may experience frustration from being unable to establish a mentoring relationship with a colleague because of gender, ethnic, or disability dissimilarities. Consequently, she may feel isolated at the workplace and become unmotivated to continue her career goals (Alston & McCowan, 1994).

INTERVENTION STRATEGIES FOR RACIALLY AND ETHNICALLY DIVERSE WOMEN WITH DISABILITIES

Rehabilitation services designed to assist individuals with disabilities appear to be less accessible to women and racially/ethnically diverse groups, although they comprise a larger percentage of persons who are disabled (Capella, 2002; Moore et al., 2002; Olney & Kennedy, 2002; Wilson, 2002). Racially and ethnically diverse women with disabilities are most likely to suffer from such exclusionary practices. Racially and ethnically diverse women are often unaware of services they are eligible to receive, in part due to limited advertising and awareness. Rehabilitation agencies could increase the number of racially and ethnically diverse women with disabilities participants by developing outreach programs designed to access this population. For example, the African American church serves as a place of spiritual and emotional support as well as a source for gaining and sharing information. By having their professional staff members address church groups, the rehabilitation agencies could increase public awareness of programs, provide a forum in which African American women with disabilities could express their concerns and needs, and demonstrate that the agency has a commitment to serving African Americans with disabilities. Paraprofessionals, community workers, and former clients also serve to enhance outreach work done by rehabilitation professionals by providing a more empathetic understanding of the issues of racially and ethnically diverse women with disabilities with regard to employment.

The tenet of centrality of work is based on the Western, Protestant work ethic that is not shared by many other cultural groups. In addition, research by Gilligan (1982) on the moral development of women has suggested that women's morality and decision-making processes are heavily based on relationships and connectiveness with others. Thus, for many women, family takes precedence over career (Lips, 1992). In addition, for many individuals with disabilities, healthcare needs take priority and may result in disrupting career development when the individual is faced with the possibility of losing health insurance by going to work. In particular, persons with disabilities are concerned about the effects of welfare reform affecting benefits and the competence of "One Stop Career Centers" to serve their needs (Coker, Flynn, Menz, & McAlees, 1998). In addition, Medicaid can become a barrier to employment due to the potential loss of benefits if the wages earned by a person with a disability exceed those that qualify for Medicaid (Sheldon, 2005).

Some counseling models may be blind to the social realities and cultural values of nonmajority group members, as well as many-majority group members (Arbona, 1996; Gysbers, Heppner, & Johnston, 1998; Leong, 1996; Szymanski, Hershenson, Enright, & Ettinger, 1996). One major risk of adhering to the values and assumptions of some models is that career counseling may contribute to the "castification" of non-majority group members. The process of castification is defined as the relegating of individuals to a lesser status based on minority group membership (Szymanski & Trueba, 1994). Examples of this castification include focusing primarily on tradition-ally female careers with women or matching functional limitations with career options when working with individuals with disabilities. These "thinking only inside the box" models contribute to the process of counseling and job placement in traditional low-wage occupations. However, both models are based on a supply-side approach. The following discussion will focus on how supply-side and demand-side approaches can be integrated for an optimal rehabilitation approach.

Supply-Side and Demand-Side Approaches

Gilbride and Stensrud (1992) differentiated between *supply-side* and *demand-side* job development approaches. Supply-side approaches include all those services designed to support and assist the person with a disability in seeking and applying for employment (i.e., providing a *supply* of applicants to employers). Research has consistently found that a core set of placement services increases the employment outcomes of people with disabilities (Gilbride, Stensrud, & Johnson, 1994;

Vandergoot, 1987). Vandergoot found that training in job-seeking skills, job-finding clubs, and interviewing skills were the key services linked to successful placement.

Demand-side techniques are services provided to employers that make the workplace more user-friendly for people with disabilities and assist employers in meeting their needs by "pulling in" (i.e., creating a *demand* for) people with disabilities. Working with this model, rehabilitation professionals act as consultants to employers. They provide services to employers traditionally purchased from other consultants by larger employers and often unavailable to smaller employers (Gilbride & Stensrud, 2003).

Gilbride and Stensrud (1993) found that employers were willing to hire people with disabilities, but were unable to recruit them. Stensrud (1999) found that employers did not know how to tap the public and private agencies that served people with disabilities. Second, many employers were uncertain about how to conduct the job selection process, and especially uncertain of their requirements under the Americans with Disabilities Act (ADA). Third, employers wanted a degree of comfort that there would be post-employment problem-solving assistance if they hired a person with a disability and confronted disability-related dilemmas. Therefore, demand-side techniques requested by employers include recruiting assistance, comfort enhancement, early employment assistance, and long-term employment assistance (Gilbride & Stensrud, 2003). To address these issues, the essential functions of a demand-side specialist include: developing consulting relationships with employers, providing consulting services to employers, providing labor market consulting services to rehabilitation counselors and agencies, and using Internet technology to enhance employment solutions. Figure 9-3 illustrates how the incorporation of both

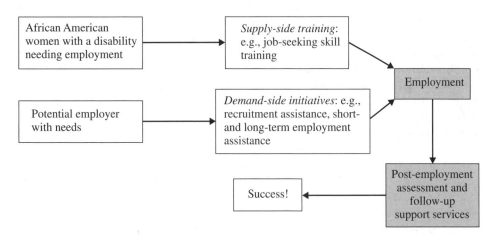

Figure 9-3 Supply-side and demand-side approaches to employment success

approaches can enhance success in employment for racially and ethnically diverse women with disabilities.

Supply-Side Strategies

According to Gilbride and Stensrud (2003), the components of supply-side strategies include job-seeking skills training, job clubs, and supportive services. When working with racially and ethnically diverse women with disabilities, some special considerations need to be made, especially with regard to support services.

For example, Wright and Leung (1993) made several recommendations for rehabilitation professionals working with racially and ethnically diverse individuals with disabilities that can also be easily applied to racially and ethnically diverse women with disabilities. A national network of employers and racially and ethnically diverse groups of persons with disabilities should be established to enable the sharing of job leads, to reduce feelings of isolation, and to provide a forum for proactively discussing employment issues. Finally, the RSA should use its existing networks to develop a national outreach program targeting racially and ethnically diverse populations in order to increase their employment levels (Wright & Leung). Rehabilitation professionals should also conduct more appropriate matching of college, adult education, and/or vocational training programs with careers in demand or careers with future demand in order to expand employment opportunities for women with disabilities.

The influence of social ties and support has been crucial for African American women (Boyd-Franklin, 1991). A support network comprised of immediate and extended family members, friends, neighbors, and fellow church members has motivated African American women and served as a coping mechanism to counter the effects of oppression. Rehabilitation professionals must be willing to expand their traditional definition of support networks in helping African American women with disabilities utilize, reclaim, or develop new support systems. For example, development of role model and mentor programs can be especially useful for racially and ethnically diverse women with disabilities (Rubin & Roessler, 1983). Initiating such programs would require rehabilitation professionals to have a readily available network of persons to serve as mentors. Former female VR consumers from racially/ethnically diverse groups could be recruited to serve as mentors and to provide job search guidance, survival tips for the workplace, and/or strategies for managing multiple roles (Alston & McCowan, 1994). Additional networking and mentoring could be provided through chat rooms on the Internet or personal sources such as MySpace or Facebook. This approach may not work for all clients as persons with low income may have limited or no access to computers.

Demand-Side Strategies

Gilbride and Stensrud (2003) also listed several steps for demand-side services including recruitment assistance, comfort enhancement, and short- and long-term employment assistance.

With regard to recruitment assistance, there should be a collaborative effort of employment programs, public education, private enterprise, and health and human services programs to enable racially and ethnically diverse women with disabilities to access employment. A national advisory body could be established with the support of the Department of Labor to address concerns related to apprenticeships, supported employment, and job restructuring to enhance access of racially and ethnically diverse persons with disabilities into labor unions.

In addressing comfort enhancement, it is important to note that there may be employers who see cultural background as being superficial or irrelevant to the rehabilitation process. One reason is that most professionals have gone through their careers without having a word mentioned about "cultural diversity." It is not necessary for employers to know everything about all cultures, but there should be development of some understanding about major values and belief systems of the people served. Rehabilitation professionals can provide education in these areas.

In addition, rehabilitation professionals have a great deal of expertise that can be used to help employers hire and accommodate employees with disabilities such as conducting job analyses to help determine essential functions, providing assistance in identifying and instituting reasonable accommodations, conducting ergonomic evaluations of work areas, and other services such as provision of assistive technology that make it easier for employers to hire, supervise, and benefit from employees with disabilities. The strength of this approach is that it is custom-made to the needs of the employees and the employers. The weaknesses are that rehabilitation professionals may need additional training in order to provide these services, as well as collaboration and referral to other professionals. Additional research as to the benefit of these approaches is necessary.

Early Employment Assistance

This type of assistance pertains to the first 90 days a person is on the job. During that time, employers look for specific work behaviors to determine whether an employee will be retained. Also, during this phase, employers expect rehabilitation personnel to be available to help resolve any problems. If they do not feel rehabilitation professionals are responsive to their needs, they will not trust their recommendations in the future (Gilbride & Stensrud, 2003). This could be especially true when dealing with women, racially and ethnically diverse populations, and persons with disabilities as many employers may be hesitant to hire employees with different needs than traditional employees. During the initial phase, the rehabilitation professional can provide key support for employers who may be hiring diverse employees for the first time.

Long-term Employment Assistance

Employers continue to expect assistance if any problems arise. During this phase, which may last for many years, employers look for employees who have appropriate job skills, good communication with coworkers and supervisors, and an apparent willingness to advance in their position. Employers expect that rehabilitation personnel should do the same for them. If counselors or contracted placement personnel do not provide long-term follow-up and problem resolution assistance, employers will not rely on them in the future as placement resources (Gilbride & Stensrud, 2003). When providing postemployment services, a case in the public VR system can be closed as Status 35 (consumer working independently and additional support is not required) or Status 37 (support is not helping consumer maintain employment). However, employers should be informed that the case may be reopened in order to protect the person from losing his/her job. Postemployment services, similar to preemployment services, are planned and mutually agreed upon between the rehabilitation consumer and his/her counselor. When postemployment goals are met, the counselor can close the case. Some specific examples would include retraining of the employee and provision of adaptive equipment or assistive technology. It must be explained to employers that the discontinuation of postemployment services does not mean that the counselor has severed his ties with the employer or rehabilitation client/customer. As stated, the case can be reopened and support services and/or intervention services could be reactivated to achieve employment stability again at any time in the future. This would reassure employers of the benefit of having a long-term relationship with the VR office.

Rehabilitation Education Issues

To be or become an effective counselor, an individual needs awareness and understanding of the complexities of the multicultural society in which we live (Brodwin, 1995). A major shortcoming of many rehabilitation counseling education programs is the lack of sufficient multicultural emphasis. Graduate programs need to provide cultural awareness and sensitivity with regard to a variety of underrepresented racial groups, as well as less recognized underrepresented groups, such as women, the elderly, persons with AIDS, and others. Each of these groups has culturally distinct characteristics, and is part of the larger culture. The trained rehabilitation counselor who is competent to work with culturally diverse populations becomes more clinically effective, culturally aware, and sensitive to a variety of specialized and individual needs, issues, and concerns (Brodwin). Existing counselors should seek out continuing education opportunities to increase their skills in working with and placing racially and culturally diverse populations of persons with disabilities.

IMPLICATIONS FOR FUTURE RESEARCH

Unfortunately, research on racially and ethnically diverse groups with disabilities has not been a priority in the national disability research agenda. The research that has been conducted in this area has often been problematic because of the way it has been managed and because the results have not always directly affected racially and ethnically diverse persons with disabilities and their communities (Wright & Leung, 1993). The identification of problems that racially and ethnically diverse persons with disabilities encounter is most advanced with respect to African Americans, Latinos, and Native Americans. Because of their relatively small numbers, there is little data on Asian Americans. Much of the research that has been conducted on minorities with disabilities has concerned mental disabilities (Brown, Stein, Huang, & Harris, 1973; Kitano, 1969; Sue & McKinney, 1975). There has been relatively little research related to physical and sensory disabilities among racially and ethnically diverse populations.

One of the key findings of the ADA Watch (a public hearing held in 1992) was that there is a lack of demographic data about people of various racial, ethnic, and cultural minorities with disabilities and their families (Wright & Leung, 1993). Research on the demographics of disability among various cultural/ethnic/racial minority groups would help facilitate the ability of government and local agencies to develop policy and to implement appropriate interventions.

VR training needs to include an emphasis on multicultural and clinical training experiences involving persons with disabilities from racially and ethnically diverse populations (Wright & Leung, 1993). Education programs should include specific courses related to multicultural experiences and service delivery. Incentives should be provided for recruitment and education of underrepresented racial/ethnic populations in vocational rehabilitation. Finally, there is a need for increased numbers of tribal-operated VR programs to meet the growing needs of Native Americans and Alaska Natives.

IMPLICATIONS FOR CAREER COUNSELING

Since a person's gender, race/ethnicity, disability status, and socioeconomic class can have significant social and psychological implications, rehabilitation counselors must consider the interconnected nature of these statuses for determining the vocational and career opportunities of minority women with disabilities (Amott & Matthaei, 1991). Many factors can influence how women with disabilities view themselves and their place in the world of work. Szymanski and Parker (2003) noted that complex experiences such as abuse, battery, rape, depression, fear, exploitation, eating disorders, childcare concerns, relationship problems, social isolation, and financial difficulties are commonplace realities in the lives of many women and may contribute to feelings of devaluation, particularly for minority women with disabilities. When a woman feels devalued by society, low self-esteem and minimal expectations for success are likely to characterize her career outlook (Gysbers et al., 1998; Szymanski & Parker), and as we learned earlier in this chapter, having a disability and being a minority often only exacerbates the negative effect of the problems.

Most models of career counseling are not applicable to ethnic minorities, women, or individuals with disabilities (Arbona, 1996; Gysbers et al., 1998; Leong, 1996). Thus, rehabilitation counselors working with minority women with disabilities have very few approaches at their disposal to offer career guidance to this population. As Gysbers et al. noted, the traditional theories of career counseling are based on the following tenets from White culture and do not hold true for persons from diverse communities: "(1) individualism and autonomy, (2) affluence, (3) structure and opportunity open to all, (4) the centrality of work, and (5) the linearity, progressiveness, and rationality of the career development process" (pp. 33–34). These tenets do not reflect the values of many minority cultures or the real experiences of persons such as minority women with disabilities who have been denied access to vocational opportunities due to systemic biases (Szymanski & Parker, 2003).

In terms of specific implications for vocational counseling and career guidance for minority women who have disabilities, rehabilitation counselors must guard against castification. Castification—similar to stereotyping—can occur in career counseling when persons from minority groups (e.g., African Americans, persons with disabilities) are relegated to a lesser status simply because of their racial or disability status, and prescriptions for vocational direction and career choice are written based primarily on group membership (Szymanski & Trueba, 1994). There is no simple application of traditional theories and models such as Super (1957) or Lofquist and Dawis (1969) to help the counselor avoid castification when the recipient of the efforts is a woman, racial/ethnic minority, and/or person with a disability. The heterogeneous nature of career needs and challenges presented by a minority woman with a disability requires the use of a broad and flexible framework or approach such as the model called INCOME: Imagining, iNforming, Choosing, Obtaining, Maintaining, and Exiting (Beveridge, Heller-Craddock, Liesener, Stapleton, & Hershenson, 2002; Szymanski & Parker, 2003). Table 9-3 provides concise definitions for the six statuses of INCOME and some applicable interventions for the model (Szymanski & Parker).

Table 9-3 Status Definitions and Interventions

Status	Potential Intervention/Aids
Imagining: Develops awareness of occupations, work, and jobs and the vast array of careers available. Expands artificial boundaries related to culture and work.	Family counseling, peer mentoring, and career awareness training
iNforming: Integration of self-identity, world of work, vocational opportunities, and cultural context.	Informational interviews, tests and assessments, computer career guidance systems (e.g., SIGI), and job shadowing
Choosing: Individual selects an occupation based on information gained from previous statuses, along with feeling of self-efficacy, outcome expectations, and job benefits (e.g., income, health care coverage).	Informed decision-making models and transferable skills analysis
Obtaining: Implementation of career decision and finding employment in chosen occupation.	Job search and placement models, labor market analysis, networking, and job fairs
Maintaining: Sustaining a career by adapting and adjusting to the demands of work and the work environment.	Performance reviews, continuing education, and career counseling follow-up interviews
Exiting: Leaving current vocational situation due to promotion, termination, or voluntary departure. The individual is in a state of transition.	Personal growth counseling, loss and grief counseling, or new career exploration

For a deeper understanding of its potential applications, the reader is encouraged to read Beveridge et al.'s (2002) original conceptualization of INCOME and to study Szymanski and Parker's review of the model in their text on work and disability.

The flexibility of the six statuses contained in INCOME allows the counselor to accommodate the cultural uniqueness of a minority woman with a disability and to tailor counseling to the career maturity and readiness of the individual. INCOME is being proposed in this chapter as one of the best conceptual frameworks for rehabilitation counselors to follow when tracking and facilitating the career development of minority women with disabilities.

CONCLUSION

In order to understand the unique issues of minority women with disabilities, one must consider how the issues of gender, race/ethnicity and disability intersect with regard to employment. Separately and collectively, women, persons with disabilities and persons of color have been discriminated against in the process of applying for jobs, compensation, promotion and/or job retention. This chapter has focused on the unique issues that make up the triple quandary of what is experienced by racially and ethnically diverse women with disabilities who seek employment opportunities and the unique challenges faced by the rehabilitation professional whose job it is to assist these consumers. Increased sensitivity and understanding is required of both the employer and the rehabilitation professional in order to appropriately place and assist these individuals to be successful in their chosen careers. Supply-side and demand-side approaches utilized by rehabilitation professionals can be customized to meet both the employer and potential employee's needs and achieve successful closure of the case. VR counselors offering direct assistance to employers could help protect jobs that would otherwise be lost due to misunderstandings or lack of knowledge about reasonable accommodations and effective ways to support the needs of women with disabilities in the workforce.

REFERENCES

Alston, R. J., & McCowan, C. J. (1994). African American women with disabilities: Rehabilitation issues and concerns. *Journal of Rehabilitation, 60*, 36–40.

Arbona, C. (1996). Career theory and practice in a multicultural context. In M. L. Savikas & W. B. Walsh (Eds.), *Handbook of career counseling theory and practice* (pp. 45–54). Palo Alto, CA: Davies-Black.

Amott, T., & Matthaei, J. (1991). *Race, gender, and work: A multicultural economic history of women in the United States*. Boston: South End.

Baldwin, M., Johnson, W. G., & Watson, S. (1993). *A double burden of discrimination: Women with disabilities*. Washington, DC: Center for the Study of Social Policy.

Beveridge, S., Heller-Craddock, S., Liesener, J., Stapleton, M., & Hershenson, D. (2002). INCOME: A framework for conceptualizing the career development of persons with disabilities. *Rehabilitation Counseling Bulletin, 45,* 195–206.

Blumrosen, A. W., & Blumrosen, R. G. (2002). *The reality of intentional job discrimination in metropolitan America—1999.* Retrieved March 12, 2007, from *http://www.eeo1.com*

Bowe, F. (1990). *Adults with disabilities: A portrait.* Washington, DC: President's Committee on Employment of People with Disabilities.

Bowe, F. (1992). *Adults with disabilities: A portrait.* Washington, DC: President's Committee on Employment of People with Disabilities.

Boyd-Franklin, N. (1991). Recurrent themes in the treatment of African American women in group psychotherapy. *Women and Therapy, 11,* 25–39.

Braddock, D., & Bacheler, L. (1994). *The glass ceiling and persons with disabilities.* Public Policy Monograph Series, No. 56. Chicago: The University of Illinois at Chicago, Institute on Disability and Human Development.

Brodwin, M. G. (1995). Barriers to multicultural understanding: Improving university rehabilitation counselor education programs. In S. Walker, K. A. Turner, I. Halle-Michael, A. Vincent, & M. D. Miles (Eds.), *Disability and diversity: New leadership for a new era* (pp. 39–44). Washington, DC: President's Committee on Employment of People with Disabilities.

Brown, R. R., Stein, K. M., Huang, K., & Harris, D. E. (1973). Mental illness and the role of mental health facilities in Chinatown. In S. Sue & N. Wagner (Eds.), *Asian Americans: Psychological perspectives* (pp. 212–231). Palo Alto, CA: Science and Behavior Books.

Burke, R. J. (1999). Disability and women's work experiences: An exploratory study. *International Journal of Sociology and Social Policy, 19,* 21–33.

Burkhauser, R. V., Haveman, R. H., & Wolfe, B . L. (1990). *The changing economic condition of the disabled: A two decade review of economic well-being.* Washington, DC: National Council on Disability.

Caiazza, A., Shaw, A. & Werschkul, M. (2004). *Women's economic status in the states: Wide disparities by race, ethnicity, and region.* Washington, DC: Institute for Women's Policy Research.

Capella, M. E. (2002). Inequities in the VR system: Do they still exist? *Rehabilitation Counseling Bulletin, 45,* 143–153.

Coker, C. C., Flynn, M., Menz, F. E., & McAlees, D. C. (1998). *Workforce development and welfare reform: Potential impact upon persons with disabilities and community rehabilitation programs.* Menomonie: University of Wisconsin-Stout, Rehabilitation Research and Training Center on Community Rehabilitation Programs.

Foo, L. J. (2003). *Asian American women: Issues, concerns, and responsive human and civil rights advocacy.* New York: Ford Foundation.

Fortune (2008, May 5). Fortune 500: WalMart's No 1. *157*(9). New York: Author.

Foucault, M. (1986). *The history of sexuality: The care of the self* (3rd ed.). New York: Vintage Books.

Frosh, S., Phoenix, A., & Pattman, R. (2000). Cultural contestations in practice: White boys and racialization of masculinities. In C. Squire (Ed.), *Culture in psychology* (pp. 47–58). Philadelphia: Routledge.

Fullerton, H. N., & Tossi, M. (2001). Labor force projections to 2010: Steady growth and changing composition. *Monthly Labor Review Online, 124.* Retrieved May 13, 2007, from *http://www.bls.gov/opub/mlr/2001/11/art2exch.htm*

Gans, H. (1979). Symbolic ethnicity: The future of ethnic groups and cultures in America. *Ethnic and Racial Studies, 12,* 1–20.

Gilbride, D., & Stensrud, R. (1992). Demand-side job development: A model for the 1990s. *Journal of Rehabilitation, 58,* 34–39.

Gilbride, D., & Stensrud, R. (1993). Challenges and opportunities for rehabilitation counselors in the Americans with Disabilities Act era. *NARPPS Journal, 8,* 67–74.

Gilbride, D., & Stensrud, R. (2003). Job placement and employer consulting: Services and strategies. In E. M. Szymanski & R. M. Parker (Eds.), *Work and disability: Issues and strategies in career development and job placement* (2nd ed., pp. 407–439). Austin, TX: PRO-ED.

Gilbride, D., Stensrud, R., & Johnson, M. (1994). Current models of job placement and employer development: Research, competencies, and educational considerations. *Rehabilitation Education, 7,* 215–239.

Gilligan, C. (1982). *In a different voice.* Cambridge, MA: Harvard University Press.

Gysbers, N. C., Heppner, M. J., & Johnston, J. A. (1998). *Career counseling: Process, issues and techniques.* Boston: Allyn & Bacon.

Habermas, J. (1984). *The theory of communicative action: Reason and the rationalization of society* (Vol. 1). Boston: Beacon.

Habermas, J. (1987). *The theory of communicative action: Vol. 2 Lifeworld and systems: A critique of functionalist reason.* Boston: Beacon.

Hamlin, N. R., Erkut, S., & Fields, J. P. (1994). *The impact of corporate restructuring and downsizing on the managerial careers of minorities and women: Lessons learned from nine corporations.* Washington, DC: U.S. Department of Labor, Glass Ceiling Commission.

Hollingsworth, D. K., & Mastroberti, C. J. (1983). Women, work & disability. *The Personnel and Guidance Journal, 61,* 587–591.

Institute for Women's Policy Research. (1995). *Research in brief: Restructuring work: How have women and minority managers fared?* Washington, DC: Institute for Women's Policy Research.

Jans, L., & Stoddard, S. (1999). *Chartbook on women and disability in the United States.* An InfoUse Report. Washington, DC: U.S. Department of Education, National Institute on Disability and Rehabilitation Research. Retrieved March 12, 2007, from *http://www.infouse.com/disabilitydata*

Johnson, W. G., & Lambrinos, J. (1985). Wage discrimination against handicapped men and women. *Journal of Human Resources, 20,* 264–277.

Kitano, H. H. L. (1969). *Japanese-Americans: The evaluation of a subculture.* Englewood Cliffs, NJ: Prentice-Hall.

Lakoff, G., & Johnson, M. (1980). *Metaphors we live by.* Chicago: University of Chicago Press.

LaPlante, M. P., & Carlson, D. (1996). *Disability in the United States: Prevalence and causes, 1992.* San Francisco: University of California-San Francisco, Disability Statistics Rehabilitation Research and Training Center.

LaPlante, P., Miller, S., & Miller, K. (1992). *People with work disability in the U.S.* San Francisco: University of California, Disability Statistics Program, Institute for Health & Aging.

Leong, F. T. L. (1996). Challenges to career counseling: Boundaries, cultures, and complexity. In M. L. Savikas & W. B. Walsh (Eds.), *Handbook of career counseling theory and practice* (pp. 333–346). Palo Alto, CA: Davies-Black.

Lips, H. M. (1992). Gender and science-related attitudes as predictors of college students academic choices. *Journal of Vocational Behavior, 40*, 62–81.

Lofquist, L. H., & Dawis, R. V. (1969). *Adjustment to work: A psychological view of man's problems in a work oriented society.* East Norwalk, CT: Appleton-Century-Crofts.

Miles, R. (1989). *Racism.* Philadelphia: Routledge.

Moore, C. L., Feist-Price, S., & Alston, R. J. (2002). VR services for persons with severe/profound mental retardation: Does race matter? *Rehabilitation Counseling Bulletin, 45*, 162–167.

Morris, J. (1991). *Pride against prejudice.* London: Women's Press.

Mpofu, E., & Conyers, L. M. (2004). A representational theory perspective of minority status and people with disabilities: Implications for rehabilitation education and practice. *Rehabilitation Counseling Bulletin, 47*, 142–151.

National Counsel on Disability. (1989). *The education of students with disabilities: Where do we stand?* Washington, DC: Author.

National Council on Disability. (1993). *Serving the nation's students with disabilities: Progress and prospects.* Washington, DC: Author.

Olney, M. F., & Kennedy, J. (2002). Racial disparities in VR use and job placement rates for adults with disabilities. *Rehabilitation Counseling Bulletin, 45*, 177–185.

Randolph, D. S. (2004). Predicting the effect of disability on employment status and income. *Work: A Journal of Prevention, Assessment and Rehabilitation, 23*, 257–266.

Randolph, D. S., & Andresen, E. M. (2004). Disability, gender and unemployment relationships in the United States from the behavioral risk factor surveillance system. *Disability & Society, 19*, 403–413.

Reid, P. T. (1984). Feminism versus minority group identity: Not for Black women only. *Sex Roles, 10*, 247–255.

Richie, B. S. (1992). Coping with work: Interventions with African-American women. *Women and Therapy, 12*, 97–111.

Rubin, S. E., & Roessler, R. T. (1983). *Foundations of the vocational rehabilitation process.* Austin, TX: Pro-Ed.

Russo, N. F., & Jansen, M. A. (1988). Women, work, and disability: Opportunities and challenges. In M. Fine & A. Asch (Eds.), *Women with disabilities: Essays in psychology, culture, and politics* (pp. 229–244). Philadelphia: Temple University Press.

Sheldon, J. R. (2005). *Policy and practice brief: Medicaid and persons with disabilities; A focus on eligibility, covered services and program structure.* Retrieved May 15, 2007, from *http://digitalcommons.ilr .cornell.edu/edicollect/60*

Smith, D. L. (2007a). The employment status of women with disabilities from the behavioral risk factor surveillance system. *Work: A Journal of Prevention, Assessment and Rehabilitation, 28*, 1–9.

Smith, D. L. (2007b). The relationship of type of disability and employment status from the behavioral risk factor surveillance survey. *Journal of Rehabilitation, 73*, 32–40.

Solomon, B. (1995). *In the company of educated women.* New Haven, CT: Yale University Press.

Staples, R. (1985). Changes in Black family structure: The conflict between family ideology and structural conditions. *Journal of Marriage and the Family, 47*, 1005–1013.

Steinmetz, E. (2006). *Americans with disabilities: 2002, Current Population Reports, P70–107*. Washington, DC: U.S. Census Bureau.

Stensrud, R. (1999). *Reasons for success and failure of supported employment placements*. Retrieved May 13, 2007, from *http://soe.drake.edu/nri/evaluation/barrierreport2.html*

Stuart, O. W. (1992). Race and disability: Just double oppression? *Disability, Handicap & Society, 7*, 177–188.

Sue, S., & McKinney, H. (1975). Asian-Americans in the community mental health care system. *American Journal of Orthopsychiatry, 45*, 111–118.

Sue, D. W., & Sue, D. (1990). *Counseling the culturally different: Theory and practice* (2nd ed.). New York: Wiley.

Super, D. E. (1957). *The psychology of careers: An introduction to vocational development*. New York: Harper & Bros.

Szymanski, E. M., Hershenson, D. B., Enright, M. S., & Ettinger, J. M. (1996). Career development theories, constructs and research: Implications for people with disabilities. In E. M. Szymanski & R. M. Parker (Eds.), *Work and disability: Issues and strategies in career development and job placement* (pp. 79–126). Austin, TX: PRO-ED.

Szymanski, E. M., & Parker, R. M. (2003). *Work and disability: Issues and strategies in career development and job placement*. Austin, TX: ProEd.

Szymanski, E. M., & Trueba, H. (1994). Castification of people with disabilities: Potential disempowering aspects of castification in disability services. *Journal of Rehabilitation, 60*, 12–20.

Thomas-Breitfeld, S. (2003). *The Latino workforce*. Washington, DC: National Council of La Raza.

Trejo, S. J. (1997). Why do Mexican Americans earn low wages? *Journal of Political Economy, 105*, 1235–1268.

Urban Institute. (2004). Unpublished calculations for the Institute for Women's Policy Research based on the 2002 and 2003 Current Population Survey March Demographic Supplements for calendar years 2001 and 2002.

U.S. Census Bureau. (2002). *Statistical abstract of the United States*. Washington, DC: Author.

U.S. Census Bureau. (2005). *2005 American Community Survey*. Retrieved March 8, 2007, from *http://factfinder.census.gov*

U.S. Department of Labor, Bureau of Labor Statistics. (2001). Table 3: Employment Status of civilian noninstitutionalized population by age, sex and race, 2000. *Employment and Earnings, 48*, 160.

U.S. Equal Employment Opportunity Commission. (2000). *Occupational employment in private industry by race/ethnic group/sex, and by industry, United States, 2000*. Washington, DC: Author.

U.S. General Accounting Office. (1993, August). *Vocational rehabilitation: Evidence for federal program's effectiveness is mixed*. Washington, DC: Author.

Vandergoot, D. (1987). Review of placement research literature: Implications for research and practice. *Rehabilitation Counseling Bulletin, 31*, 243–272.

Vernon, A. (1996a). A stranger in many camps: The experience of disabled Black and ethnic minority women. In J. Morris (Ed.). *Pride against prejudice* (pp. 47–68). London: Women's Press.

Vernon, A. (1996b). Fighting two different battles: Unity is preferable to enmity. *Disability & Society, 11*, 285–290.

Vernon, A. (1996c). Deafness disability and simultaneous oppression, a conference paper to the PSI and ADSUP conference, *Deaf and disabled people: Towards a new understanding*, December 1996.

Vernon, A. (1999). The dialectics of multiple identities and the disabled people's movement. *Disability & Society, 14*, 385–398.

Vinje, C. L. (1996). Native American economic development on selected reservations: A comparative analysis. *American Journal of Economics and Sociology, 55*, 427–442.

Waters, M. (1996). Optional ethnicities: For Whites only? In S. Pedraza & R. Rumbault (Eds.), *Origins and destinies: Immigration, race and ethnicity in America* (pp. 145–167). Belmont, CA: Wadsworth.

Wilson, C. (1996). *Racism: From slavery to advanced capitalism.* Thousand Oaks, CA: Sage.

Wilson, K. B. (2002). Exploration of VR acceptance and ethnicity: A national investigation. *Rehabilitation Counseling Bulletin, 45*, 168–176.

Wilson, K. B., Alston, R. J., Harley, D. A., & Mitchell, N. A. (2002). Predicting VR acceptance based on race, gender, education, work status at application, and primary source of support at application. *Rehabilitation Counseling Bulletin, 45*, 132–142.

Wirth, L. (1945). The problem of minority groups. In R. Linton (Ed.), *The science of man (woman) in the world crisis* (pp. 347–372). New York: Columbia University Press.

Wright, T. J. (1988). Enhancing the professional preparation of rehabilitation counselors for improved service to ethnic minorities with disabilities. *Journal of Applied Counseling, 19*, 4–10.

Wright, T. J., & Leung, P. (1993). *Meeting the unique needs of minorities with disabilities: A report to the President and Congress.* Washington, DC: National Council on Disability.

CHAPTER 10

Cross-Cultural Issues for Asian Pacific Americans with Disabilities in the Vocational Rehabilitation System

Rooshey Hasnain, EdD;
Paul Leung, PhD

INTRODUCTION

Asian Pacific Americans (APAs), or more inclusively "Asians and Native Hawaiians/Pacific Islanders," are growing in both numbers and diversity. Thus, they are posing new challenges for the state and federal vocational rehabilitation (VR) system. In particular, those who have disabilities remain severely underserved and difficult for VR providers to reach.

Although APAs are America's fastest growing ethnic group and comprise 5% of the U.S. population (U.S. Census Bureau, 2007), service providers in rehabilitation tend to pay little attention to them. Notwithstanding occasional attention in the vocational rehabilitation literature (Hampton, 2000; Chan, Lam, Wong, Leung, & Fung, 1988; Leung, 1993; Leung, 1996), the intersection between disability and citizens of APA descent remains largely unexplored (Kim-Rupnow, Park, & Starbuck, 2005).

Given the rapid growth and lack of information on APAs, this chapter has four primary objectives: (1) to define APAs and highlight the complexity of this racial and geographically diverse category; (2) to review research that has identified disparities in service access and outcomes for APAs; (3) to identify limitations of prior research on and services for APAs; and (4) to present implications for future research and practice.

ASIAN PACIFIC AMERICANS ARE A DIVERSE AND COMPLEX GROUP

According to the United States Census Bureau (2007), the APA population in the United States is projected to grow proportionately more than any other American minority group, from about 12.1 million (5% of the U.S. population) in 2004, to more than 41 million (11% of the U.S. population) by 2050. Of the 12.1 million APAs in the United States today, about 13% have some type of disability (Park, Kim-Rupnow, Stodden, & Starbuck, 2005; U.S. Census Bureau, 2002). But the APA population is very complex and different in multiple dimensions. The following are some of the main reasons for the diversity of the APA population.

Diversity in Terms of Country of Origin

Perhaps more than any other ethnic category APAs are particularly diverse and complex, differing both between groups and within the larger group due to a number of factors including language, socioeconomic class, immigration status, length of time in the United States, acculturation, and cultural ties to their homelands. In fact, the APA census category itself was created as an artificial device via Executive Order (Wright, 1994) and used in the 1990 census to include Asian Americans "having origins in any of the original peoples of the Far East, Southeast Asia, or the Indian subcontinent including, for example, Cambodia, China, India, Japan, Korea, Malaysia, Pakistan, the Philippine Islands, Sri Lanka, Thailand, and Vietnam" (U.S. Census, 2002, p.1). Importantly, these countries also represent about 60% of the world's population (U.S. Census Bureau, 2008, December) encompassing large cultural and linguistic group differences.

Overall, APAs may include more than 50 disparate ethnic groups and over 100 language and dialect groups (President's Advisory Commission on Asian Americans and Pacific Islanders, 2001). It should be noted that these groups have little in common in terms of history, culture, language, religion, or governance. In addition, relationships between some of these countries have been characterized more by conflict than by cooperation. Despite these differences however, in the United States the APA category has been more or less accepted by persons of Asian or Pacific origin primarily because it provides the numbers they need to gain more political influence.

The category Asian does not refer to a homogeneous group. While each ethnic group may have some similarities that are descriptive in a general way, each group also has significant differences that must be considered. The combination of Native Hawaiians and Pacific Islanders in this demographic group may also cause misunderstanding and confusion, given that these two groups are not that similar to the other Asian groups in many ways (Palafox, Buenconsejo-Lum, Riklon, & Waitzfelder, 2002). These two groups—Native Hawaiians and Pacific Islanders—are included in this chapter because until the 2000 U.S. Census, they were categorized with Asian Americans.

Diversity in Terms of Migration Experiences

Further adding to the diversity of the APA population are other variables or precursors that affect behavior and outcomes, including the individuals' or families' initial experiences of migration to the United States, generational issues, degree of acculturation, geographic location, identity, language, educational level, and living arrangements (enclaves such as Chinatowns as well as the increasing number of suburban enclaves; Chung, 1995). Historically, APAs have arrived in diverse immigration streams that include highly skilled and affluent immigrants, as well as unskilled refugees with limited or no savings, limited English proficiency, and few job skills. These diverse streams create wide socioeconomic variations (Zhan, 2003). Additionally, APA immigrants and refugees have come to the United States in different time periods and for vastly different reasons: some need to escape religious and ethnic oppression, war, and poverty, while others seek political asylum and still others pursue educational and economic opportunities. Those who come as refugees are likely to be quite different from those who come as immigrants to seek specific educational and/or professional opportunities. These many variables may also determine how comfortable individuals of APA origin are with the majority population and the use of governmental services and whether or not they know what services are available to them.

Diversity in Terms of Ethnic Identification

Of all the ethnic populations in the United States, APAs most often check off as "other" in reporting ethnicity since they may refer to their ethnicity rather than their race (i.e., one may think of her/himself as Vietnamese rather than Asian). This approach to data gathering, along with self-report forms that are sometimes difficult to understand, leads to inaccurate projections of what APAs with disabilities may or may not need; as a result, insufficient funds and resources have been allocated since this group is often not counted in population reports. Finally, growing numbers of APAs are of mixed race or ethnicity (U.S. Census Bureau, 2007), adding to the uncertainty about the needs and assets of the diverse ethnic groups that are clustered together in this category.

ASIAN PACIFIC AMERICANS LACK ACCESS TO VR AND OTHER SERVICES

Despite their growing numbers, APAs remain relatively invisible in the VR system. Many APAs seeking VR services encounter a confusing and fragmented system known for its lengthy application process and complex eligibility-determination procedures. APAs who do access the system quickly discover that services are limited, that agencies have long waiting lists, or that some publicized services are not even available (Hart, Zimbrich, & Whelley, 2002). These barriers result from a variety of bureaucratic and financial factors that include: (a) inconsistent organizational procedures and services across agencies; (b) excessive paperwork and incomprehensible jargon primarily in English; (c) differing application procedures for eligibility or entry portals; and (d) limited enrollment for programs due to varying fiscal cycles and service capacity constraints (Hasnain, 2001). A lack of centralized service delivery further widens the access gaps for this group of APAs with disabilities. As a result, APAs are underrepresented in the public VR programs in 48 of the 50 states, (Kim-Rupnow, Park, & Starbuck, 2005), making it urgent to improve service access.

Researchers have found that racial and ethnic minorities, especially APAs with disabilities, are less likely than their White peers to apply or gain access to the VR service system (Dziekan & Okocha, 1993; Kim-Rupnow et al., 2005; Wilson, Alston, Harley, & Mitchell, 2002) and they receive VR services at lower rates (Kim-Rupnow et al.). In addition, many APAs are less likely to be eligible for state or federal VR services due to relatively high income levels (Wilson et al.), and/or to receive relevant information about rehabilitation and related services such as personal care attendants, postsecondary education, or vocational training options (Zhan, 2003). Finally, even when APA individuals are accepted into the system, their services are often terminated prematurely (Hampton, 2003; Kim-Rupnow et al.) due to linguistic and/or cultural barriers or institutional bias. In the case of recent immigrants, many VR offices lack access to translators for many of the Asian languages and dialects spoken in the countries of origin.

Given these experiences, APAs with disabilities are less likely to gain access to supported employment and independent living services compared with their White counterparts (Kim-Rupnow et al., 2005). In fact, Hampton (2003) indicated that in the 1990 annual report of the Rehabilitation Services Administration (RSA), APAs constituted only 1% of total clients served by state independent living centers and 1.3% of clients in rehabilitation assistance programs. These rates remain similarly low today. In addition, for APAs, the Americans with Disabilities Act (ADA) may be a greater cultural hurdle than for other groups (Leung, 1993) because of their cultural reluctance to draw attention to personal vulnerabilities. Finally, APAs, like some other multicultural groups, have yet to receive culturally and linguistically tailored VR services and supports within their communities in an equitable and accessible manner.

If the APA population grows as projected, it will likely continue facing access barriers to needed services (Wilson et al., 2002). Recent changes in federal policy have prompted efforts to reduce barriers to accessing the VR system by focusing more on culturally diverse populations. Section 21 of the Rehabilitation Act Amendments of 1992 requires increased participation of ethnic minority individuals with disabilities in VR programs and independent living centers, yet 16 years after the passing of Section 21, the participation of APAs in the VR system has not improved. Moreover, this finding extends beyond the VR system. For example, the U.S. Surgeon General's report on mental health conducted by the U.S. Department of Health and Human Services (2001) cited three comprehensive studies on the use of mental health services by APAs, all finding that this group used fewer services per capita compared to other ethnic groups. The report also suggested that those APAs who did use mental health services were more severely ill and/or received a lower quality of care than their White counterparts.

FACTORS LIMITING ATTENTION TO ASIAN PACIFIC AMERICANS WITH DISABILITIES

Too often, APAs are lumped together as a single group in quantitative studies. Similarly, in qualitative studies individual groups are considered representative of all APAs (Chung, 1995). Some researchers (e.g., Yang, Leung, Wang, & Shim, 1996) suggest that available incidence and prevalence data on disability may not accurately reflect the reality for APA rates given the differing procedures used to assess disability rates in this population (Chin, Mio, & Iwamasa, 2006).

Researchers use aggregate data to make overgeneralizations as they describe the vocational rehabilitation process of various APA individuals without recognizing the ethnic and socioeconomic diversity within this group (Kim-Rupnow et al., 2005; Chin et al., 2006). Moreover, the problematic lack of meaningful data on the VR status of APAs has given rise to the assumption that APAs with disabilities, as a group, actually have less or no need for rehabilitation supports such as transportation or assistive technology provisions, mobility training, and other services. Of course this assumption is inaccurate and misleading, particularly in the case of poor immigrants from remote rural areas in their countries of origin. Therefore, it is essential to use disaggregated data for subgroups within the APA populations. In addition, the little information that is available is sometimes misinterpreted because of definitional differences regarding disability, ethnicity, or race. For example, Chung (2005) explored some questions on health and disability rates among Asian Americans in Massachusetts. He found that APAs are an underserved population in terms of disability needs and are dealing with difficult circumstances (e.g., hurdles such as access to health care, high costs of medications, and lack of health insurance). Moreover, researchers often fail to find representative samples of this group for their surveys, creating further difficulties for both policymakers and direct service providers who aim to be inclusive and responsive to this group's needs and challenges. For example, Minkler, Fuller-Thomson, and Guralnick (2006) found that disability rates are linked to education (more education, less disability), income (less income, more disability) and working in manual and service-related jobs (the higher the amount of occupational risk, the higher the disability rate). They have also found that APA immigrants and their families who have a longer history in the United States are more likely to have higher levels of education and income. In addition, more recent immigrants/refugees are more often employed in jobs that involve a higher risk of acquiring a disability, compared to those who have lived here longer.

In summary, several factors lead us to suspect that the research-based incidence and prevalence rates of disability for APAs may understate the reality of their actual rates. Even when the data are accurate, the diverse nature of APA ethnic groups suggests that between-group differences are significant. Including well-educated fifth-generation Japanese Americans with first-generation refugees from Southeast Asia may be convenient for demographers, but it increases the chances of inaccurate representation of both groups. This substantial variation makes it difficult to understand the vocational rehabilitation needs of a subgroup of APAs with disabilities and their families. There are several contextual and cultural factors that can play a role in influencing APA's utilization of VR services. These include common misperceptions, limited resources, and various types of cultural biases. The next two sections examine these issues in more detail.

CONTEXTUAL FACTORS THAT HELP EXPLAIN POOR UTILIZATION OF VOCATIONAL REHABILITATION SERVICES

Asian Pacific Americans are Considered a "Model Minority"

The first factor that may keep APAs with disabilities from receiving VR services is their overall reputation as the "model minority." This stereotyping term implies that this minority group achieves a higher degree of success and its members are healthier and wealthier in comparison to other immigrant ethnic groups. What flows from this stereotype is the belief that APAs do not need assistance or social services because they are ostensibly doing well. As a result, APAs have been excluded from important research studies, population reports, and service planning often due to limited resources and funding constraints concerning health and disability issues (Chin et al., 2006; Zhan, 2003).

Since the mid-1960s, Asian Americans have long been portrayed as a group of ethnic, racial, or religious people that the majority of Americans believe are successful based on merit alone (Brightman, Kim-Rupnow, & O'Brian, 2005). In essence, APAs are seen as having "made it" in American society. Although this may be true for Asian immigrants with several generations in this country, it is not the case for refugees or recent immigrants. This stereotype reflects false and dangerous assumptions regarding education, income, social status, disability, and need for services. These inaccurate assumptions obscure disparities in APA health and disability, making it difficult for service providers and policymakers to address the inequities. In addition, this stereotype can mislead providers of VR services to assume that APAs have less need for services compared to other applicants (Park et al., 2005) because they have fewer or less-pressing disabilities or because they as a group have the means and resources to care for those in need.

Lack of Bilingual, Bicultural Vocational Rehabilitation Providers of Asian Pacific American Descent

A second issue is the lack of culturally responsive providers. The current workforce within the VR system lacks racial, ethnic, and linguistic diversity (Flowers, Crimando, Forbes, & Riggar, 2005; Flowers, Edwards, & Pusch, 1996). A lack of bilingual, bicultural VR providers of APA descent may be keeping many APAs with disabilities from using VR services and programs. For example, a needs assessment done by the Oregon Health Science University found ignorance, disrespect, and disregard among service providers to be common systemic barriers (Community Solutions, 1999). Similarly, several of the service recipients that participated in the Oregon survey indicated that they were treated by mainstream service providers in ways that they found intimidating, embarrassing, frustrating, and demeaning.

Community Influences on Utilization of Vocational Rehabilitation Services

Communities constitute a third important factor. Some APAs with disabilities may be living in isolated, rural/urban communities and their parents or other responsible family members may have little education or limited English proficiency skills, preventing them from learning about VR services and programs (U.S. Department of Health and Human Services, 2001). APA representation in VR programs has not changed despite state and federal diversity initiatives (Niemeier, Burnett, & Whitaker, 2003). This shortcoming is well-documented by Hampton (2003) who identified concerns of Chinese Americans, aged 35–81 years of age, with physical disabilities from arthritis, diabetes, cancer, and polio, who lived in low-income housing, did not speak English, or did not own a car, and expressed concerns about their difficulties in accessing health care and rehabilitation services.

In recent years, increased attention has focused on APAs' underutilization of VR services and programs (NCD, 2003). Yet little is known about VR outcomes or means of accessing and utilizing services for racial and ethnic groups, particularly among APAs with disabilities (Thomas, Rosenthal, Banks, & Schroeder, 2002). The factors leading to this underutilization cited in the mental health literature may provide some clues. Most of the research on APA groups has mainly focused on "community needs or cultural differences (attitudes towards Western style health care) which have mainly reflected the passive aspects of APA lives" (Chung, 1995, p.78) with little focus on disability status, VR experiences, and outcomes. The few studies (Hampton, 2003; Pi, 2001) about the VR process indicate that various factors, such as gender, poverty, generational differences, premigration traumas, and/or belief systems, can influence vocational training outcomes in various ways. These factors can hinder or facilitate the VR process for a service provider and keep an APA with a disability from having a positive experience or outcome.

Several other socioenvironmental factors contribute to the sizable disparity among various APAs with disabilities. For instance, researchers have found evidence that disabilities are disproportionately concentrated in more vulnerable populations such as those who live in poor housing conditions, lack easy access to local rehabilitation services, and experience difficult lifestyles due to financial problems and lack of access to health insurance or work incentives (Laveist, 2006). Living in neighborhoods with higher exposure to crime and lack of transportation (public or private) are likely to put APAs with disabilities at further disadvantage. Researchers (Hasnain, 2001; Niemeier et al., 2003) have identified factors that reduce a person's chance of receiving VR services. These include geographic inaccessibility, lack of familiarity with the U.S. service system, low levels of education, lack of legal U.S. immigration status, and minimal English language skills. Discrimination and the inadequate number of trained rehabilitation professionals of APA backgrounds also result in fewer resources being available for members of these cultural groups (Chin et al., 2006).

CULTURAL FACTORS THAT HELP EXPLAIN POOR UTILIZATION OF VOCATIONAL REHABILITATION SERVICES

Beliefs about Disability

Cultural factors also affect access to VR services and options among APAs with disabilities, including cultural and religious beliefs and attitudes about disabilities. In exploring culture and its influence on disability and rehabilitation, one must consider the complexity of a specific cultural or ethnic context. Too often we turn to an individual's country of origin to identify values, attitudes, and traditions without realizing that individuals who have immigrated to a new location make adaptations that essentially create or bring about a "culture" that may differ somewhat from their home culture.

The term *disability* does not translate well into the language of some Asian groups, possibly resulting in misinterpretations and misunderstandings. For example, Chinese speakers translate disability into a term meaning "useless" which reflects the way a society sees a person with a disability rather than a condition or function. Some APAs' perception of what disability means also affects the way they may respond to interviewers or complete forms and surveys. Likewise, terms such as cognitive disability (i.e., developmental disability, autism) do not exist in some APAs' native language or are not easily translatable into a native language. Even when researchers use specific and functional terminology, there is room for misinterpretation. For example, if the ability to prepare meals is used as a functional criterion for disability, the type of cooking facility or its location may be more of a barrier than the functional ability itself.

As is true for all ethnicities and cultures, the view that a person or community holds about disability can lead to a variety of actions or a lack thereof. That is, some families may identify the cause of disability with biomedical factors as defined by disability professionals and physicians, while others may link the cause of the disability with personal actions, or religious or folk explanations. Although little research has been conducted on the attitudes that members of various APA groups hold toward various disabilities (e.g., Down syndrome, deafness, polio, or diabetes), a few studies suggest that in some cultures disability may be interpreted in various negative ways. For instance, some APA families may think disability results from disobeying a Higher Power or God, or is the work of the devil, or in some instances due to evil spirits. For other APA individuals and communities, disability may be seen as bad luck or a punishment for an ancestor's past sins or indiscretions (karma), while yet others may see it as a sign of good fortune or a blessing (Zhan, 2003).

Whatever the cause of the disability, "many APAs tend to rely on family members for support before seeking professional help and they tend to mistrust governmental agencies and therefore may not seek assistance from state VR systems" (Park & Starbuck, n.d.). Hampton (2003) cites the example of a 42-year-old Chinese woman who immigrated to the United States from a small village 22 years earlier. She decided not to come back to the VR office after she was told that she needed to take several tests in order to determine her eligibility. Because no one explained the procedure to her in detail, a communication breakdown occurred between the VR counselor and the Chinese woman who feared that she had done something wrong and the governmental agency would be coming after her for it.

Other aspects that should be considered include using culturally-based definitions and meanings of the term disability and/or service jargon. For example, among many South Asian Muslim families of a particular social class or of modest educational level, the functionality of a person—cognitively, physically, or emotionally—with a disability is given more weight than the specific label of disability, whether it affects the person's cognitive, physical, or mental abilities. In other words, the disability terms may be meaningless to them as long as the individual can function in his or her community.

These perceptions can influence or reinforce the way a person with a disability or his/her family perceives it. Some individuals may not even think of themselves as having a disability or a significant health issue, given the way that the issue is seen within their culture or family. For example, a young Cambodian man with a cognitive disability who works at his family's restaurant may not be viewed as having a disability since he is functional and able to perform his duties. Clearly, these variables can influence whether or not a person or family seeks rehabilitation services and/or supports.

Stigma and Shame

Stigma and shame can also play a significant role in how a cultural or ethnic group perceives a disability and assists members in gaining services and supports. For example, Simpson, Mohr, and Redman (2000) found that among the Vietnamese they studied, the shame of a traumatic brain injury or other kinds of disabilities or health conditions goes beyond the individual and brings shame onto the entire family, reflecting the emphasis on family (e.g., collectivism) over individuals in some APA cultures. Shame within a family also relates to how an individual or family is perceived by society, which is linked to the practice of "saving face" (Hasnain, Shaikh, & Shanawani, 2008). Saving face is a broad term linked with various cultural values such as family honor and its opposite, humiliation and disgrace.

Saving face may carry different levels of meaning to an individual with a disability or his/her family, but it most often involves keeping disability hidden within the family or the APA community. Such differing perceptions and cultural beliefs may prevent an individual and his/her family from seeking needed rehabilitation training and supports. Many families from such backgrounds are not aware of many VR services available, such as vocational training, guidance counseling and job referral, independent living skills development, and/or transportation assistance. As a consequence, "these stigmatic responses can take a toll in outcomes for APAs with disabilities such as in employment, education, and community living" (Saetermoe, Scattone, & Kim, 2001, p.1).

Reliance on the Family

A third issue is the level of reliance on family members. Many APAs with disabilities rely on their families or other resources in their ethnic community before seeking mainstream professional or public help (Hampton, 2000). In fact, members of large APA families and communities may use fewer VR services because they tend to distrust the U.S service systems (Park & Starbuck, 2002).They may believe that the government may try to send them back to their home country or jeopardize their immigration status for permanent residency. Another important cultural factor is the way an APA individual, family, and/or community defines success. For example, traditional American culture views employment and advanced schooling as indicators of success. However, in other cultures a family member's role in the community, including civic participation or work ethic, such as being a good homemaker, a farmer, or security guard for a corporation may be equally or even more highly valued. It is also important to note that the cultural tendencies mentioned here vary based on the ethnic group, along with a family's place of residence, social class, profession, educational level, and other related individual factors such as gender or birth order in a family.

Degree of Acculturation

The degree of acculturation to U.S. society may also influence VR outcomes for APAs with disabilities. Since acculturation is a process that varies across individuals and families, an acculturated person can be defined in a variety of ways. For many individuals it is one way, that is, people bend their traditional patterns in the direction of the surrounding dominant culture in which they live. In other cases, individuals may interact with the dominant or mainstream culture on its terms, yet continue to hold the beliefs of their cultural group or enclave and conduct most of their activities in accordance with those beliefs. Other individuals may adhere to American practices and routines in some areas of living, such as their views of education and work, and, yet differ radically in their views of disability or rehabilitation (Zhan, 2003). Given the complexity of acculturation issues, factors such as time spent in the United States and proximity to the traditional culture and social class can greatly influence behavior and beliefs. All of these factors may have a positive or negative effect on VR outcomes yet few researchers have explored them in part because these issues (e.g., values, perspectives) are often hard to identify, define, and measure. Yet, Barry (2001) has done a considerable amount of research on measuring acculturation (i.e., The East Asian Acculturation Scale [EAAS]) and has studied these issues in contexts outside of VR. The findings of this study suggest that the EAAS may be a useful tool for rehabilitation researchers and providers to examine the acculturation patterns of East Asian immigrants.

Although VR services may seem abundant and readily accessible from the viewpoint of the mainstream service provider, differences in culture and worldviews prevent APAs from understanding and grasping the range of services and supports available to them. For instance, U.S. culture is highly individualistic and places particular value on personal autonomy and independence (Hampton & Marshall, 2000; Sue & Sue, 1999); as a result, the VR system has embraced these values in its mission and goals. The notion of independence, a concept deeply rooted in American culture, contrasts strongly with the beliefs of many APA groups that emphasize family, collectivism, and interdependence (Hong, 1997). Because the concepts of self-determination, independent living, and self-advocacy are often emphasized by VR specialists and independent living center programs, APAs with disabilities could become discouraged from utilizing such services if staff members do not identify and translate these terms and assumptions in culturally tailored ways.

In fact, the majority of U.S. VR programs are driven by values of autonomy and independence which may be foreign or even offensive to some APAs, especially to those who have recently immigrated to the United States. For example, when APAs with disabilities enter the VR system, an independent living center, or community work program, they may be confused by the self-directed decision-making process expected of them. The few APA consumers who are part of the VR system may be upset over the lack of direction from their counselors (Hampton, 2003). In other words, American rehabilitation counselors, program directors, and policymakers may believe that individuals with a disability function best when becoming independent of family and other supports. However, APAs with disabilities may see this independence as aversive and experience it as a lack of caring or concern for them. They may even want to live with and be part of their entire extended family and expect the family to make decisions and take responsibility for them (NCD, 1999). On the other hand, while the extended family is traditionally seen as a valued asset in APA cultures, rehabilitation professionals may overlook the extended family's traditional role. Instead, rehabilitation staff should recognize and encourage kinship contributions when family members develop and carry out rehabilitation plans for APAs (Hampton, 2000), which could make a difference in achieving outcomes for APAs with disabilities. The following scenario illustrates the need for effective communication and understanding of worldviews between service providers and people of APA cultures (Hasnain et al., 2008; see Exhibit 10-1).

Exhibit 10-1
Case Scenario

A Pakistani Muslim father explained that he had approached a VR service agency for assistance because his 19-year-old son with a developmental disability needed more support as he grew older. The agency offered a personal care attendant, but could not guarantee that the attendant would be of Pakistani and Muslim descent. The father explained that it was not acceptable to him to have a non-Pakistani working in his home because his family expected the son to follow certain cultural practices such as daily prayers and rituals with which a non-Pakistani would not be familiar. The agency worker's response was that this was the only service that they could offer. The father at that point refused any service from

continued

the agency and contacted his parents living in the area who now help respond to some of their grandson's needs.

The scenario described could have been handled in several more culturally appropriate and positive ways. For example, an agency could have offered to employ the grandfather or some other male relatives (e.g., cousins, siblings) to work as the young man's personal care attendants (PCAs) or the family could have suggested it. Another option is that the worker could have said that while the agency did not have Pakistani PCAs available, it would try to recruit some or search for some within other agencies. She/he could also have asked the father if Muslim PCAs of other cultural groups would be suitable. Given such scenarios, it is clear that the shortage of ethnically diverse professionals in the disability field reduces the likelihood of APAs with disabilities utilizing such services. Such limitations in the system can combine with differences in cultural values and worldviews to reduce desired outcomes. It also suggests that rehabilitation providers "may need to learn to recognize and acknowledge Eurocentric biases they may have in addition to those inherent in the VR system" (Park et al., 2005, p. 36).

IMPLICATIONS FOR RESEARCH

To address disparities in access and outcomes, we suggest several ways to improve research on APAs. The VR system needs data collection methods that recognize the complexity of APAs as a cultural group. Efforts must include APAs with disabilities both as an aggregate as well as divided into specific categories that reflect the diversity of this broad population. While data collection methods may not seem to impact VR service delivery, APAs with disabilities will continue to remain invisible if appropriate data are not available about their population clusters and ethnicity.

Central questions must also be explored in future research. For example, what ways of approaching outreach and services are most successful in addressing the issues of APAs with disabilities and their families? Do APAs respond to outreach and services similarly to, or differently from, other underserved ethnic/racial groups? Are they more likely to drop out of the VR process earlier? If so, why? What commonalities exist within the general APA population, if anything? What groups and subgroups fall into this category? It is also important to differentiate among subethnic groups clustered within the APA category, given their high level of cultural and linguistic variability. Answers to these and similar questions can only come from data and the analysis of data that includes APAs with disabilities. Policy and procedures must flow from a solid foundation of data.

To reduce disparities in service availability and outcomes for APAs with disabilities, disability professionals and researchers must continue to work to determine the prevalence of disability and service needs of the APA segment of society. Without accurate research data and sound findings, it is difficult to convince policymakers to increase funding for programs to better serve APAs with disabilities, to train service providers to better identify their needs, and to adequately serve this growing population in a culturally sensitive manner, especially in the VR system.

Research studies that incorporate cultural and linguistic competency in all stages of development and implementation can help us to better understand the mindset of APAs with disabilities and their families. Researchers, policymakers, VR counselors, and others who assist the APA population need to follow strength-based principles and researchers must employ culturally appropriate measures. This approach includes adequate sampling processes that capture the diversity within APA populations, including their various worldviews and cultural histories. In addition, we need to explore ways that the family and community can be included in studies of APAs with disabilities so that we can provide a clearer picture of their needs and service desires. A more family-centered approach may shape policy and funding in culturally appropriate ways for the often overlooked APA group.

IMPLICATIONS FOR PRACTICE

The combined effects of poverty and ethnicity, compounded by language and communication barriers, are associated with lower levels of service utilization. Another contributing factor is the diverse sociodemographic characteristics of APAs with disabilities and their families and the lack of rehabilitation providers of APA backgrounds (National Center for Dissemination of Disability Research, 1999). For all these reasons, it is critical that the VR system make an effort to learn about and support APAs with disabilities. The following are some strategies that appear promising.

Cultural Brokering

Cultural brokering has proven to be an effective practice to bridge gaps between ethnic groups and community and human services programs (Brightman, 2006; Jezewski & Sotnik, 2005). Because language and cultural factors can make interactions between APAs and formal service systems difficult and frustrating, and because service providers may hold negative attitudes towards APA consumers and often lack adequate training in cultural and linguistic competency to address the needs of this diverse population, service providers must offer cross-cultural training and technical assistance to their staff members and run culturally sensitive outreach programs in order to reach marginalized and/or underserved populations like APAs (Marshall, Sanderson, Johnson, Du Bois, & Kvedar, 2006). In cultural brokering interventions, a "middleman" or "go-between" works with the individual and the family on one side, and the service providers on the other, to ensure that both sides understand the required procedures in regard to their worldview. Service providers may have the basic attributes needed to act as brokers but could benefit from training in using these elements more intentionally in their interaction and procedures when working with APA consumers and their families.

Outreach Efforts

Second, considering outreach, it may be more effective to use nontraditional outreach methods that cater to the cultural needs of a population rather than approaches that have only succeeded with the majority population. While little research has been conducted, observations suggest that VR programs are in such demand that they see little payoff in catering to new or underserved populations. Therefore, incentives or additional resources are needed if VR offices are to provide adequate culturally sensitive outreach. Given the need to increase the diversity of APA research samples, VR researchers and service providers should form relationships with APA communities not only to recruit research participants and service recipients but to work in developing a trusting partnership that is mutually beneficial for both parties, especially for those in most need of VR services and supports. It would also help if APA-specific organizations could be offered resources for training, consultation, and technical assistance in this area. Working with education and training programs to recruit APAs into this field is critical to "grow" personnel for future needs, as described in more detail below. In addition, documentation of success stories and promotion of APAs with disabilities who have achieved positive VR outcomes need to be shared with stakeholders and policymakers as well as with the APA community.

Bilingual Collaboration and Support

Third, bilingual collaboration and support are crucial (Brightman et al., 2005). Partnering with local community and faith-based organizations that incorporate a family or a collective decision-making model may be a particularly effective approach in communities with existing VR programs and relatively larger numbers of APAs. During the 1980s and 1990s, several innovative VR programs were developed that catered specifically to new immigrants and refugees. A good example of such a partnership is the Vietnamese Boat People SOS (2008), a program located in Falls Church, Virginia. The established ties and language capacity of these programs and agencies, along with their acceptance by APAs make them logical partners for the VR process. Another example is the use of a telephone-based language support line by health and rehabilitation professionals at a health clinic in Chicago in order to communicate with recently arrived APA refugees with physical disabilities, since their staff interpreters did not speak Burmese, Nepal Bhasa, Lao, Gujarati, Tongan, or Samoan, among others.

Increase Representation of Asian Pacific Americans as Vocational Rehabilitation Providers

Finally, it is necessary to increase the cross-cultural competency of VR personnel through on-going training and staff development. One step is to increase the visible presence of APAs in VR programs, especially in states and localities where they comprise a significant proportion of the population. Specific outreach efforts are also needed to recruit and retain staff from APA populations including those who are bilingual. Doing so increases cultural and linguistic competence, and will also allow programs to visibly demonstrate their cultural awareness and welcome APAs with disabilities through the presence of persons to whom APAs can relate.

A first step towards creating a welcoming environment is often what is most noticeable to persons with little knowledge or understanding of the VR process. New community-based participatory action models and related outreach activities can focus on using a community rather than a standardized traditional Eurocentric approach as a way to serve APAs with disabilities in relevant and meaningful ways. Unfortunately, this tailoring to distinctive cultures can be particularly difficult when agencies face pressure to produce outcomes quickly, but it is essential if agencies are to meet the needs of APA populations that have been underserved. In sum, we must first incorporate the concepts of family, culture, and community into research and practice, which have traditionally focused on individuals; only then can the current VR system actually increase the participation of APAs with disabilities and serve them effectively.

CONCLUSION

This chapter concludes that VR research and services for APAs are inadequate. In order for access and VR outcomes to improve for APA individuals with disabilities, researchers and service providers must understand APA immigration and acculturation status. This view has been echoed for years in the social service delivery arena and yet the situation has scarcely improved. Given the long history of APAs and the multiple generations of APA families in the United States today, it is imperative that they be included in research and policy development.

Service providers need to develop an understanding of the individual's history and cultural background. Rehabilitation efforts tailored to the cultural needs of APAs with disabilities may bring about better outcomes, including greater access to job training and educational and work options. In fact, considering the limited training and employment options available for the APA group, the rehabilitation provider needs to be especially resourceful and persistent in doing outreach, forming ties with APA consumers, and finding good job and vocational education/training matches (Hong, 1997).

Recognizing the diversity of APAs is important for tailoring research protocols specific to the VR processes and outcomes of multiple APA populations. Although many studies have examined how cultural differences play a role in VR service outcomes, the bulk of the existing literature focuses on other ethnic and racial groups with disabilities—particularly African Americans and Latinos—essentially ignoring APAs with disabilities. Thus, a greater focus on APAs is clearly needed given the steadily rising number of this population and the failure of the current U.S. VR system to adequately reach out to and serve them. Such a forward-thinking agenda would only help to increase the representation of APAs with disabilities in social services, vocational systems, and in the community.

REFERENCES

Barry, D. T. (2001). Development of a new scale for measuring acculturation: The East Asian Acculturation Measure [EAAM]. *Journal of Immigrant Health, 3*(4), 193–197.

Boat People SOS (2008). *Humanitarian Resettlement Program.* Retrieved April 4, 2008, from *http://www.bpsos.org/node/290*

Brightman, J. D. (2006). Promising practices brief: Cultural brokering. *NTAC-AAPI Promising Practices Brief Series, (7)*4, 1–4.

Brightman, J. D., Kim-Rupnow, W. S., & O'Brien, M. D. (2005). Promising practices brief: bilingual support. *NTAC-AAPI Promising Practices Brief Series, (7)*1, 1–4.

Chan, F., Lam, C. S., Wong, D., Leung, P., & Fung, X. S. (1988). Counseling Chinese Americans with disabilities. *Journal of Applied Rehabilitation Counseling, 19*(4), 21–25.

Chin, J. L., Mio, J., & Iwamasa, G. Y. (2006). Ethical conduct of research within Asian and Pacific Islander American populations. In J. E. Trimble & C. B. Fisher (Eds.), *The Handbook of Ethical Research with Ethnocultural Populations and Communities.* Thousand Oaks, CA: Sage.

Chung, T. L. (1995). Asian American in enclaves—They are not one community: New modes of Asian American settlement. *Asian American Policy, 5*, 78–94.

Chung, T. L. (2005). *Asian health and disability issues in Malden, Massachusetts.* The Malden Asian Disability Advocacy Coalition.

Community Solutions (1999). Barriers facing minority youth in transition. Portland: Oregon Health Sciences University.

Dziekan, K. I. & Okocha, A. A. G. (1993). Accessibility of rehabilitation services: Comparison by racial-ethnic status. *Rehabilitation Counseling Bulletin, 36*(4), 183–189.

Flowers, C. R., Crimando, W., Forbes, W. S., & Riggar, T. F. (2005). A regional survey of rehabilitation cultural diversity within CILs: A ten-year follow-up. *Journal of Rehabilitation, 71*(2), 14–21.

Flowers, C. R., Edwards, D., & Pusch, B. (1996). Rehabilitation cultural diversity initiative: A regional survey of cultural diversity within CILs. *Journal of Rehabilitation, 62*(3), 22–28.

Hampton, N. Z. (2000). Meeting the unique needs of Asian Americans and Pacific Islanders with disabilities: A challenge to rehabilitation counselors in the 21st century. *Journal of Applied Rehabilitation Counseling. 31*(1), 40–44.

Hampton, N. Z. (2003). Asian Americans with disabilities: Access to education, health care, and rehabilitation services. In L. Zhan (Ed.), *Asian Americans: Vulnerable populations, model interventions, and clarifying agendas* (pp.69–88). Sudbury, MA: Jones and Bartlett.

Hampton, N. Z. & Marshall, A. (2000). Culture, gender, self-efficacy, and life satisfaction: A comparison between Americans and Chinese people with spinal cord injuries. *Journal of Rehabilitation, 66,* 21–31.

Hart, D., Zimbrich, K., & Whelley, T. (2002). Challenges in coordinating and managing services and supports in secondary and postsecondary options. National Center on Secondary Education and Transition Issue Brief, 1(6). Minneapolis: University of Minnesota.

Hasnain, R. (2001). *Entering adulthood with a disability: Individual, family, and cultural challenges.* Unpublished doctoral dissertation, Boston University, Boston.

Hasnain, R., Shaikh, L. C., & Shanawani, H. (2008). *Disability and the Muslim perspective: An introduction for rehabilitation and health care providers* (CIRRIE Monograph Series). University at Buffalo, The State University of New York, Center for International Rehabilitation Research & Exchange.

Hong, G.K. (1997). *Rehabilitation counseling for Asian Americans: Psychological and social considerations.* Retrieved January 1, 2008, from: *http://www.dinf.ne.jp/doc/english/Us_Eu/ada_e/pres_com/pres-dd/hong.htm*

Jezewski, M. & Sotnik, P. (2005) Disability service providers as culture brokers: In J. Stone (Ed.), *Culture and Disability* (pp. 31–64).Thousand Oaks, CA: Sage.

Kim-Rupnow, W. S., Park, H. C., & Starbuck, D. E. (2005). Status overview of vocational rehabilitation services for Asian Americans and Pacific Islanders with disabilities. *Journal of Vocational Rehabilitation, 23,* 21–32.

Laveist, T. A. (2006). *Minority populations and health: An introduction to health disparities in the United States.* San Francisco: Jossey-Bass.

Leung, P. (1993). Minorities with disabilities and the American with Disabilities Act: A promise yet to be fulfilled. *Journal of Rehabilitation Administration, 16,* 92–98.

Leung, P. (1996). Asian Pacific Americans and section 21 of the Rehabilitation Act amendments of 1992—includes related information. *American Rehabilitation, 22*(1) 2–6.

Marshall, C. A, Sanderson, P. R., Johnson, S. R., Du Bois, B., & Kvedar, J. C. (2006). Considering class, culture, and access in rehabilitation intervention and research. In K. J. Hagglund and A. W. Heinemann (Eds.), *The handbook of applied disability and rehabilitation research* (pp. 25–44). New York: Springer.

Minkler, M. Fuller-Thomson, E. & Guralnik, J. M. (2006). Gradient of disability across the socioeconomic spectrum in the United States, *The New England Journal of Medicine 355*(7), 695–704.

National Center for the Dissemination of Disability Research (1999). Disability, diversity, and dissemination: A review of the literature on topics related to increasing the utilization of rehabilitation research outcomes among diverse consumer groups. *Research Exchange, 4*(2), 2–15.

National Council on Disability [NCD]. (1999). *Lift every voice: modernizing disability policies and programs to serve a diverse nation.* Washington, DC: Author.

National Council on Disability.[NCD]. (2003). *People with disabilities on tribal lands: Education, health care, vocational rehabilitation, and independent living.* Washington, DC: Author.

Niemeier, J. P., Burnett, D. M., & Whitaker, D. A. (2003). Cultural competence in the multidisciplinary rehabilitation setting: Are we falling short of meeting needs? *Archives of Physical Medicine & Rehabilitation, 84*(8), 1240–1245.

Palafox, N. A., Buenconsejo-Lum, L., Riklon, S., & Waitzfelder, B. (2002). Improving health outcomes in diverse populations: Competency in cross-cultural research with indigenous Pacific Islanders populations. *Ethnicity & Health, 7*(4), 279–285.

Park, H. C., Kim-Rupnow, W. S., Stodden, R., & Starbuck, D. E. (2005). Disparity of closure type in vocational rehabilitation services. *Journal of Vocational Rehabilitation, 23,* 33–38.

Park, H. C. & Starbuck, D. E. (2002). Information brief: Asian Americans and Pacific Islanders, National Technical Assistance Center for Asian Americans and Pacific Islanders with Disabilities. Honolulu University of Hawaii at Manoa.

Pi, E. H. (2001). *Asians and Pacific Islanders with disabilities.* White Paper–Pacific regional conferences on Asians and Pacific Islanders with disabilities. 1–15. California Governor's Committee for Employment of Disabled Persons.

President's Advisory Commission on Asian Americans and Pacific Islanders (2001). *Asian Americans and Pacific Islanders: A people looking forward-action for access and partnerships in the 21st century. Interim Report to the President and the Nation.* Washington DC: White House Initiative on Asian Americans and Pacific Islanders.

Rehabilitation Act Amendments of 1992, Pub. L. 102-569, 29 U.S.C. U701 et seq (1992).

Saetermoe, C. L., Scattone, D., & Kim, K. H. (2001). Ethnicity and the stigma of disabilities. *Psychology and Health, 6*(6), 699–713.

Simpson, G., Mohr, R., & Redman, A. (2000). Cultural variations in the understanding of traumatic brain injury and brain injury rehabilitation, *Brain Injury, 14*(2) 125–140.

Sue, D. W. & Sue, D. (1999). *Counseling the culturally different.* New York: Wiley.

Thomas, D. F., Rosenthal, D. A., Banks, M. E., & Schroeder, M. (2002, September). *Diversity in Vocational Rehabilitation: People, practice, and outcomes.* Paper presented at Community-Based Rehabilitation: Research for Improving Employment Outcomes Conference, Washington, DC.

U.S. Census Bureau (2002). *The Asian Population: 2000, Census 2000 Brief.* Retrieved October 30, 2008, from *http://www.census.gov/prod/2002pubs/c2kbr01-16.pdf*

U.S. Census Bureau (February, 2007). *The American Community–Asians: 2004. American Communtiy Service Reports.* Retrieved October 30, 2008, from *http://www.census.gov/prod/2007pubs/acs-05.pdf*

U.S. Census Bureau (2008, December). International Database. Retrieved March 5, 2009, from *http://www.census.gov/ipc/www/idb/*

U.S. Department of Health and Human Services. (2001). *Mental health: A report of the Surgeon General, Mental health care for Asian Americans and Pacific Islanders.* Rockville, MD: Author.

Wilson, K. B., Alston, R. J., Harly, D. A., & Mitchell, N. A. (2002). Predicting VR acceptance based on race, gender, education, work status at application and primary source of support at application. *Rehabilitation Counseling Bulletin, 45*(3), 132–142.

Wright, L. (1994, July 25). One drop of blood. *The New Yorker*, 46–55.

Yang, H., Leung, P., Wang, J., & Shim, N. (1996). Asian Pacific Americans: the need for ethnicity specific data. *Journal of Disability Policy Studies, 1*(7), 33–54.

Zhan, L. (2003). *Asian Americans: Vulnerable populations, model interventions, and clarifying agendas.* Sudbury, MA: Jones and Bartlett.

Models to Improve Rehabilitation Services for Multicultural Popuations with Disabilities

(A) MODELS FOR REHABILITATION TRAINING

CHAPTER 11

Cultural Competence Education in Rehabilitation

Mary A. Matteliano, MS, OTR/L;
John H. Stone, PhD

INTRODUCTION

High immigration rates in the United States have resulted in cultural differences between the recipients of rehabilitation services and those who provide such services. Thirty years ago approximately 1 in 20 persons in the United States were born in another country. Today the ratio is more than 1 in 10 (Stone, 2004). Increasingly, service providers are called upon to provide services to persons whose culture may differ from their own. Culture often influences our understanding of disability and the goals and methods of rehabilitation, which can affect communication between service providers and consumers (Groce, 2004). Consequently, the theme of cultural competence has assumed an increasingly important role in the delivery of services in the United States, as well as in other countries with large immigrant populations. While there may be no universally accepted definition of the term "cultural competence," the delivery of effective services to persons from other cultures requires an understanding of the ways in which culture may affect one's views of disability.

The purpose of this chapter is to identify educational approaches that will be effective in preparing future service providers to work with clients from other cultures. First, we will review data on the ethnoracial composition within the rehabilitation professions. Next, we will review the general literature on cultural competence, as well as the specific literature on cultural competence in rehabilitation. We will then review literature on the teaching of cultural competence and ways to measure or evaluate it. Finally, we will describe one of the current projects of the Center for International Rehabilitation Research Information and Exchange (CIRRIE) that has developed a cultural competence training curricula for university programs in physical therapy, occupational therapy, speech therapy, and rehabilitation counseling. Because of CIRRIE's funding mandate from the National Institute on Disability and Rehabilitation Research, its focus in the area of cultural competency are the cultures of persons who have come to the United States from other countries. Consequently, the main focus of this chapter is on the cultures of recent immigrant groups, rather than U.S.-born persons of different cultures. However, in some cases the issues they face may be analogous to those faced by Latinos, African Americans, and Native Americans that will also be included in this chapter.

PURPOSE AND DOMAIN

Other chapters in this book have presented recent data on immigration, including growth trends and the principal countries of origin for immigration. This section contains information on the racial/ethnic composition of the workforce in the rehabilitation professions.

Leavitt (1999) points out that although ethnic minorities constitute approximately 30% of the U.S. population, they make up less than 8% of health and rehabilitation professionals. The majority of rehabilitation service providers in today's workforce are U.S.-born persons of European ancestry. In occupational therapy for example, "More than 90% of occupational therapy practitioners are European Americans. Only 76% of the United States population is European American. African Americans, Hispanic and Latino Americans, and Native Americans are underrepresented in our profession" (McGruder, 2003, p. 85). In audiology and speech-language pathology the situation is similar.

As of year-end 2004, approximately 7.7% of audiologists, 7.0% of speech-language pathologists, and 8.0% of those with dual certification were members of a racial/ethnic minority group. These percentages have remained relatively constant over the years and are well below their distribution within the general population (Slater, 2007, p. 144). The pattern is similar for physical therapy.

In contrast to the statistics depicting the growing diversity of the United States, the statistics on the ethnicities of recent physical therapy graduates demonstrate greater homogeneity. According to the Commission on Accreditation in Physical Therapy Education (CAPTE), the ethnicities of the 2003–2004 graduates of physical therapy programs are as follows: 80.9% Caucasian, 6.1% Asian, 4.5% Hispanic/Latino; 5.2% African American, 0.5% Native American, 1.7% other, and 1.1% unknown (Lattanzi & Purnell, 2006, p. 7).

In VR counseling, over 93% of VR counselors and approximately 92% of VR administrators classify themselves as White (Wilson, Whittaker, & Black, 2007). As a consequence, most foreign-born persons in the United States receive rehabilitation services from persons whose culture is often quite different from theirs. Why does this matter? Because culture influences people's understanding of the nature of disability, its causes, what to do about it, treatment compliance, role of family, and the concept of independence (Stone, 2004). Groce (1999) points out that,

> *Understanding sociocultural models of disability is of more than academic interest. . . .*
> *The intent is not to catalogue every known variation in disability beliefs, but rather to*

alert the practitioners to the fact that the ways in which disability and rehabilitation are conceptualized will have an impact on the manner in which rehabilitation professionals are received, regarded and able to serve their patients. (p. 38)

In the next few sections we will review literature on cultural competence, how it is taught and how it is evaluated.

LITERATURE REVIEW

Cultural Competence in the Provision of Rehabilitation Services

Rehabilitation services, including occupational therapy, physical therapy, speech-language therapy, and rehabilitation counseling, are services used to remediate or compensate for a person's loss of ability to participate in daily activities.

Those who have emigrated from Central America, South America, and Mexico may have experienced torture, threats, executions, and forced disappearances in their country of origin. Eisenman, Gelberg, Liu, and Shapiro (2003) assessed Latino immigrants in three community-based primary care clinics and found that those that were exposed to political violence were more likely to suffer from post-traumatic stress disorder (PTSD), mental health problems, and depression. They also reported more limitations in physical functioning, worse perceptions of general health, chronic pain, and decreased participation in their daily occupations compared to those who did not report exposure to political violence. The rehabilitation specialist should be aware that other migrant groups from Africa, Asia, and Eastern Europe may have also experienced political oppression and torture (Amnesty International, 2006; Polgreen 2007). Unless trust is developed between the client and the provider, pertinent information that is vital to the individual may not surface (Aceron & Savage, 2004; Ayonrinde, 2003; Whiteford, 2005). If left untreated, the recent immigrants' symptoms of depression and PTSD may be expressed as chronic pain, alcoholism, or other forms of self-abuse (Pernell-Arnold, 1998).

Religious views may also affect the rehabilitation process (Aceron & Savage, 2004). For example, certain orthodox Jewish or Muslim beliefs do not allow contact between members of the opposite sex unless they are married (Hasnain, Shaikh, & Shanawani, 2008). Many rehabilitation procedures require personal contact such as instruction in bathing and dressing techniques and close physical contact to assess and monitor physical limitations. Rehabilitation professionals may need to modify their contact with members of the opposite sex for cultural or religious reasons (Ahmad, Alsharif, & Royeen, 2006; Ayonrinde, 2003). Some persons may believe that intervention from rehabilitation professionals is unnecessary and interferes with a fatalistic belief system that is associated with the disability (Groce & Zola, 1993). Other groups may see disability as a punishment or a curse (Jacobson, 2004; Lopez-De Fede, 2004). Healing beliefs and cultural practices may be misunderstood and professionals may suspect abuse unless they become familiar with certain healing techniques and rituals. *Coining* or *cupping* is a technique used in some Asian cultures. Heat is used to banish impurities and this technique produces welts on the body (Ayonrinde; Pachter, 1994). Latino people may consult traditional healers, *curanderos*, who may contradict the advice of rehabilitation professionals and physicians (Juckett, 2005). Negotiating with persons who represent the family and their beliefs may become an addition to the rehabilitation program (Bonder, 2001; Pachter; Santana-Martin & Santana, 2004).

Somatization is frequently encountered across different cultures when either the language or culture does not provide an adequate explanation of a psychological condition (Ayonrinde, 2003; Juckett, 2005; Thompson & Blasquez, 2006). An interesting interview with a family physician resulted in this case example of a Bantu-Somali woman and depression.

> . . . I took care of this Somali woman and at some point I realized there was no physical cause for these complaints, she kept coming in and at some point you have to think about depression. It was pretty obvious to me she was depressed and you have to start thinking this is the cause of her symptoms that the interpreter and I . . . there is no word for depression in their language so how do you even begin to get at that? In that situation the closest we could get to was the word "to break my heart" and we tried, we tried to get there you know. Eventually you come to some sort of an agreement. (M. Glick, personal communication, December 2006)

The agreement that was negotiated in this example demonstrates that the healthcare provider's unique role with persons from diverse backgrounds must include client advocacy. The process of culture-brokering creates an atmosphere of understanding that will result in conflict resolution and the provision of culturally competent services.

Teaching Cultural Competence

Under the rubric of appropriate training to achieve cultural competency, professionals are expected to be educated on the causes and consequences of disparities and to understand how stereotyping, cultural bias, and clinical uncertainty influence assessment and treatment (Ayonrinde, 2003). Proponents of cultural competency argue that universities and colleges that train professionals are responsible for providing culturally competent educational programs (Institute of Medicine, 2002).

Although professional accreditation standards require this, the evidence suggests that most teaching institutions fall short in providing substantive cultural competence training for service providers (Agency for Healthcare Research and Quality [AHRQ], 2004; Jones, Cason, & Bond, 2004).

There may be several reasons for the lack of cultural content in rehabilitation curricula. Faculty may find it challenging to add additional content to their already overburdened curricula and to do this in a timely manner (Leal-Idrogo, 1997). Another problem is that achieving multicultural competence calls for a developmental approach. Cultural competence is a process and not an event (Campinha-Bacote, 2002). Students acquire skills if cultural content is infused in many different courses using a variety of methods over a period of time (Hughes & Hood, 2007; Patternson & Spry, 2007). Therefore, in order for students to develop cultural competence it requires a united effort among all faculty that teach in rehabilitation programs.

There are several models that can be used to guide curriculum planning. The Campinha-Bacote model outlines a process that is similar to the Institute of Medicine (IOM) recommendations for teaching cultural competency (Campinha-Bacote, 2002). The Campinha-Bacote model consists of five constructs: cultural awareness, cultural knowledge, cultural skill, cultural encounters, and cultural desire (Campinha-Bacote, 2002). Cultural awareness, the ability to understand one's own culture and perspective as well as stereotypes and misconceptions regarding other cultures is a first step (Campinha-Bacote, 2007; Hunt & Swiggum, 2007). Although introductory courses will sensitize students by providing information that promotes cultural awareness and knowledge, a comprehensive program would necessarily emphasize a continuum of cultural competence that would be threaded throughout the curriculum (Campinha-Bacote 2002; Kripaiani, Bussey-Jones, Katz, & Genao, 2006).

The Purnell model for cultural competence assumes that all healthcare professionals need culture-specific information, as well as general information about the many cultures that influence beliefs about illness and disability (Purnell & Paulanka, 2003). This model offers an organizing framework for teaching cultural competence in healthcare professions and shows utility for use in rehabilitation programs (Black & Purnell, 2002). This model is depicted as a circle with the macro aspects on the four outside rims of the circle. They include the global society, community, family, and the person. In many non-Western societies, "the individual is defined in relation to the family, including ancestors or another group rather than a basic unit of nature" (Purnell & Paulanka, p.10). Several of the micro constructs provide a framework that considers the influence of the immediate environment on beliefs and attitudes toward illness and disability. The micro constructs include: "inhabited localities, communication, family roles and organization, workforce issues, biocultural ecology, high-risk behaviors, nutrition, pregnancy and childbearing practices, death rituals, spirituality, healthcare practices, and healthcare practitioners" (Purnell & Paulanka, p. 11). For example, when serving a person who has just arrived in the United States, the rehabilitation specialist must consider the macro circumstances that affect that person's health status including: country of origin, reasons for immigration, current community of residence, and the individual's social, economic, and human capital (Alba & Nee, 2003). The micro influences: perceptions of practitioners, use of folk practitioners, religious practices, language, gender roles, and use of touch may influence the rehabilitation process (Purnell & Paulanka). The provision of culturally competent services should address belief systems at the macro and micro level, thus considering the global community influence as well as the behavior of the individuals within their local context.

Self-efficacy, the belief that one can achieve competence in a specific area, motivates the individual to overcome obstacles and embrace the learning experience (Jeffreys, 2006). A model that emphasizes the development of self-efficacy in the area of cultural competence has been developed by Jeffreys (2006). This model addresses the cognitive, practical, and affective domains of learning and was first developed as an educational model for training nursing students in cultural competence (Jeffreys, 2006). The student gains knowledge about different cultural backgrounds and achieves skill by learning verbal and nonverbal communication techniques. Affective learning is developed through experiences that help the student to become self-aware and appreciate cultural differences, thus developing acceptance and advocacy (Jeffreys).

Affective components of this model, the development of empathy and the appreciation for the other's viewpoint, combined with the cognitive and practical domains, can be achieved through structured cultural encounters. Griswold, Zayas, Kernan, and Wagner (2007) discuss the development of empathy and cultural humility among medical students who have participated in refugee clinics. During an encounter with an elderly Vietnamese woman, a medical student tossed his checklist aside as the patient began to cry and tell him about the loss of her family members. The student discusses a transformation in his approach: ". . . I was going through the checklist. . . as she started to cry it shook me. . . I stopped the interview. . . as the empathy kicked in, the checklist started to fall out of my head" (Griswold et al., p. 59).

The cultural brokering model is a theoretical model developed by Jezewski (1990) for health services. The culture brokering model was adapted by CIRRIE for rehabilitation systems (Jezewski & Sotnik, 2004), and a training workshop was designed based on the model. It has shown to be very useful in training rehabilitation personnel in how to identify culturally related problems and devise solutions for those problems. There is a body of literature on the concept of culture brokering that can inform service providers on how to broker for consumers (National Center for Cultural Competence, 2004). The Jezewski model has three stages: (1) Problem identification, (2) Intervention strategies, and (3) Outcomes. *Problem identification* includes a perception of a conflict or breakdown in communication, *Interventions* are aimed at establishing trust and rapport, and maintaining connections. *Strategies* to implement interventions include mediating, negotiating, advocating, and networking. Stage three is evaluating *Outcomes*, both successful or unsuccessful. Success is achieved if connections are established between consumers and the rehabilitation system, as well as across systems.

What makes this brokering model a *culture*-brokering model is a fourth component, *Intervening Conditions*. These are culturally-based factors that must be considered at all three stages: analyzing the problem, devising appropriate strategies, and evaluating outcomes. The intervening conditions include type of disability, communication, age of the consumer, culture-sensitivity, time, cultural background, power or powerlessness, economics, bureaucracy, politics, network, and stigma. The model is not a set of rules or steps to follow. Rather, it is a conceptual framework that can guide the service provider in analyzing problems and devising culturally appropriate solutions. The culture broker must understand both the culture of the client as well as the culture of the service system. For disability services, the brokers most often will be a person within the agency because the delivery system may be far too complex for the lay person to negotiate and mediate in most conflict/problem situations.

Several contradictions are inherent in the role of culture broker. If brokers are people who function as go-betweens, with whom do they align themselves? Does the broker represent one of the two parties, or is the broker acting on behalf of both parties? If the broker is an employee of the system, might there be a tendency to represent the interests of the system more than those of the consumer? The answer is yes in some respects, but there are also attributes of a successful culture broker, such as, a willingness to be a risk taker, the ability to tolerate ambiguous situations, and a degree of comfort functioning at the boundaries of different systems. Such attributes may be acquired through years of experience, but the learning process should begin as students. (For a more detailed description of this culture brokering model, including its applications to case studies, see Jezewski and Sotnik, 2004.)

Cultural competence training, if it lives up to its promise of improving the provision of services, will be a step toward relieving the disparities that exist in the current system (Giger et al., 2007). However, caution within training programs should be exercised. Knowledge of various cultures and their practices, if not considered within the context of individuals and their unique circumstances, can result in destructive stereotyping. Stereotypes that are associated with particular cultures may affect service provision in adverse ways. Therefore, although knowledge of cultures is important, service providers must refrain from stereotyping and be constantly aware of the heterogeneity of persons within cultural groups (Campinha-Bacote, 2002; Juckett, 2005).

In our experience, we have found that courses that emphasize communication and therapeutic interaction offer opportunities for exploration and an understanding of one's own culture. These courses are usually taught to students prior to acceptance into a professional program or during the first year. Assignments that are specific to cultural awareness may include a class exercise in which students write about their individual ethnicity/racial background. This leads to a class discussion about cultural awareness, stereotyping, and variations among cultures. Several classroom activities may also be used to help students develop an appreciation of their cultural awareness. Self-assessment questionnaires and surveys encourage student self-reflection and lead to group discussions and the development of cultural awareness, cultural sensitivity, and an appreciation for diversity (Spence-Cagle, 2006). Several activities that enhance student self-awareness include the self-test questionnaire: "Assessing your transcultural communication goals and basic knowledge" and the "Cultural Values Questionnaire" (Luckman, 2000). The Village of 100 (Meadows, 2005); the Implicit Association Test in which the student selects a test on skin tone, race, religion, Arab-Muslim, or Asian (Project Implicit, 2007); Body Ritual Among the Nacirema, (American Anthropological Association, 1956); and the Multicultural Sensitivity Scale (MSS; Jibaja, Sebastian, Kingery, & Holcomb, 2000) are classroom activities that target students' awareness of their cultural backgrounds and lead to lively discussions.

After cultural awareness exercises, students can progress to the development of knowledge about other cultures. Encounters in nontraditional settings offer opportunities for students to try out new skills with clients from diverse cultures with guidance and feedback from their instructors (Hunt, 2007; Luckman, 2000; Purnell & Paulanka, 2003). Students may increase their knowledge about different cultures by visiting ethnically diverse neighborhoods, exploring ethnic supermarkets and restaurants, attending religious services that are different from their own religious backgrounds, and observing programs in ethnically and racially diverse neighborhood community centers (Hunt & Swiggum, 2007; Jeffreys, 2006; Luckman). These introductory observational opportunities should be set up as nonthreatening encounters that lead to self-reflection through written assignments and group discussions (Hunt & Swiggum). A by-product of this self-reflective process is the development of an appreciation for ethnic diversity, religious practices, food preferences, family values, health beliefs, and neighborhood/community programs (Griswold et al., 2007). Furthermore, encounters in ethnically and racially diverse settings allow the student to develop confidence when encountering clients from diverse backgrounds (Hunt & Swiggum).

The acquisition of knowledge about specific cultures can be approached in several ways. Students can access an online monograph series (Stone, 2001-2003). The monographs focus on the top 10 countries of origin of the foreign-born population in the United States according to the U.S. Census Bureau: Mexico, China, Philippines, India, Vietnam, Dominican Republic, Korea, El Salvador, Jamaica, and Cuba. There is an additional monograph on the culture of Haiti. Assignments can be provided using a case study format with the monograph series as a resource.

Prior to the clinical encounters, the use of case studies are also helpful in developing clinical decision making, self-reflection, and examining ethical dilemmas

(Spence-Cagle, 2006). The case study format has been used to help students to process, problem-solve, and apply strategies that will enhance their knowledge of culturally competent service (Lattanzi & Purnell, 2006; Stone, 2004). Therefore, case studies encourage the examination of the professionals' explanatory model and the client's explanation of their disability experience and help to develop culture-brokering skills and allow for the appreciation of various belief systems (Jezewski & Sotnik, 2004; Kleinman, 1988).

Students must then be provided with clinical encounters that allow for the development of skills when working with clients from diverse cultures (Campinha-Bacote, 2002). Neighborhood community centers, schools, and adult day care facilities are several examples of potential sites that may offer diversity and contribute to students' fieldwork experiences (Griswold et al., 2007; Hunt & Swiggum, 2007).

Through observations and clinical encounters, students develop and expand on their interviewing techniques, including the use of interpreters, the ability to become flexible with traditional assessment procedures, and an appreciation for the client's narrative (Hunt & Swiggum, 2007). The personal narrative and listening to the client's story are best learned through clinical encounters (Griswold et al., 2007; Kripaiani et al., 2006). Students must learn when to leave aside traditional assessment procedures and encourage clients to describe their disability experience in their own words (Griswold et al.; Kleinman, 1997). The person's view of disability does not necessarily surface when using standardized assessments that are popular among professionals (Ayonrinde 2003; Becker, Beyene, Newsom, & Rodgers, 1998).

In order to understand the participant's perception of disability, interviewers can use a modified version of Kleinmans' eight questions and incorporate them into their interview schedule. The questions help the provider understand the clients' explanatory model by asking what caused their disability and what it means to them (Kleinman, 1988).

There are many factors that should be considered by rehabilitation providers in culturally diverse settings, and a number of these should be elaborated on and examined in depth in the academic setting. Examples are:

- Cultures vary on their expectation of formality in clinical situations. For example, Asian Americans may be more formal, especially elders (Liu, 2004; Wells & Black, 2000). Thus, clinical encounters should reflect this style of interaction.
- Some cultural groups communicate in ways that are different from the direct style of communication favored by Americans. For example, some cultures communicate in a less direct manner and rely on the context and subtleties in style to get their message across (Jezewski & Sotnik, 2004).
- Many Latin and Middle Eastern cultures do not value time in the same way as Americans. They may prioritize personal commitments over time commitments

in business encounters or in adherence to clinical appointments (Sotnik & Jezewski, 2004).

- Some cultures, for example those of the Middle East, expect long greetings and inquiries about family members and their states of health. They may also expect offerings of food and drink (Ahmad et al., 2006).

- The assistance of an interpreter should be used to facilitate communication; however, family members should not be used in this role, if possible. The dual role of family member and interpreter may cause conflict, and valuable information may be omitted (Dyck, 1992). Clinicians must become familiar with techniques on how to use an interpreter and seek interpreters who are well-trained and artful in the subtle negotiation process between client and provider (Ayonrinde, 2003).

- In some cultures, such as the Hmong, a husband or oldest son will make decisions for all members of the clan. The individual's wishes are deferred to a designated member in the clan (Leonard & Plotnikoff, 2000). Thus, it is important to ascertain who the primary decision maker in the family is and enlist his or her help in the diagnostic and rehabilitation process.

- Certain occupations and daily activities may be defined in ways that are not familiar to the provider. For example, some cultures prioritize certain daily activities (e.g., hygiene, dressing, and eating) whereas others do not (Zemke & Clark, 1996).

- Assessment tools that evaluate individual differences and preferences, including the personal narrative, should be included in the rehabilitation process (Clark, 1993).

Measurement of Cultural Competence

Although the Campinha-Bacote model, the Purnell model, Jeffrey's model of self-efficacy and the cultural-brokering model offer guidelines for cultural competence curricula, the literature on outcomes related to cultural competence training in rehabilitation is sparse. In order to ensure that the curriculum is reflecting the diverse and changing needs of the population, rehabilitation programs must find a way to evaluate the content of their programs (Black & Purnell, 2002; Lie, Boker, & Cleveland, 2006). In this section we will identify assessment tools that are used to measure cultural competence across various disciplines and are suitable for use in rehabilitation preservice programs (refer to Table 11-1 for a summary of the assessment tools).

Table 11-1 Models and Measures of Cultural Competence

Model	Assessment	Summary of Assessment Measures
Campinha-Bacote model *Description:* Cultural competence consists of five constructs: cultural awareness, cultural knowledge, cultural skill, cultural encounters, and cultural desire.	Inventory for Assessing the Process of Cultural Competence Among Health Care Professionals-Revised (IAPCC-R; Campinha-Bacote, 2003)	The IAPPC-R consists of 25 items that measure these cultural constructs. The IAPPC-R uses a 4-point Likert scale. The IAPCC-R takes approximately 10–15 minutes to complete. The IAPCC-R is copyrighted and permission to use the tool is required. It can be ordered through the website, *www.transculturalcare.net*
Jeffrey's Cultural Competence and Confidence model (CCC) *Description:* Cultural competence is an ongoing process, integration of cognitive, practical, and affective domains develop transcultural self-efficacy (confidence).	Transcultural Self-Efficacy Tool (TSET; Jeffreys, 2006)	The TSET is an 83-item pencil and paper assessment. Students rate their confidence on a Likert scale ranging from 1 = no confidence to 10 = totally confident. The TSET takes approximately 25 minutes to complete. Different methods can be used to rate scores to reflect high, medium, or low self-efficacy.
Purnell's model for cultural competence *Description:* The macro aspects of this model consider the global society, community, family, and person. Micro aspects of this model include 12 domains common to all cultures including: communication, healthcare practices, family roles, heritage, and spirituality.	No specific tool	

(continued)

Table 11-1 Models and Measures of Cultural Competence (continued)

Model	Assessment	Summary of Assessment Measures
Culture brokering model *Description:* Identifies three stages—Problem identification, intervention strategies, and evaluating outcomes. Intervention strategies include: advocating, negotiating, and mediating. Must consider intervening conditions during analysis of the problem and when developing strategies to evaluate outcomes.	No specific tool. Outcomes are accomplished when connections between consumers and the rehabilitation system are achieved.	
No model	Tool for Assessing Cultural Competence Training (TACCT)	Student's knowledge, attitudes, and skills are defined across five domains: cultural competence rationale, context, and definition; key aspects of cultural competence; impact of stereotyping on decisions; and health disparities and cross-cultural clinical skills. A binary response, "yes" or "no" is recorded by each participant for all 67 items. The approximate time allotted for completion is about 20 minutes. The TACCT is available through the Web site *http://www.aamc.org/meded/tacct/*
No model	Cultural Awareness Questionnaire (CAQ; Cheung, Shah, & Muncer, 2002)	The assessment consists of 4 sections: (1) demographic information; (2) 10 statements relating to cultural issues, education, and fieldwork, scored on a 5-point Likert scale; (3) students perceived degree of cultural competence (rated on a continuum of 1–12), and (4) student comments. The CAQ has been used to assess occupational therapy students' awareness of cultural issues and their educational experiences.

Table 11-1 Models and Measures of Cultural Competence (continued)

Model	Assessment	Summary of Assessment Measures
Cultural competence model Description: The model encompasses four interrelated but separate elements (cultural identity, cultural awareness, cultural sensitivity, and cultural competence).	Cultural Competence Assessment (CCA; Schim, Doorenbos, Miller, & Benkert, 2003)	The self-report questionnaire has 25 items with two subscales, cultural awareness and cultural sensitivity (CAS), and cultural competence behaviors (CCB). The CCA is scored using a 5-point Likert scale; scores can range from 25–125. Higher scores indicate a higher degree of cultural competence.

One study used The Tool for Assessing Cultural Competence Training (TACCT) to compare faculty and third year medical students' perception of cultural competence training (Lie et al., 2006). The TACCT

> ... encompasses content items representing students' knowledge, attitudes, and skills for five domains: cultural competence rationale, context, and definition; key aspects of cultural competence; the impact of stereotyping on medical decision-making; health disparities and factors influencing health; and cross-cultural clinical skills. (Lie et al., p. 558)

A binary response, "yes" or "no" is recorded by each participant for all 67 items under the 5 specified domains on the TACCT. The approximate time allotted for completion of the TACCT is about 20 minutes (Lie et al., 2006). Lie et al. found that faculty and medical students' responses were similar in that they agreed on the amount and content of cultural competence instruction that was taught. Researchers concluded that TACCT is a useful tool in helping to identify gaps in curricula that address cultural competence training.

The Transcultural Self-Efficacy Tool (TSET) was developed to measure nursing students' confidence in performing nursing duties for culturally diverse patients (Jeffreys, 2006). After an extensive review of the literature and item assessment (Jeffreys & Smodlaka, 1996), the TSET was divided into three subscales: cognitive (25 items), practical (30 items), and affective (28 items) with a total of 83 items. Students rate their confidence on a Likert scale ranging from 1 = no confidence to 10 = totally confident. Approximately 25 minutes should be allotted to complete the TSET. Different methods can be used to rate participant's scores to reflect high, medium, or low self-efficacy. The most common method is to calculate the mean score for the subscale item responses to assess self-efficacy strengths (Jeffreys).

Content and construct validity was established for TSET (Jeffreys & Smodlaka, 1996), and a factor analysis showed that all items contribute to the conceptual framework of self-efficacy further verifying the construct validity of the instrument (Jeffreys, 2006). High estimates of reliability (internal consistency) were found for the whole instrument and the identified factors across several studies (Cronbach's alpha ranging from 0.92 to 0.98; Jeffreys). The TSET, with minor adaptations for rehabilitation professionals, shows value and can be used to measure confidence in areas of knowledge (cognition), application of assessment skills, and the development of self-awareness and acceptance.

The Inventory for Assessing the Process of Cultural Competence Among Healthcare Professionals-Revised (IAPCC-R) was developed by Campinha-Bacote (2003) and is designed to measure the level of cultural competence among students in the health professions. It consists of 20 items that measure confidence on the 5 cultural constructs associated with the Campinha-Bacote model: cultural awareness, cultural knowledge, cultural skill, cultural encounters, and cultural desire. The IAPCC-R is a pencil and paper test that takes approximately 15 minutes to administer. Students rate their answers using a 4-point Likert scale. Responses range from "strongly agree" to "strongly disagree." High scores depict a higher level of confidence.

Several reliability studies of the IAPCC-R have been conducted among a variety of health professionals. Gulas (2005) conducted a study among physical therapy students and the results showed a Cronbach's alpha of .78 and a Gutman split-half of .77. Stephen (2006) examined the responses of 52 providers including occupational therapists, physical therapists, social workers, and other disciplines prior to a multicultural panel discussion at 2 and 6 months later. Reliability results were Cronbach alpha of .72, pretest, and .87, 6 months posttest. Luquis and Perez (2005) found the reliability coefficient were Cronbach's alpha of .849 and a Guttman split-half of .829 among 455 health educators using a modified version of the IAPCC-R.

Cheung et al. (2002) developed the Cultural Awareness Questionnaire (CAQ) to assess occupational therapy students' perceptions of cultural issues and their level of cultural awareness. The questionnaire consists of four sections. The first section includes questions on demographic data, the second section consists of 10 statements, and students rate their responses on a 5-point Likert scale. The third section requires the participant to rate their degree of cultural awareness on a continuum from 1–12, and the fourth section has a "further comments" section that can be used for qualitative analysis. Section Two statements are divided into three categories: occupational therapy trends, the impact of cultural influences, and student beliefs about their occupational therapy education. The majority of students in this study, 88%, stated they had limited awareness of other cultures and limited resources about other cultures. The students were aware of the growth of cultural influences but were concerned about their own lack of cultural exposure (Cheung et al.). Rasmussen, Lloyd, and Wielandt (2005) report low reliability, Cronbach alpha .69, on statements

2 through 5 on the scale. Further investigation is needed on the reliability and validity of this tool for use among other rehabilitation disciplines. Although this study was conducted in England and replicated in Australia, it shows value and has the potential to be used in the United States, especially since all three countries have large influxes of immigrant populations in common.

The Cultural Competence Assessment (CCA) was developed by Schim et al. (2003) and was based on their model of cultural competency. Four elements of the model (cultural identity, cultural awareness, cultural sensitivity, and cultural competence) are joined together to form an analogous jigsaw puzzle (Doorenbos, Schim, Benkert, & Borse, 2005). The CCA is a pencil and paper survey that takes about 20–30 minutes to complete. The subscales of the CCA rate responses differently. The subscale for cultural diversity asks the respondent to identify various groups that they have encountered within the past 12 months and record this on a single-item index. Cultural awareness and cultural sensitivity (CAS) subscales and cultural competence behaviors (CCB) are measured using a 5-point Likert scale. Reliability and validity testing was conducted with 113 hospice providers. Internal consistency ratings were .92, internal consistency for subscales of cultural competence behaviors were .93, and cultural awareness and sensitivity were .75. Construct validity was established by factor analysis. In addition, there were significant moderate correlations when CCA scores were compared to the IAPCC scores, thus establishing validity between two instruments that have similar key constructs (Doorenbos et al.).

The CCA was also found to be sensitive enough to capture differences in cultural competence training among hospice workers and among healthcare workers from different disciplines (Schim et al., 2003). Doorenbos et al. (2005) found the CCA to show a high correlation for test-retest reliability ($r = .85$, $p = .002$) when examining responses from 405 healthcare providers. They also found the CCA to show strong reliability, Cronbach's alpha was .89, using items from the CAS and CCB subscales. This assessment was developed for use among various healthcare professions and shows possibilities for use in rehabilitation preservice programs.

In conclusion, scales that identify provider confidence and that assess the results of cultural instruction will help to identify whether service provider curricula have been successful in cultural competence training. The TACCT is useful for assessing cultural competence in educational programs and identifying gaps. Reliability studies using the CAQ across other rehabilitation disciplines will contribute to the usefulness of this assessment. The TSET is unique in that it measures not only the student's awareness of their own cultural background; it also assesses the student's awareness and understanding of the client's cultural background. In addition the TSET measures the student's level of confidence within a variety of cultural situations (Jeffreys, 2006). An advantage of the TSET, IAPCC-R, and CCA is that they are associated with a model that provides a theoretical basis and a guiding framework for the use of the assessment. Both the TSET and the TACCT are currently being used to assess cultural competence training for the CIRRIE project.

IMPLICATIONS FOR FUTURE RESEARCH

The measurement of cultural competence training in preservice rehabilitation programs is of the utmost importance. We must be able to answer the question, "Have we effectively prepared students for the diversity that they will encounter as entry level professionals?" Our programs should provide a realistic link between education and clinical practice. This can be done by first identifying gaps in the curricula. Such gaps in the curricula should be the concern of all teaching faculty. Information on students' and faculty's perception of cultural competence instruction can be identified by using the TACCT. The measurement of students' confidence with persons from other cultures can be investigated by using the TSET. Students' perception of their cultural competence training and its implications for future practice can be measured though the use of the IAPCC-R and the CAQ. Since most rehabilitation programs offer various levels of fieldwork experience, many of the assessments, the TSET, CAS, CAQ, and the IAPCC-R, can be administered after this experience.

Data that are collected and analyzed should be distributed to other rehabilitation programs through publications in peer-reviewed journals and presentations at national and international conferences. Continued growth in areas of assessment and outcome measurement for cultural competence training will improve the quality of our rehabilitation programs.

IMPLICATIONS FOR EDUCATIONAL PRACTICE

Teaching Cultural Competence in University Rehabilitation Programs

This section describes an approach to incorporating cultural competence training in university programs that prepare professionals in rehabilitation counseling, physical therapy, occupational therapy, and speech therapy. The CIRRIE developed and is testing curricula and curriculum materials for these fields. The current work with preservice university training, complements previous CIRRIE publications; most notably a 13-volume monograph series, *The Rehabilitation Service Provider's Guide to the Cultures of the Foreign Born* (Stone, 2001–2003) and a book that summarized the series (Stone, 2004).

The CIRRIE approach to cultural competence at the university level includes four main principles: (1) integrating cultural competency into existing courses, rather than creating new courses; (2) developing cultural competence curricula that is profession-specific, rather than generic; (3) providing multidisciplinary case studies; and (4) making materials available to instructors.

Integrating Cultural Competency into Existing Courses, Rather than the Creation of New Courses

Although the academic credentialing standards for programs in the rehabilitation professions now require cultural competence, the curricula of most programs are already overloaded. This makes it difficult to add new courses. More importantly, a separate course on cultural competence makes the topic appear to students to be isolated from the "real" set of professional skills that they are required to master. Students may consider it an interesting topic but one of little practical importance. Moreover, by separating cultural competence from courses that develop practice skills, it becomes abstract and difficult to relate to practice.

Another reason for integrating cultural competence into existing courses is that students have an opportunity to see its implications and apply its principles in a variety of contexts. They also see that it is not just a special interest of one faculty member, but an integral part of many aspects of their future practice. As it reappears in their coursework each semester, their knowledge, attitudes, and skills in this area develop and deepen. The CIRRIE curriculum development effort has identified specific courses in the curricula of these programs where cultural competence is most relevant, and CIRRIE is working with faculty to develop activities and materials that are appropriate for each course.

Developing Cultural Competence Curricula that is Profession-Specific, Rather than Generic

CIRRIE's prior experience with providing cultural competency workshops for in-service training strongly suggested that an off-the-shelf generic approach is less effective than training that is specific to the profession in which the competence is to be applied. Generic training must be understandable by all the rehabilitation professions, so the specific terminology or concepts of each profession must be avoided. As a result, cultural competence becomes more abstract. With profession-specific training, students are better able to see its relevance and applicability to their profession, not as something outside its mainstream. Consequently, CIRRIE's approach is to work with faculty from each profession to analyze their curriculum and incorporate cultural competence into it in ways that seem most relevant to that profession.

Providing Multidisciplinary Case Studies

Although CIRRIE's general approach is profession-specific, we have found that studies developed in one program can sometimes be adapted for use in other programs. For example, a case scenario developed for a course in physical therapy may be useful in courses in occupational therapy, speech therapy, or rehabilitation counseling. The general facts of the case may be presented to students from each program, but many of the problems, questions, and assignments related to the case may be different for each of the professions. The use of common case studies provides an opportunity to analyze cultural factors from a multidisciplinary perspective, which is often the type of setting in which rehabilitation is practiced.

Making Materials Available to Instructors

Most instructors realize the need for the infusion of culture into their curricula but they may be reticent to incorporate culture into their current classroom structure if the burden of creating new materials is added to their course preparation. CIRRIE has approached this dilemma through specific strategies to allow instructors easy access to cultural content. A Web site was created in order to organize cultural materials into interdisciplinary and discipline-specific assignments, case studies, lectures, reference materials, and classroom activities. Faculty representatives from four rehabilitation professions contributed to the Web site and information is exchanged across disciplines and is available for other faculty members. CIRRIE has published curriculum guides for cultural competence within the curricula of physical therapy, occupational therapy, and speech therapy, as well as rehabilitation counseling. These guides may be accessed at *http://cirrie.buffalo.edu/curriculum/*.

CONCLUSION

It is sometimes questioned whether cultural competence can be taught or whether it can be acquired only through experience. It is true that cultural competence instruction is much different than much of the rehabilitation curricula, which are quite technical. Much of rehabilitation practice, especially in the therapeutic professions, focuses on the application of scientific knowledge. Cultural competence is less straightforward and does not yet have a strong evidence base. Teaching cultural competence can be challenging for several reasons. First, most instructors did not receive instruction in cultural competence when they were students, so they do not have a clear model. Second, cultural competence is not defined or assessed with the same precision as other areas of the curriculum. It is our position that students can begin to acquire cultural competence in their university programs, even when instruction may not be ideal. It is hoped that some of the discussion and resources mentioned in this chapter will be useful to instructors as we attempt to better develop this challenging aspect of our rehabilitation curricula.

REFERENCES

Aceron, S., & Savage, T. A. (2004). Factors affecting the adjustment to disability for new immigrants. *Topics in Stroke Rehabilitation, 11*(3), 67–75.

Agency for Healthcare Research and Quality. (2004). *Setting the agenda for research on cultural competence in healthcare.* Washington, DC: U.S. Department of Health and Human Services, Retrieved March 11, 2007, from *http://www.ahrq.gov/research/cultural2.htm*

Ahmad, O. S., Alsharif, N. Z., & Royeen, M. (2006). Arab Americans. In M. Royeen & J. L. Crabtree (Eds.), *Culture in rehabilitation* (pp. 181–202). Upper Saddle River, NJ: Pearson Education.

Alba, R., & Nee, V. (2003). *Remaking the American mainstream.* Cambridge, MA: Harvard University Press.

American Anthropological Association. (1956). Body ritual among the Nacirema. *American Anthropologist, 58*(3), 503–507.

Amnesty International. (2006, June). *Chad/Sudan: Sowing the seeds of Darfur: Ethnic targeting in Chad by Janjawid militias from Sudan.* Retrieved April 29, 2007, from *http://web.amnesty.org/pages/sdn-290606-editorial-eng*

Ayonrinde, O. (2003). Importance of cultural sensitivity in therapeutic transactions: Considerations for healthcare providers. *Disability Management and Health Outcomes, 11*(4), 234–246.

Becker, G., Beyene, Y., Newsom, E., & Rodgers, D. (1998). Knowledge and care of chronic illness in three ethnic minority groups. *Family Medicine, 30,* 173–178.

Black, J. D., & Purnell, L. D. (2002). Cultural competence for the physical therapy professional. *Journal of Physical Therapy Education, 16*(1), 3–10.

Bonder, B. R. (2001). Growing old in the United States. In B. R. Bonder, & M. Wagner (Eds.), *Functional performance in older adults* (2nd ed., pp. 7–27). Philadelphia: F. A. Davis.

Campinha-Bacote, J. (2002). The process of cultural competence in the delivery of healthcare services: a model of care. *Journal of Transcultural Nursing, 13*(3), 181–184.

Campinha-Bacote, J. (2003). *The process of cultural competence in the delivery of healthcare services* (4th ed.). Cincinnati, OH: Transcultural CARE Associates Press.

Campinha-Bacote, J. (2007). The process of cultural competence in the delivery of healthcare services (5th ed.). Retrieved September 20, 2008, from *http://www.transculturalcare.net/Resources.htm*

Cheung, Y., Shah, S., & Muncer, S. (2002). An exploratory investigation of undergraduate studentsí perceptions of cultural awareness. *British Journal of Occupational Therapy, 65*(12), 543–550.

Clark, F. (1993). Occupation embedded in a real life: interweaving occupational science and occupational therapy. *American Journal of Occupational Therapy, 47*(12), 1067–1078.

Doorenbos, A. Z., Schim, S. M., Benkert, R., & Borse, N. N. (2005). Psychometric evaluation of the cultural competence assessment instrument among healthcare providers. *Nursing Research, 54*(5), 324–331.

Dyck, I. (1992). Managing chronic illness: an immigrant womanís acquisition and use of healthcare knowledge. *American Journal of Occupational Therapy, 46*(8), 696–705.

Eisenman, D., Gelberg, L., Liu, H., & Shapiro, M. (2003). Mental health and health-related quality of life among adult Latino primary care patients living in the United States with previous exposure to political violence. *Journal of the American Medical Association, 290*(5), 627–634.

Giger, J., Davidhizar, R. E., Purnell, L., Harden, J. T., Phillips, J., & Strickland, O. (2007). American academy of nursing expert panel report: developing cultural competence to eliminate health disparities in ethnic minorities and other vulnerable populations. *Journal of Transcultural Nursing, 18*(2), 95–102.

Griswold, K., Zayas, L., Kernan, J. B., & Wagner, C. M. (2007). Cultural awareness through medical student and refugee patient encounters. *Journal of Immigrant and Minority Health, 9,* 55–60.

Groce, N. (1999). Health beliefs and behavior towards individuals with disability cross-culturally. In R. Leavitt (Ed.), *Cross-cultural rehabilitation: An international perspective* (pp. 37–47). Philadelphia: W. B. Saunders.

Groce, N. (2004). Immigrants, disability and rehabilitation. In J. H. Stone (Ed.) *Culture and disability: Providing culturally competent services* (pp. 1–14). Thousand Oaks, CA: Sage.

Groce, N. E., & Zola, I. K. (1993). Multiculturalism, chronic illness, and disability. *Pedicatrics, 91*(5), 1048–1055.

Gulas, C. (2005). *Establishing the reliability of using The Inventory For Assessing The Process of Cultural Competence Among Healthcare Professionals with physical therapy students.* Unpublished doctoral dissertation, Saint Louis University, Saint Louis, MO.

Hasnain, R., Shaikh, L., & Shanawani, H. (2008). Disability and Islam: an introduction for rehabilitation and healthcare providers. *Monograph series for the Center for International Rehabilitation Research Information and Exchange (CIRRIE).* Buffalo, NY: CIRRIE.

Hughes, K. H., & Hood, L. J. (2007). Teaching methods and an outcome tool for measuring cultural sensitivity in undergraduate nursing students. *Journal of Transcultural Nursing, 18*(7), 57–62.

Hunt, R. (2007). *Beyond relativism: Comparability in cultural anthropology.* Lanham, MD: Rowman Altamira.

Hunt, R., & Swiggum, P. (2007). Being in another world: Transcultural experiences using service learning with families who are homeless. *Journal of Transcultural Nursing, 18*(2), 167–174.

Institute of Medicine. (2002). *Unequal treatment: What healthcare providers need to know about racial and ethnic disparities in health-care.* Washington, DC: National Academy Press.

Jacobson, E. (2004). An introduction to Haitian culture for rehabilitation service providers. In J. H. Stone (Ed.), *Culture and disability: Providing culturally competent services* (pp. 139–159). New York: Sage.

Jeffreys, M. R. (2006). *Teaching cultural competence in nursing and healthcare: Inquiry, action, and innovation.* New York: Springer.

Jeffreys, M., & Smodlaka, I. (1996). Steps of the instrument design process: An illustrative approach for nurse educators. *Nursing Education, 21*(6), 47–52.

Jezewski, M. A. (1990). Culture brokering in migrant farm worker healthcare. *Western Journal of Nursing Research, 12*(4), 497–513.

Jezewski, M. A., & Sotnik, P. (2004). Disability service providers as culture brokers. In J. H. Stone (Ed.), *Culture and disability: Providing culturally competent services* (pp. 31–64). New York: Sage.

Jibaja, M. L., Sebastian, R., Kingery, P., & Holcomb, J. D. (2000). The multicultural sensitivity of physician assistant students. *Journal of Allied Health, 29*(2), 79–85.

Jones, M. E., Cason, C. L., & Bond, M. L. (2004). Cultural attitudes, knowledge, and skills of a health workforce. *Journal of Transcultural Nursing, 15*(4), 283–290.

Juckett, G. (2005). Cross-cultural medicine. *American Family Physician, 72*(11), 2267–2275.

Kleinman, A. (1988). *The Illness narratives; Suffering, healing, and the human condition.* New York: Basic Books.

Kleinman, A. (1997). "Everything that really matters": social suffering, subjectivity, and the remaking of human experience in a disordered world. *The Harvard Theological Review, 90*, 315–335.

Kripaiani, S., Bussey-Jones, J., Katz, M. G., & Genao, I. (2006). A prescription for cultural competence in medical education. *Journal of General Internal Medicine, 21*(11), 1116–1120.

Lattanzi, J., & Purnell, L. (2006). Introducing cultural concepts. In J. Lattanzi & L. Purnell (Eds.), *Developing cultural competence in physical therapy practice* (pp. 2–20). Philadelphia: F. A. Davis.

Leal-Idrogo, A. (1997). Multicultural rehabilitation counseling. *Rehabilitation Education, 11*(3), 231–240.

Leavitt, R. (1999). Introduction. In R. Leavitt (Ed.), *Cross–cultural rehabilitation: An international perspective* (pp. 1–7). London: W.B. Saunders.

Leonard, B. J., & Plotnikoff, G. A. (2000). Awareness: the heart of cultural competence. *American Association of Critical Care Nurses, Clinical Issues, 11*(1), 51–59.

Lie, D., Boker, J., & Cleveland, E. (2006). Using the tool for assessing cultural competence training (TACCT) to measure faculty and medical student perceptions of cultural competence instruction in the first three years of the curriculum. *Academic Medicine, 81*, 557–564.

Liu, G. Z. (2004). Best practices: Developing cross-cultural competence from a Chinese perspective. In J. H. Stone (Ed.), *Culture and disability: Providing culturally competent services* (pp. 65–86). New York: Sage.

Lopez-De Fede, A. (2004). An introduction to the culture of the Dominican Republic for disability service providers. In J. H. Stone (Ed.), *Culture and disability: Providing culturally competent services* (pp. 187–201). New York: Sage.

Luckman, J. (2000). *Transcultural communication in healthcare.* Albany, NY: Delmar Thompson Learning.

Luquis, R. R., & Perez, M. A. (2005). Health educators and cultural competence: Implications for the profession. *American Journal of Health Studies, 20*(3), 156–163.

McGruder, J. (2003). Culture, race, ethnicity, and other forms of human diversity. In E. Crepeau, E. Cohn, & B. A. Schell (Eds.), *Willard & Spackmanís Occupational Therapy* (10th ed., pp. 81–95). Philadelphia: Lippincott Williams & Wilkins.

Meadows, D. (2005). State of the village report. Retrieved June 15, 2007, from *http://www .sustainer.org/dhmdhm_archive/index.php?display_article=vn338villageed*

National Center for Cultural Competence. (2004). *Bridging the cultural divide in healthcare settings: the essential role of culture broker programs.* Washington, DC: Georgetown University National Center for Cultural Competence.

Pachter, L. M. (1994). Culture and clinical care: folk illness beliefs and behaviors and their implications for healthcare delivery. *The Journal of the American Medical Association, 271*(9), 690–694.

Patternson, J. B., & Spry, J. (2007). Ethical issues in diversity. In P. Leung, C. R. Flowers , W. B. Talley, & P. R. Sanderson (Eds.), *Multicultural issues in rehabilitation and allied health* (pp. 45–63). Linn Creek, MO: Aspen Professional Services.

Pernell-Arnold, A. (1998). Multiculturalism: myths and miracles. *Psychiatric Rehabilitation Journal, 21*(3), 224–230.

Polgreen, L. (2007, April 15). Militia talks could reshape conflict in Darfur. *The New York Times*, pp. 1–4.

Project Implicit. (2007). *The Implicit association test.* Retrieved May 30, 2007, from *https://implicit .harvard.edu/implicit/demo/takeatest.html*

Purnell, L. D., & Paulanka, B. J. (2003). *Transcultural healthcare: A culturally competent approach.* Philadelphia: F. A. Davis.

Rasmussen, T. M., Lloyd, C., & Wielandt, T. (2005). Cultural awareness among Queensland under-graduate occupational therapy students. *Australian Occupational Therapy Journal, 52*, 302–310.

Santana-Martin, S., & Santana, F. O. (2004). An introduction to Mexican culture for service providers. In J. H. Stone (Ed.), *Culture and disability: Providing culturally competent services* (pp. 161–186). New York: Sage.

Schim, S. M., Doorenbos, A. Z., Miller, J., & Benkert, R. (2003). Development of a cultural compe-tence assessment instrument. *Journal of Nursing Measurement, 11*(1) 29–40.

Slater, S. (2007). Workforce issues in communication sciences and disorders. In R. Lubinski, L. C. Golper, & C. Frattali (Eds.). *Professional issues in speech-language pathology and audiology* (3rd ed., pp. 141–157). Clifton Park, NY: Thomson.

Sotnik, P., & Jezewski, M. A. (2004). Culture and disability services. In J. H. Stone (Ed.), *Culture and disability: Providing culturally competent services* (pp. 15–30). New York: Sage.

Spence-Cagle, C. (2006). Student understanding of culturally and ethically responsive care: impli-cations for nursing curricula. *Nursing Education Perspectives, 27*(6), 308–314.

Stephen, J. (2006). *The effect of a multi-cultural panel discussion on cultural competence of health system employees.* Forth Worth, TX: Cook Childrenís Medical Center.

Stone, J. (Ed.). (2001–2003). *The rehabilitation service provideris guide to the cultures of the foreign born* (monograph series). Buffalo, NY: CIRRIE.

Stone, J. (2004). Understanding immigrants with disabilities. In J. H. Stone (Ed.), *Culture and dis-ability: Providing culturally competent services* (pp. 225–230). New York: Sage.

Thompson, T., & Blasquez, E. (2006). The smorgasbord of the Hispanic cultures. In M. Royeen & J. L. Crabtree (Eds.), *Culture in rehabilitation* (pp. 218–241). Upper Saddle River, NJ: Pearson Education.

Wells, S. A., & Black, R. M. (2000). *Cultural competency for health professionals.* Bethesda, MD: AOTA.

Whiteford, G. E. (2005). Understanding the occupational deprivation of refugees: A case study. *Canadian Journal of Occupational Therapy, 72*(2), 78–88.

Wilson, K., Whittaker, T., & Black, V. (2007). Case management and vocational rehabilitation coun-seling. In P. Leung, C. Flowers, W. Talley, & P. Sanderson. (Eds.), *Multicultural issues in rehabilita-tion and allied health.* Linn Creek, MO: Aspen Professional Services.

Zemke, R. F. C., & Clark, F. (1996). Defining and classifying. In R. F. C. Zemke and F. Clark (Eds). *Occupational Science: the evolving discipline* (pp. 43–46). Philadelphia: F. A. Davis.

CHAPTER 12

A Three-Dimensional Model for Multicultural Rehabilitation Counseling

Allen N. Lewis, PhD, CRC;
Aisha Shamburger, MS, CRC

INTRODUCTION

This chapter introduces the Three-Dimensional Model,[1] which is a conceptual framework of multicultural counseling. The Three-Dimensional Model is a tool that counselors develop for themselves to help them determine where to go, what to look for, and what to do in order to provide effective services to people with disabilities who are culturally different from the counselor, making no assumptions about the counselor's cultural orientation. The point is that this tool should be useful when counselor and client are culturally different, a point that arguably could be made about every counselor–client dyad given that each person has a unique cultural orientation based on individualized life experience.

In the public vocational rehabilitation (VR) system, the imperative to effectively serve culturally diverse populations is now a matter of law. The Rehabilitation Act Amendments of 1992 (Section 21) require the state–federal program to become more effective in serving underserved and culturally diverse populations (Rehabilitation Act Amendments). As such, we offer the Three–Dimensional Model as a tool that counselors, within the VR system as well as in other areas of rehabilitation, can use to guide and inform their cross-cultural work with individuals with disabilities from

[1]Adapted with permission from Lewis, A. N. (2006). The Three-factor Model of multicultural counseling for consumers with disabilities. *Journal of Vocational Rehabilitation*, 24(3), 151–159, with permission from IOS Press.

different cultural backgrounds. This chapter is divided into eight primary sections that present: (1) purpose and origins of the Three-Dimensional Model; (2) domains of the Three-Dimensional Model; (3) rationale of the Three-Dimensional Model; (4) understanding how the model works (four components); (5) development of the Three-Dimensional Model (six steps); (6) strengths of the Three-Dimensional Model; (7) implications for future research; and (8) conclusion.

PURPOSE AND ORIGINS OF THE THREE-DIMENSIONAL MODEL

In simple terms, the Three-Dimensional Model requires counselors to develop their own model for considering: (a) who the person with a disability is in terms of cultural identification, (b) where the person with a disability is developmentally, and (c) how the person with a disability defines optimal adjustment to the disability and where he/she is relative to such optimal adjustment. Once developed, the model is applied in each counseling situation. Such application is aimed at understanding the unique qualities that each person with a disability brings to the counseling situation. While the model offers its user a systematic process for exploration, the outcome of such exploration will be driven by the unique attributes of the service recipient. So, this model's intent is to facilitate the illumination of those unique attributes by ensuring that the counselor has a process that guarantees that such exploration will occur.

The model is predicated on the lead author's experience as a counselor educator and his perspective that two critical components to counselor preparation for multicultural counseling exist: (a) to equip the counselor with a personal awareness of his/her own readiness to counsel across cultural lines, and (b) to encourage counselors to review three critical aspects of the person with a disability's status (cultural identity, stage of development, and adjustment to disability) early in the counseling process. The Three-Dimensional Model is a means to facilitate the counselor's development and use of a thorough and competent approach to the second of these two critical components, the three-part review. If, for either component, the counselor determines that he/she is not equipped to work with a particular person with a disability, enhanced supervision or referral to another counselor can be arranged. If counseling continues, the information derived from this review process will be valuable to counselors in expediting the working alliance that is highly related to positive counseling outcomes (McMahon, Shaw, Chan, & Danczyk-Hawley, 2004).

The Three-Dimensional Model evolved several years ago when the lead author was tasked with developing a course that exposed graduate-level rehabilitation counseling students to two areas: cultural diversity and human development. In the course development process, the author pondered a myriad of options on how to make such a broad topical focus into an experience that would be meaningful for students. Rather than taking an approach that would have resulted in a cursory examination of many topics, and at the end of the course have students attempt to make logical sense of a large mass of information in two broad subject matter areas, the course was designed to focus on exploring the influence of cultural diversity factors and human development on the process of adjusting to a disability. With this focus, it made sense to design a culminating course experience that required students to build their own three-dimensional conceptual model for conducting an adequate assessment of who a person with a disability is in terms of cultural identity, stage of development, and adjustment to disability, all from the person with a disability's point of view. The exploration process for each counselor may be systematic as a starting point, but each counseling assessment situation will progress in a unique manner with the outcome of the process revealing the uniqueness of who the specific person with a disability is in each of the three domains.

DOMAINS OF THE THREE-DIMENSIONAL MODEL

The Three-Dimensional Model is intended to stimulate early consideration of (a) cultural identity, (b) stage of development, and (c) adjustment to disability, when working with people with disabilities who are culturally different from the counselor. The model serves as a conceptual prompt that invokes an intentional and systematic interview process in which a counselor explicitly explores and evaluates these three domains of a person with a disability. The model is flexible in that each counselor is encouraged to develop a unique assessment approach and then adjust it, in terms of sequencing and use of specific techniques, in order to accommodate the uniqueness of each person with a disability and varied professional applications. For example, if the goals or setting relate primarily to career advancement in persons who have a relatively stable and adjusted disability status, developmental considerations may be more important early on than adjustment to disability concerns. If a person with a disability has recently experienced a point-in-time trauma that resulted in a severe functional impairment, the model might suggest more attention be focused on adjustment to disability early on, since fluctuations in relative adjustment may be apparent from one meeting to the next. However, in most situations where a counselor sees a new person with a disability of a different culture, there will be a need to get acquainted with the individual in all three domains.

The Three-Dimensional Model is consistent with current multicultural counseling literature in a manner that is evolutionary, not revolutionary. It explicitly endorses and relies on two of the core multicultural counseling competencies identified by Sue, Arredondo, and McDavis (1992): (a) the counselor understands the worldview of people with disabilities who are culturally different without imposing negative judgments, and (b) the counselor is able to practice appropriately with the person with a disability. The model also draws heavily upon the "common factor" multicultural counseling theory that posits that certain factors cut across all counseling models and are suitable for all cultures (Harper & McFadden, 2003). Among such factors are congruent expectations and a solid working alliance between the counselor and the person with a disability (Harper & McFadden; McMahon et al., 2004).

In addition, the Three-Dimensional Model, with its focus on the counselor getting acquainted with the person with a disability in the three domains, can positively affect the four factors that facilitate rapport between a client and counselor according to Sue et al. (1998). Those four factors are: (a) positive relationship between the person with a disability and the counselor, (b) understanding of the person with a disability's worldview by the counselor, (c) the expectation of a positive outcome of services held by the person with a disability, and (d) the provision of services that respect the worldview and culture of the person with a disability. Some have criticized the relevance of multicultural counseling competencies (Patterson, 2004; Thomas & Weinrach, 2004), but even these researchers maintain that everyone is a multicultural being and that emphasis upon individual-specific uniqueness is important. Thus, the Three-Dimensional Model is consistent with much of the literature, as noted above.

Why are the three domains in the Three-Dimensional Model important in multicultural counseling of persons with disabilities? There is no prior empirical or conceptual work that directly integrates these three concepts (cultural identity, stage of development, and adjustment to disability), which underscores the innovation inherent in this approach. Relatedly, Livneh and Antonak (1997) have proposed an ecological framework that begins to show the interaction between: (a) variables associated with disability, (b) the sociodemographic attributes of the individual, (c) personality characteristics of the individual, and (d) factors associated with physical and social environments. This ecological framework begins to approximate interactions between factors that are somewhat similar to the domains explicit in the Three-Dimensional Model. Specifically, the domain of cultural identity in the Three-Dimensional Model considers factors similar to Livneh and Antonak's sociodemographic attributes of the individual. The domain of stage of development in the Three-Dimensional Model is somewhat related to Livneh and Antonak's (1997) factors associated with physical and social environments. The domain of adjustment to disability in the Three-Dimensional Model takes into account factors similar to Livneh and Antonak's variables associated with disability.

Cultural Identity

Taking each of the three domains separately, cultural identity is important in rehabilitation. The aforementioned legal mandate (i.e., Section 21 of the Rehabilitation

Act Amendments of 1992) is based on the recognition that an individual's race and ethnicity can predict access to public VR services as well as outcomes. The rehabilitation literature contains several authors highlighting the importance of culture in the overall disability experience (e.g., Mpofu & Conyers, 2004; Tower, 2003). Also, current changes in the American demography reflect greater cultural diversification, providing even more reason for understanding the influence of culture on the disability experience. For example, national population data estimates indicate that in the 10 years between the year 2000 and the year 2010, the White population in the United States will increase by 7.2% compared to increases of 12.9% for African Americans, 33.3% for Asians, and 34.1% for Latinos (U.S. Census Bureau, 2004).

Stage of Development

The occurrence of disability is a non-normative event that is unanticipated in normal human development. The *when* of disability, or age of onset, has enormous implications for the ability of an individual to learn and adjust, thus underscoring the importance of human development (Papalia & Olds, 2004). One's development status provides an indication of an individual's ability to respond to predictable life tasks and challenges, which offers a hypothesis about how the individual might respond to the challenge of a disability. Herein is the crux of the importance of the stage of development domain in the Three-Dimensional Model. A developmental perspective adds context to the true impact of the disability (Quinn, 1998), and it requires an ecological orientation that is consistent with rehabilitation principles.

This ecological orientation is exemplified by the concept of the person–environment fit that is integral to the social model of disability, which attributes many of the handicapping effects of disability to structural and attitudinal barriers that are external to the individual (Quinn, 1995; French, 1993; Funk, 1987). Some of these barriers (e.g., pejorative attitudes, biases, and stereotypes) also negatively impact persons who are culturally diverse (Chesler, 1965; Rubin & Roessler, 2001; Yuker, 1965), thus linking cultural identity and stage of development. As such, the inclusion of the role of stage of development in the disability experience in the Three-Dimensional Model makes strong intuitive sense.

Adjustment to Disability

Adjustment to disability is important since the goal of the rehabilitation process is to maximize adjustment (Dell Orto & Power, 2007). All counseling of people with disabilities is intended to advance adjustment not only as a goal in its own right, but to optimize the involvement of persons with disabilities in our society (Gandy, Martin, Hardy, & Cull, 1987; Rubin & Roessler, 2001). The domain of adjustment has been central to the discussion about the disability experience (i.e., Kendall & Buys, 1998; Lustig, Rosenthal, Strauser, & Haynes, 2000; Mpofu & Bishop, 2006; Rothrock, 1999).

RATIONALE OF THE THREE-DIMENSIONAL MODEL

The rationale underlying the Three-Dimensional Model goes beyond the independent value of each of the three domains and fills a void in the current multicultural counseling literature. The multicultural counseling literature contains frameworks and models that primarily speak to multicultural counseling theory (e.g., Harper & McFadden, 2003); multicultural counseling strategy (e.g., Atkinson, 2004); multicultural counseling competency (e.g., Reynolds, 1999; Sue et al., 1992); and the various roles counselors play in successfully counseling across cultural lines (e.g., Atkinson, Thompson, & Grant, 1993; Stone, 2005). However, these contributions of the multicultural counseling literature tend to understate the person with a disability's perspective on his/her stage of development or current level of adjustment to the disability. This understatement is evidenced by the fact that there is no model in the current literature that addresses multicultural counseling theory, strategies, competency, the various roles counselors can play, and also attends to stage of development of the person with a disability and adjustment to disability. The Three-Dimensional Model values each domain (cultural identity, stage of development, and adjustment to disability), and confers equal importance on their interaction and integration. Moreover, the authors found no model in the literature with the inherent flexibility to allow the rehabilitation counselor to develop a model that is customized to his or her own personal counseling style and that has the specific purpose of assessing who the culturally diverse person with a disability is in terms of his/her cultural identity, stage of development, and adjustment to disability. The profile that results is unique to the person with a disability, and the Three-Dimensional Model merely helps to ensure that the counselor has an approach to pursuing this exploration that is pre-planned, systematic, integrated into one's counseling style, and likely to be used because the counselor has developed it. Ultimately, the Three-Dimensional Model helps to improve the quality and effectiveness of the counseling relationship.

Individualization, a fundamental tenet within rehabilitation, is endemic to the Three-Dimensional Model as it affords rehabilitation counselors the opportunity to develop a tool based on specifying the particular content a counselor deems to be important to know in assessing culturally diverse people with disabilities. In the Three-Dimensional Model, no a priori assumption is made about the preeminence of any domain, rendering them all of equal importance as a starting point. This attribute of the model encourages each counselor to assign an importance to each of the three domains based upon his/her own intuition, experience, and professional expertise. This process of individualizing the model may promote "buy in" from the counselor and increase the probability that the model will be used. Thus, in application, the model requires a steadfast focus on the three key areas, yet it influences the counseling process in a flexible and emergent manner, addressing specific concerns as they surface naturally. In other words, as long as the counselor is vigilant and mindful of all three dimensions, he/she can exhibit considerable individualization and flexibility in the application of specific strategies and techniques. Of course, this same individualization is inherent in the picture of the person with a disability that emerges from the model, given that each individual's uniqueness will influence the resulting profile. Part of what is distinctive about this model is that it places cultural identity in the context of counseling along with other important dimensions of the client and in the client–counselor relationship.

UNDERSTANDING HOW THE MODEL WORKS: FOUR COMPONENTS

To understand how the model actually works in the context of multicultural counseling, the process is divided into the four components: Starting Resources, Key Activities, Goals, and Supporting Mechanisms. Using these four components to illustrate how the model works in the context of multicultural counseling is based in part on characteristics of a logic model, which explicitly uses the Starting Resources (also called Inputs) and Key Activities components. The logic model is a program evaluation tool designed to clarify how programs work for evaluation purposes originally developed by McNamara (Kellogg Foundation, 2001; Kirkpatrick, 2001; Lambur & Mayeske, 2000).

Starting Resources

Each counselor begins the counseling process with raw materials, or Starting Resources (e.g., unique perceptions, experience, knowledge, skills and abilities the counselor brings to the counseling process). These counselor characteristics include:

- worldview and stereotypes (or cognitive schemas)
- appreciation for limitations, including with whom the counselor can and cannot work effectively
- life experience with culturally diverse individuals
- skill proficiency and "toolbox" of interventions (i.e., usual counseling strategies, techniques, and approaches)

Key Activities

Starting Resources make it possible for Key Activities to take place. Key Activities include:

- establish a positive relationship with the person with a disability
- learn who the person with a disability is
- determine the fit between the person with a disability and the counselor

Goals

Key Activities occur in pursuit of Goals which include:

- Goal 1: Predict who the person with a disability is in terms of race, ethnicity, etc. based on physically identifiable attributes (arguably happens to some extent automatically based on initial judgments about what the counselor perceives).
- Goal 2: Predict who the person with a disability is with respect to the domains of cultural identity, stage of development, and adjustment to disability based on physical attributes and the counselor's subjective reality.
- Goal 3: Understand who the person with a disability really is from the perspective of the person with a disability (the model helps to develop this) and regroup to make needed adjustments to initial counselor perceptions about the person with a disability.
- Goal 4: Assess appropriately the fit in understanding between the person with a disability and the counselor.
- Goal 5: Proceed with counseling in a manner that serves the person with a disability's best interest.

Supporting Mechanisms

For each Goal there is an accompanying supporting mechanism. The Supporting Mechanism is the underlying process that facilitates the goal attainment (i.e., a mechanism of action). For example, Goals 1 and 2 are facilitated by the counselor's stereotypes and worldview. Goals 1 and 2 are somewhat automatic based upon the natural inclination of human beings (i.e., human nature) to make judgments and generalizations, some of which may be stereotypical about persons who are visibly different in the absence of more specific individuating information (Fiske, Neuberg, Beattie, & Milberg, 1987). Piaget's work (1972) related to judgments based on cognitive schemas is also relevant here as an underlying theoretical foundation for the supporting mechanism. The Three-Dimensional Model itself, active listening, and gentle probing are examples of supporting mechanisms for Goal 3, along with a willingness of the counselor to modify his or her own worldview (Sue et al., 1992). Counselor self-awareness and knowledge of the person with a disability through the use of the Three-Dimensional Model and objectivity are the supporting mechanisms for Goal 4 (Sue et al., 1992). Genuineness, respect, positive regard (i.e., what is best for the person with a disability—the concept of beneficence), and codes of ethics (e.g., the Code of Ethics for the national Commission of Rehabilitation Counselor Certification) are the supporting mechanisms for Goal 5. Ethical conduct may include referral to another counselor if and when the working alliance is not possible. See Table 12-1 for a visual representation of the flow of Starting Resources, Key Activities, Goals, and Supporting Mechanisms.

DEVELOPMENT OF THE THREE-DIMENSIONAL MODEL: SIX STEPS

In developing an individualized Three-Dimensional Model, each counselor determines how he/she will consider and explore the three domains of cultural identity, stage of development, and adjustment to disability in each counseling situation. As such, the Three-Dimensional Model is different for each counselor. This distinctiveness is a strength that accommodates the mandate for individualization in rehabilitation philosophy required by legislation (Rehabilitation Act of 1973). In addition, each counselor has the ability to develop a model consistent with intuitive and conceptual understanding of the three domains, preferred counseling style, and intended use (population or setting). Adherence to using the model increases the likelihood that these three domains will be explored in each new multicultural counseling situation. So, the important question is not how a review of the three domains is conducted, but that it is conducted in a manner that encourages true exploration of each domain, deliberately taking into account the perspectives of both the counselor and the person with a disability as outlined in the components presented above.

Six key steps exist for each counselor to develop his or her own Three-Dimensional Model for a multicultural counseling application.

Step 1

Decide how broadly or narrowly to apply the model. Typically, a single general model is preferred for efficiency, but there may be compelling reasons to have several models to allow for customization to specific populations of persons with disabilities (e.g., deafness, mental illness, or traumatic brain injury) or contexts (e.g., work adjustment, psychosocial rehabilitation, psychotherapy, family counseling). It

Table 12-1 Three-Dimensional Model Applied to Multicultural Counseling Process

Starting Resources	Key Activities	Goals	Supporting Processes
• Human nature (HN) (i.e., counselor's cognitive schemas and worldview)	• Establish relationship with consumer	1. Identify who consumer is based on physically identifiable attributes	1. HN (i.e., counselor's cognitive schemas and worldview)
• Counselor's understanding of whom he/she can work with effectively	• Learn who consumer really is	2. Predict who consumer is in the three domains of disability adjustment, development, and cultural identity	2. HN (i.e., counselor's cognitive schemas and worldview)
• Counselor's skill/experience with culturally diverse individuals	• Evaluate fit between counselor and consumer and make the best decision about forming a therapeutic alliance OR making a referral	3. Understand who consumer really is in all three domains and regroup to make needed adjustments to initial perceptions of the consumer (i.e., modify as needed predictions made in Goal 2)	3. Look, listen, gently probe, and learn by invoking the Three-factor Model (i.e., use pre-determined questions/conceptual prompts in all three areas to get to know the consumer, and then willingly modify own), HN (i.e., cognitive schemas and worldview as needed)
• Counselor's usual tools and approaches		4. Assess appropriately the fit between counselor and consumer	4. Knowledge of self, consumer (from Three-factor Model), and objectivity
• Three-factor Model		5. Act in a way that suits the consumer's best interest	5. Concern for what is best for consumer and code of ethics
			Options: *Develop* Rehabilitation Plan OR *Refer*

Source: Lewis, A. N. (2006). The three-factor model of multicultural counseling for consumers with disabilities. *Journal of Vocational Rehabilitation, 24*(3), 151–159, reprinted with permission from IOS Press.

is important to remember that all counseling must be conducted in the appropriate cognitive and sensory mode.

Step 2

Consider each of the three domains separately and determine which theoretical orientation is best for each. With this consideration, one or more theoretical or conceptual frameworks will need to be explored in each of the three domains. The decided-upon framework for each domain may be based on a single or on multiple (i.e., a blended approach) theoretical or conceptual frameworks. In each of the three domains are examples of theoretical or conceptual frameworks that might be considered. The actual pool of potential frameworks to be considered is much larger than the small sample that follows. Counselors will consider theoretical/conceptual frameworks that they are already familiar with or those they feel compelled to investigate.

- Regarding cultural identity frameworks: the counselor may favor a "layers of diversity" framework (Gardenswartz & Rowe, 1998), a personal dimensions of identity framework (Arredondo & Glauner, 1992), an assimilation framework (Helms, 1990), an acculturation framework (Cross, 1995), a whole person framework (Wegscheider-Cruse, 1981), or an identity development framework (Cass, 1979).
- Exploring stage of development: the counselor may favor a psychoanalytic framework (Erikson, 1963; Freud, 1959), a mechanistic framework (Bandura, 1977; Skinner, 1976; Watson, 1913), an organismic perspective (Piaget, 1972), a humanistic framework (Maslow, 1970), a generic continuum of adjustment to disability (comprised of the three phases of awareness, acceptance, and adjustment developed by this author, and influenced in part by the two-staged acceptance-adjustment continuum developed by Gandy et al., 1987), or a lifespan development framework (Papalia & Olds, 2004; Quinn, 1998).
- Adjusting to disability: the counselor may consider such frameworks as the psychosocial adaptation to disability framework (Livneh & Antonak, 1991), the stages of change/transtheoretical framework (Prochaska & DiClemente, 1984), a generic continuum of adjustment to disability (comprised of the three phases of awareness, acceptance, and adjustment developed by this author, and influenced in part by the two-staged acceptance-adjustment continuum developed by Gandy et al., 1987), or again, the whole person framework (Wegscheider-Cruse, 1981).

Ultimately the decision on which framework(s) to use will be based upon such considerations as counselor training, experience, expertise, and preference as well as the characteristics of the target population of people with disabilities (i.e., cultural relevance and meaning).

Step 3

Sketch the model. First, decide on a graphic format for the model that is appealing to the counselor (e.g., flow chart, geometric shapes, etc.). This model-making may require several drafts. The goal is to have a visual representation of the model that includes the three domains of cultural identity, stage of development, and adjustment to disability on a single sheet of paper that the counselor can easily commit to memory. Arnheim (1972) argued that visioning is a primary medium of thought and recall. Therefore, drawing a sketch that is meaningful to the counselor may help to integrate the tool into one's personal counseling style in a manner that does not foster a reliance on written notes or text.

Step 4

Test the model for conceptual integrity. Do this by writing a brief narrative describing each of the three domains and their relationships to each other using only the graphic representation of the model (no notes, books, or other references).

Step 5

Test the model for applied integrity. Do this by using it to practice interviewing real people with disabilities who are culturally different from the counselor.

Step 6

Revise the model based upon the results of Steps 4 and 5, and continue to do so at regular intervals so that the counselor can continually improve and refine his or her approach to deliberately considering the cultural identity, stage of development, and adjustment to disability of the person with a disability in a multicultural counseling situation.

An Illustration of Individualized Model Development

The following Three-Dimensional Model is intended for use with adults with any type of chronic illness or disability. The six-step model development process just described is invoked as follows.

Step 1: Specify a Population of Interest

This is a generic model that could be used with many populations of adults with disabilities.

Step 2: Consider the Three Domains Separately

Step 2.1: Consider Cultural Identity The framework of Wegscheider-Cruse (1981) provides a whole person perspective that is typically applied to adjustment to disability. This model is entirely consistent with every major tenet of rehabilitation philosophy and the "whole person" concept in particular. However, Wegscheider-Cruse's framework also has application in understanding a person with a disability's cultural identity. If total adjustment to a disability involves achieving balance in the realms of physical, mental, emotional, spiritual, social, and volitional functioning, then understanding who a person with a disability is culturally might be enhanced in consideration of these same six realms. Using this orientation would suggest the following points of discussion between the counselor and person with a disability in exploring the person with a disability's perspective on his/her cultural identity:

- What does the person with a disability know about the meaning and importance of physical health and appearance, mental health and functioning, emotional health and functioning, spiritual health and functioning, social functioning, and volition?
- How does the person with a disability prioritize and balance these life realms?

Step 2.2: Consider Stage of Development Where is the person with a disability in terms of stage of developmental functioning? Is the person with a disability functioning in a manner consistent with age-based developmental milestones as addressed, for example, in the lifespan development framework of Papalia and Olds (2004)? Such a consideration would lead to questions such as, is the person with a disability encountering life challenges and tasks commensurate with typically occurring experiences at this point in the lifespan based on chronological age, or is this individual ahead of or behind the typical normative curve? Maslow's (1970) hierarchy of needs provides one framework for determining what needs the person with a disability is attempting to meet, and counseling will succeed only to the extent that it is relevant to those needs. The following interview questions might follow using Maslow's framework:

- Do you have any pressing needs regarding food, clothing, or shelter?
- Do you feel generally safe and secure as you go about your daily activities?

- Who is important and active in your life?
- What three or four things are most important in your life?
- What two or three things appear to be important to most people, but do not matter very much to you?

Step 2.3: Consider Adjustment to Disability Several theoretical frameworks from rehabilitation and psychology appear to have potential here. First, there is the generic three-phase continuum of adjustment developed by this author and influenced in part by Gandy et al. (1987). This framework provides some sense of where the person with a disability is with respect to the adjustment continuum (i.e., awareness, acceptance, or adjustment), while concurrently clarifying what the person with a disability defines as an ideal level of adjustment. Personal assets or residual capabilities of the person with a disability are other fertile areas for exploration (Livneh & Antonak, 1991). Third, knowing the person with a disability's personal commitment to active involvement in counseling and rehabilitation processes is highly recommended (Prochaska & DiClemente, 1984). In the aggregate, these frameworks suggest the following examples of interview questions to understand the person's adjustment to disability:

- How aware are you of the medical and psychosocial aspects of your disability? Please describe them.
- How does your disability limit you with respect to major life activities? How does it benefit you?
- How would you describe your current degree of acceptance of the limitations imposed by your disability? How would you describe the opportunities it offers?
- How have you demonstrated your positive adjustment to the disability in the pursuit of specific life goals? How have you demonstrated your less than positive adjustment?
- If everything goes well, how will you be different when our work together (i.e., the rehabilitative process) is complete?
- What are you especially good at that has not been affected by your disability?
- What are you really good at that has been affected by your disability? Can these barriers be removed, minimized, compensated for, or accommodated?
- What are you willing to invest to ensure that our work together is successful?

Step 3: Sketch Your Model

Figure 12-1 illustrates a sketch of this particular generic Three-Dimensional Model. The sketch uses graphic attributes and symbolism to provide an easily remembered

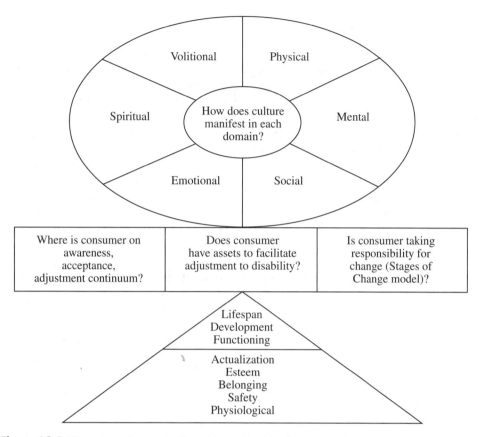

Figure 12-1 Illustration of a generic Three-Dimensional Model

conceptual prompt for its model developer regarding what must be explored in each new multicultural counseling situation. Viewed in total, Figure 12-1 resembles a human body. Note the oval shape at the top of the figure is analogous to a "head on a body" and is the location of a person with a disability's cultural identity, symbolizing that cultural experience resides in one's memory, i.e., the brain. Stage of development, the sum total of one's life experiences and associated responses up to the present time, is the base of the model at the bottom of the figure, depicting the "legs on a body." Accordingly, adjustment to disability involves a prominent emotional component, in addition to the obvious cognitive aspects, and is located in the middle of the figure, symbolizing the "torso of a body" where one's heart is located to portray that emotional connection.

Step 4: Write a Narrative

Stage of development, represented by the triangle in Figure 12-1, is the base of the model—a bedrock component reflecting both current developmental challenges as understood through Maslow's (1970) framework (bottom portion of triangle) as well as the person with a disability's lifespan development functioning (top portion of triangle). Adjustment to disability is represented by a rectangle that teeters precariously on the triangular foundational base of stage of development and reflects adjustment concerns associated with the three-phased generic adjustment to disability continuum (left third of rectangle), an assets-based view on adjustment to disability (middle third of rectangle), and the person with a disability's degree of investment in own adjustment to disability as per the stages of change framework (right third of rectangle); all symbolizing the instability and challenge involved in achieving balance or total adjustment to disability. Cultural identity is represented by the oval at the top of the figure that portrays the six dimensions of a whole person—each of which must be understood through the person with a disability's cultural lens. The oval shape symbolizes an ability to tilt left or right to interact with the aspects of adjustment to disability represented by the rectangle that supports the cultural identity oval, keeping in mind that both cultural identity and adjustment to disability either balance or do not balance on the triangular stage of development base. All three domains (cultural identity, stage of development, and adjustment to disability) exist in a unique, delicate, and precarious balance within an individual.

Step 5: Pilot the Model

In order to test the model in an applied manner, the counselor engages in several structured interviews with new people with disabilities who are culturally different from the counselor. The goal is to discuss all or most of the questions (i.e., conceptual prompts) deriving from the model in the first one to three meetings. Good counseling practice suggests that these questions not necessarily be posed directly, which may have the effect of being perceived as a judgmental interrogation, but rather should serve as prompts for areas the counselor must strategically explore in a manner consistent with his or her own unique counseling style and the interpersonal style of the interviewee.

Step 6: Evaluate and Revise the Model Periodically

On an intermittent basis, the model must be revisited and revised in the interest of both professional development and continuous refinement. To accomplish this, repeat any of Steps 1 through 5 as needed, and then revisit and refine the model as in this Step (Step 6).

Another Illustration of Model Development

Figure 12-2 is another illustration of a Three-Dimensional Model to be used with persons who experience brain injury. This model is based on looking at the three phases of adjustment to disability (Gandy et al., 1987) as they correlate with a framework for understanding disability acceptance based on the three post-injury (in the case of an acquired disability like traumatic brain injury) stages of reactions (Livneh & Antonak, 1991). The interface between these two frameworks maps the adjustment phase of awareness (the main task is gaining information and understanding) to the post-injury acceptance stages of early and intermediate reactions (where the prominent emotions are shock, denial [early reactions] and anger, depression [intermediate reactions]). The adjustment phase of acceptance (the main tasks are gaining peace with post-injury function with the assistance of family supports and

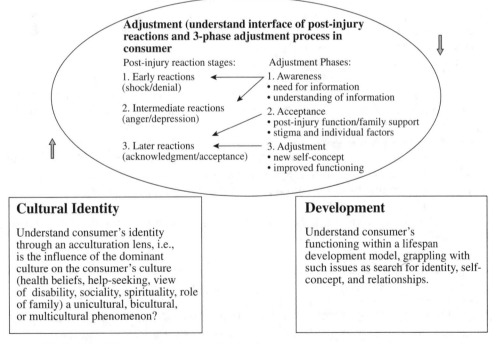

Figure 12-2 Illustration of a Three-Dimensional Model to be used with persons who experience brain injury

minimizing stigma), along with the actual adjustment phase (the main tasks are developing a new self-concept and achieving improved functioning), both correlate with the later reactions stage, where acknowledgement and true acceptance of the disability occur.

In this example model, the cultural identity domain is addressed and understood using an acculturation framework where one can see the influence of the dominant culture on the individual's indigenous culture in terms of specific health beliefs and behavior, help-seeking patterns, views of disability, and the role of key factors such as family and spirituality in worldview. Ultimately, the cultural identity domain examines whether the individual embraces a unicultural, bicultural, or multicultural response in the interaction between the two cultural points of view (Cross, 1995).

The exploration of stage of human development in this example model is based on using a lifespan development approach (Papalia & Olds, 2004) where the goal is to address developmental functioning over the course of one's life. The ebbs and flows of such functioning over a lifespan would be characterized by and understood through such task-related struggles as the search for identity and self-concept, and fulfillment in key life relationships. Notice the visual symbolism and inherent dynamism in this example model's graphic depiction indicated by the fact that the oval shape that represents adjustment to disability has the ability to teeter back and forth, right to left within the cradle-like structural base as conveyed by the arrows proximal to both cultural identity and stage of development. This provides an opportunity for an interaction between cultural identity and stage of development through adjustment to disability (see Figure 12-2).

Figure 12-3 offers yet another example of a Three-Dimensional Model, to be used generally for all individuals with a disability encountered in a vocational context. This example model can be used when working with individuals with varying backgrounds, ages, and disabilities that are returning to work after an acquired disability. When working with this population, it is imperative that the person with a disability move toward adopting a working knowledge of the disability and reach some level of acceptance or adjustment to be able to go to work, therefore, the adjustment to disability domain should be initially assessed. Note its position in the middle of the visual as the anchor to the boat, Figure 12-3. In addition, the cultural identity and stage of development domains can vary, with the exploration of both offering critical information about the person with a disability.

This example model is helpful in vocational counseling because it fully acknowledges that the individual has a disability and allows the counselor to identify what progress the person has made in adjusting to the disability as a first step. In the initial phase of the counseling process, the counselor can seek to elevate the person with a disability's knowledge and promote self-advocacy. Subsequently, the counselor allows the person to share information about him/herself relative to factors that affect all people regardless of disability status such as gender, age, race, ethnicity,

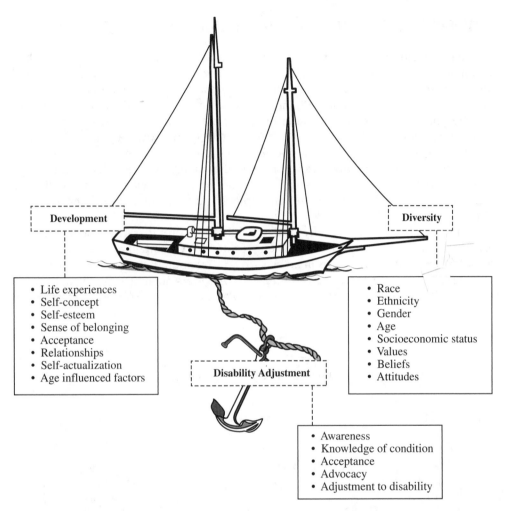

Figure 12-3 Illustration of a Three-Dimensional Model to be used with individuals with a disability in a vocational context

class, the ability to utilize one's gifts and talents, a sense of being connected or belonging to something, and how the person views him/herself. This is an important phase for both the person with a disability and the counselor. Although the person with a disability is primarily coming to the counselor to address matters relating to how disability affects work, the person is viewed from a holistic perspective and multiple factors that have helped to shape and influence who he/she is can be identified and addressed by utilizing this example model (Figure 12-3).

STRENGTHS OF THE THREE-DIMENSIONAL MODEL

There is a business argument for the Three-Dimensional Model. In this new millennium, it is clear that human service and rehabilitation providers face unprecedented demands related to accountability. These demands take on four primary forms: (1) limited and uncertain funding, (2) increasing demands for services, (3) an insistence on the part of people with disabilities that services meet their needs, and (4) a requirement imposed by payers (citizens, legislative, and governmental bodies) that funds be expended responsibly and in ways that maximize the reach of such resources. In effect, together these four types of demands or stressors constitute a set of countervailing forces that encroach upon human service and rehabilitation providers and can be termed the "multiple source accountability demands" (see Figure 12-4).

The idea that human service and rehabilitation providers face such multiple sources of accountability demands seems particularly compelling these days, as it raises a clear imperative for human service and rehabilitation providers: "Do more with less." Doing more with less requires that providers not engage in the delivery of services that either lack or have questionable effectiveness (Lewis, Armstrong, & Karpf, 2005). Therefore, it behooves all rehabilitation service providers to have an

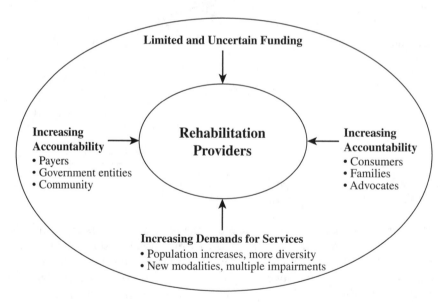

Figure 12-4 Influence of demands or stressors on human service and rehabilitation providers

explicit framework to guide efforts and promote efficiency, while affording the versatility to serve a variety of individuals with disabilities who seek counseling services.

The rehabilitation system in this country cannot fully meet the imperative of doing more with less and offering programs that are efficacious, unless the system knows what works with every segment of the service population. Inherent in this goal is the need for counselors to work effectively and ethically with persons who are culturally diverse. Therefore, the charge to engage in effective multicultural counseling is heightened significantly these days given the demands and stressors that we as professionals face.

In the context of counselors increasingly being expected to do more with less, reconciling the requirements for individualization and efficiency, suggests that a systematic and integrative model is likely to best meet both requirements. For example, if counselors working across cultural lines review the three domains early on, then biases can be identified (Rosenthal, 2002; Rosenthal & Kosciulek, 1996) and remediated in supervision or obviated through reassignment before time and resources are wasted. In this manner, the Three-Dimensional Model is intended to promote sound business and ethical interests by offering a solid assessment process at the beginning of the multicultural counseling endeavor (see Figure 12-4).

There is also an argument for the Three-Dimensional Model based on it having key model properties. First, the model is comprehensive in that the three included domains together offer a holistic description of the person with a disability. Second, the model is parsimonious in that it involves three major domains (cultural identity, stage of development, and adjustment to disability) and six development steps. Model propositions are confined to those that serve to both manifest the uniqueness of each person with a disability and enhance the working alliance between the person with a disability and the counselor. Third, the model is internally consistent. Its elements are logically related to each other, and no element is contradictory to another. These three dimensions (comprehensiveness, parsimony, and internal consistency) are important in evaluating other models in social science (Lave & March, 1975).

IMPLICATIONS FOR FUTURE RESEARCH

The Three-Dimensional Model is intended to serve as a conceptual prompt to assist counselors in assessing multicultural counseling situations. Models are not true or false, but have utility in illustrating social phenomenon and identifying new points of exploration (Linde, 2003). Future research will help determine the range of acceptability of the relationships among the Three-Dimensional Model elements and may provide the ultimate indication of its efficacy. More than 300 students have been trained on the model in the context of a graduate rehabilitation multicultural counseling course at Virginia Commonwealth University, yielding positive anecdotal evidence to date on the utility and efficacy of the Three-Dimensional Model. Therefore, future research could focus on empirically evaluating whether and how the use of the Three-Dimensional Model is effective in multicultural counseling. Use of this model could be compared to "practice as usual," similar to Garcia's evaluations of ethics models presented in Chapter 13. In addition, future research could empirically identify critical factors in effective multicultural counseling relationships to assess the degree to which these map onto the domains included in the Three-Dimensional Model.

CONCLUSION

The Three-Dimensional Model, when used in a multicultural counseling scenario, is intended to promote a counselor's efficient and keen understanding of the cultural identity, stage of development, and adjustment to disability of a culturally different person with a disability. In turn, this understanding can enable the counselor to estimate the probability of an optimal and ethical match between the profile of the person with a disability and the biases, worldview, stereotypes (generalizations about individuals based on category membership; Hogg & Abrams, 1988), and experience of the counselor and can guide effective counseling practices leading to positive outcomes. The model accommodates diverse perspectives in multicultural counseling while furthering the bedrock tenet of individualization that is part and parcel of rehabilitation legislation and philosophy.

REFERENCES

Arnheim, R. (1972). *Visual thinking*. Berkeley: The University of California Press.

Arredondo, P. & Glauner, T. (1992). *Personal dimensions of identity model*. Boston: Empowerment Workshops.

Atkinson, D. R. (2004). *Counseling American minorities*. Boston: McGraw Hill.

Atkinson, D. R., Thompson, C. E., & Grant, S. K. (1993). A three-dimensional model for counseling racial/ethnic minorities. *Counseling Psychologist, 21*(2), 257–277.

Bandura, A. (1977). *Social learning theory*. Englewood Cliffs, NJ: Prentice-Hall.

Cass, V. C. (1979). Homosexual identity formation: A theoretical model. *Journal of Homosexuality, 7*(2/3), 219–235.

Chesler, M. A. (1965). Ethnocentrism and attitudes toward the physically disabled. *Journal of Personality and Social Psychology, 2*(6), 877–882.

Cross, W. E. (1995) The psychology of nigrescence: Revising the Cross Model. In J. G. Ponterotto, J. M. Casas, L. A. Suzuki, & C. M. Alexander (Eds.), *Handbook of multicultural counseling* (pp. 93–122). Thousand Oaks, CA: Sage.

Dell Orto, A. E. & Power, P. W. (2007). *The psychology and social impact of illness and disability*. New York: Springer.

Erikson, E. H. (1963). *Childhood and society*. New York: Norton Press.

Fiske, S. T., Neuberg, S. L., Beattie, A. E., & Milberg, S. J. (1987). Category-based and attribute-based reactions to others: Some informational conditions of stereotyping and individuating processes. *Journal of Experimental Social Psychology, 23*, 399–427.

French, S. (1993). Disability, impairment or something in between? In J. Swain, V. Finkelstein, S. French, & M. Oliver (Eds.), *Disabling barriers: Enabling environments* (pp. 17–25). London: Sage.

Freud, S. (1959). An autobiographical study. In J. Strachey (Ed.), *The standard edition of the complete psychological works of Sigmund Freud* (p. 20). London: Hogarth. (Original work published 1925.)

Funk, R. (1987). *Disability rights: From caste to class in the context of civil rights*. New York: Praeger.

Gandy, G. L., Martin, E. D., Hardy, R. E., & Cull, J. G. (1987). *Rehabilitation counseling and services: Profession and process*. Springfield, MA: Charles C. Thomas.

Gardenswartz, L. & Rowe, A. (1998). *Managing diversity in health care*. San Francisco: Jossey-Bass.

Harper, F. D. & McFadden, J. (2003). *Culture and counseling: New Models*. New York: Macmillan.

Helms, J. (1990). Toward a model of White racial identity development. In J. Helms (Ed.), *Black and White racial identity* (pp. 49–66). Westport, CT: Greenwood.

Hogg, M. A. & Abrams, D. (1988). *Social identifications*. London: Routledge.

Kellogg Foundation. (2001). *Logic model development guide: Logic models to bring together planning, evaluation & action*. Battle Creek, MI: W. K. Kellogg Foundation.

Kendall, E. & Buys, N. (1998). An integrated model of psychosocial adjustment following acquired disability. *The Journal of Rehabilitation, 64*(3), 16–20.

Kirkpatrick, S. (2001). *The program logic model: What, why and how?*, Retrieved March 20, 2007, from CharityVillage.com Web site: *http://www.charityvillage.com/cv/research/rstrat3.html*

Lambur, M. & Mayeske, G. (2000). *Logic modeling: A process for enhancing program effects and evaluation results* (Facilitator training manual). Crofton, MD: The Program Design Institute.

Lave, C. A. & March, J. G. (1975). *An introduction to models in social sciences*. New York: Harper and Row.

Lewis, A. N. (2006). The Three-factor Model of multicultural counseling for consumers with disabilities. *Journal of Vocational Rehabilitation, 24*(3), 151–159.

Lewis, A. N., Armstrong, A. J., & Karpf, A. (2005). Using data to improve outcomes in rehabilitation practice. *Journal of Rehabilitation Administration, 29*(1), 43–56.

Linde, G. (2003). The use of two-dimensional models in social science: An auto critical review. *European Journal of Teacher Education, 26*(1), 37–45.

Livneh, H. & Antonak, R. F. (1991). A hierarchy of reactions to disability. *International Journal of Rehabilitation Research, 14*, 13–24.

Livneh, H. & Antonak, R. F. (1997). *Psychosocial adaptation to chronic illness and disability*. Gaithersburgh, MD: Aspen.

Lustig, D. C., Rosenthal, D. A., Strauser, D. R., & Haynes, K. (2000). The relationship between sense of coherence and adjustment in persons with disabilities. *Rehabilitation Counseling Bulletin, 43*(3), 134–141.

Maslow, A. (1970). *Motivation and personality*. New York: Harper & Row.

McMahon, B. T., Shaw, L. R., Chan, F., Danczyk-Hawley, C. (2004). "Common factors" in rehabilitation counseling: Expectancies and the working alliance. *Journal of Vocational Rehabilitation, 20*(2), 101–105.

Mpofu, E. & Bishop, M. (2006). Value change and adjustment to disability: Implications for rehabilitation education practice and research. *Rehabilitation Education, 20*(3), 147–161.

Mpofu, E. & Conyers, L. (2004). A representational theory perspective of minority status and people with disabilities: Implications for rehabilitation education and practice. *Rehabilitation Counseling Bulletin, 47*(3), 142–151.

Papalia, D. E. & Olds, S. W. (2004). *Human development.* New York: McGraw Hill.

Patterson, C. H. (2004). Do we need multicultural counseling competencies? *Journal of Mental Health Counseling, 26*(1), 67–73.

Piaget, J. (1972). *The psychology of the child.* New York: Basic Books.

Prochaska, J. O. & DiClemente, C. C. (1984). *The transtheoretical Model: Crossing the traditional boundaries of therapy.* Melbourne, Australia: Krieger.

Quinn, P. (1995). Social work and disability management policy: Yesterday, today and tomorrow. *Social Work in Health Care, 20*(3), 67–82.

Quinn, P. (1998). *Understanding disability: A lifespan Model.* Thousand Oaks, CA: Sage.

Rehabilitation Act of 1973, 29 U.S.C., as amended in 1992, Title I, Section 21, Pub. L. No. 102–569, § 701–744.

Rehabilitation Act Amendments of 1992, Pub. L. No. 102–569, 106 Stat. (1992).

Reynolds, A. L. (1999). Working with children and adolescents in the schools: Multicultural counseling implications. In R. H. Sheets & E. R. Hollins (Eds.), *Racial and ethnic identity in school practices: Aspects of human development* (pp. 213–229). Mahwah, NJ: Lawrence Erlbaum.

Rosenthal, D. A. (2002). Racial bias in rehabilitation: A response to Thomas and Weinrach. *Rehabilitation Education, 16*(3), 307–311.

Rosenthal, D. A. & Kosciulek, J. F. (1996). Clinical judgment and bias due to client race or ethnicity: An overview with implications for counselors. *Journal of Applied Rehabilitation Counseling, 27*(3), 30–36.

Rothrock, J. A. (1999). A personal experience of acceptance and adjustment to disability. In G. L. Gandy, E. D. Martin, & R. E. Hardy (Eds.), *Counseling in the rehabilitation process: Community services for mental and physical disabilities* (2nd ed.; pp. 204–217). Springfield, IL: Charles C. Thomas.

Rubin, S. E. & Roessler, R. T. (2001). *Foundations of the vocational rehabilitation process.* Austin, TX: ProEd.

Skinner, B. F. (1976). *About behaviorism.* New York: Vintage.

Stone, J. S. (2005). *Culture and disability: Providing culturally competent services.* Thousand Oaks, CA: Sage.

Sue, D. W., Arredondo, P. & McDavis, R. (1992). Multicultural counseling competencies and standards: A call to the profession. *Journal of Multicultural Counseling and Development, 20*(2), 64–88.

Sue, D. W., Carter, R. T., Casas, J. M., Fouad, N. A., Ivey, A. E., & Jensen, M. (1998). *Multicultural counseling competencies: Individual and organizational development.* Thousand Oaks, CA: Sage.

Thomas, K. R. & Weinrach, S. G. (2004). Mental health counseling and the AMCD Multicultural counseling competencies: A civil debate. *Journal of Mental Health Counseling, 26*(1), 41–43.

Tower, K. D. (2003). Disability through the lens of culture. *Journal of Social Work in Disability and Rehabilitation, 2*(2/3), 5–22.

U.S. Census Bureau. (2004). *Population projections: U.S. Interim projections by age, sex, race and Hispanic origin.* Retrieved June 15, 2007, from *http://www.census.gov/ipc/www/usinterimproj*

Watson, J. (1913). Psychology as a behaviorist views it. *Psychological Review, 20,* 158–177.

Wegscheider-Cruse, S. (1981). *Another chance: Hope and help for the alcoholic family.* Palo Alto, CA: Science and Behavior Books.

Yuker, H. (1965). Attitudes as determinants of behavior. *Journal of Rehabilitation, 31,* 15–16.

CHAPTER 13

Ethical Decision-Making Models in Multicultural Rehabilitation Counseling

Jorge Garcia, Ph.D.

INTRODUCTION

Imagine you have a client named Maria who came to see you as a counselor because she learned that she is infected with the HIV virus and needs your help to be able to deal with its emotional and vocational consequences. She discloses to you that she still engages in unprotected sex with her boyfriend and has not informed him about her condition. Since there is a high risk of infection, an identifiable potential victim, and your client refuses to disclose her condition to her boyfriend, you proceed to tell her that you may have to disclose this information to him since this would be consistent with your ethical obligations. Then she proceeds to tell you that she fears retaliation since her boyfriend has a history of violence and carries a gun, which she is quite sure he would use against her. This is a serious dilemma for you as the counselor since both courses of action (disclosure or the decision not to disclose) are supported by the ethical principle of nonmaleficence (prevention of harm to others). What should you do in this circumstance? What would be the best ethical decision?

As the theoretical and professional foundations of multicultural counseling have progressed, ethical standards to help regulate the practice of multicultural counseling have evolved. Ibrahim and Arredondo (1986) authored a proposal to develop specific ethical standards regarding multicultural counseling in the areas of education, research, assessment, and practice. LaFromboise and Foster (1989) extended this discussion by bringing attention to other issues related to ethics in multicultural counseling, such as the use of participants in research and right to treatment.

Responding to this need, in the 2006 revision of the ethical standards, the American Counseling Association (ACA) included specific excerpts requiring counselors to respect diversity, avoid discrimination, and demonstrate cultural sensitivity when engaging in direct client services, research, education, testing, computer applications, public communications, and relationships with employers and employees (Herlihy & Corey, 2006). Moreover, within the section on professional competence, it requires counselors to show a commitment to gain knowledge, awareness, and skills related to serving a diverse clientele. Diversity is defined in the ACA code in terms of age, culture, disability, ethnic group, gender, race, religion, sexual orientation, marital status, and socioeconomic status.

Furthermore, researchers have stated the need to prepare professionals to become more skillful in dealing with ethical dilemmas, particularly those involving multicultural issues in the areas of rehabilitation (Falvo & Parker, 2000), mental health services (Remy, 1998), and gender issues (Steiner, 1997). Baruth and Manning (1999) alluded to this need by stating that the ethical dilemmas faced by counselors are complex and become even more so when working with persons who have different worldviews. Readers interested in more specific examples of ethical dilemmas can find them in the ACA ethical standards casebook (Herlihy & Corey, 2006). As stated by LaFromboise and Foster (1989), the challenge then becomes to develop ethical decision-making models that reflect a convergence of our current knowledge about multicultural counseling theory and ethical reasoning.

This chapter describes theoretical ethical decision-making models and summarizes empirical research geared toward evaluating or testing these models from a multicultural perspective. It also discusses potential applications of these models, particularly the transcultural integrative model recently developed by the author. Finally, this chapter addresses the implications of the current research for educators and practitioners, as well as the need to conduct research that expands the knowledge about this subject.

ETHICAL DECISION-MAKING MODELS

In examining the available ethical decision-making models published in the field, the author found minimal references to culture, or how to integrate culture into the ethical decision-making process systematically. Moreover, empirical research aimed at validating or evaluating these models is lacking in the literature. The following is a review of the current models and the presentation of a model that can be used by counseling practitioners facing ethical dilemmas involving clients from diverse backgrounds. Adapted primarily from the original Integrative Model developed by Tarvydas (1998), while also drawing from the Social Constructivist Model (Cottone, 2001) and the Collaborative Model (Davis, 1997), this proposed model is titled the Transcultural Integrative Ethical Decision-Making Model. In terms of ethical theory, the proposed model is founded in both principle (or rational) ethics (Kitchener, 1984), and virtue ethics (Freeman, 2000; Jordan & Meara, 1995). These models and theories are discussed in the following section.

Rational Model

This type of model is based primarily on principle ethics (Kitchener, 1984). This means that once the principles in conflict have been identified, the professional chooses the best course of action. This choice is based on a rational evaluation of the advantages and disadvantages of choosing one course of action over another. In following this model, a professional must use rational justification to choose one course of action over another (Bersoff, 1996). The essentials of this model have been described by Forrester-Miller and Davis (1995) in these seven steps: (1) identify the problem, (2) refer to the code of ethics and professional guidelines, (3) determine the nature and dimensions of the dilemma, (4) generate potential courses of action, (5) consider the potential consequences of all options and then choose a course of action, (6) implement the course of action, and (7) evaluate the course of action. An examination of the narrative under each of these steps yields the conclusion that no cultural variables are included in the analysis of a dilemma under this model. The assumption may be that one set of values applies to all cultures, as stated by Pedersen (1997).

Welfel (2002) offers a similar extended nine-step model of rational ethical decisionmaking. This model serves its purpose as a general model, but for specific dilemmas involving clients from diverse cultures, professionals would either have to fill in the gaps or adapt the model to suit their cultural perspectives, as a cultural analysis is not provided.

Virtue Ethics Model

Advocates for a virtue ethics model, Jordan and Meara (1995) rely on the personal characteristics and wisdom of the professionals making an ethical decision rather than on the ethical principles involved. Proponents of this model claim that it is very difficult to reach an agreement when different principles are in conflict in a particular situation. Instead, they state that the primary factor in arriving at a decision is the professionals' moral or personal beliefs. Central virtues mentioned under this model include integrity, prudence, discretion, perseverance, courage, benevolence, humility, and hope. This approach has not been developed into a format with specific steps and, again, cultural analyses or implications have not been included in this model.

Freeman (2000) defined virtue ethics as addressing "who one is, what one ought to become, and what form of action will bring one from the present to the future" (p. 90). The virtue of self-understanding based on honesty, openness, and willingness to take responsibility for one's life would allow counselors to determine who they are in terms of character. Self-understanding, symbolization, and imagination would allow counselors to decide who they ought to become in terms of a conceptualization of change. Finally, Freeman stated that prudent judgment would allow counselors to change or become the person they ought to be. Thus, virtue ethics represents a shift from appraisal of the act to the appraisal of the one acting. This would mean that an action is right when it reflects what a counselor with virtuous character would do in a particular situation. Freeman describes the need to define human goods and virtuous traits before a determination is made about what is the right thing to do in a given set of circumstances.

It does not appear possible to determine a definite number of virtue traits that counselors need to have because the traits needed seem to depend on the specific situation. For example, Tarvydas (1998) determined that reflection, balance, collaboration, and attention to context were counselor-essential virtues working within the framework of the Integrative Model. Freeman (2000) emphasized other virtues such as self-understanding, openness, honesty, and prudent judgment. Since none of these authors addressed specific dilemmas involving differing cultural worldviews, the virtues they mentioned do not necessarily reflect all the ones needed for cases of that nature. Therefore, the transcultural model proposed in this article involves the virtue of tolerance, which means accepting diverse worldviews, perspectives, and philosophies (Welfel, 2002).

Social Constructivism Model

Cottone (2001) proposed a social constructivism model that crosses both the psychological and systemic-relational paradigms of mental health services. It is based on Maturana's (1970) biology of cognition theory, which states that what is real evolves through personal interaction and agreement as to what is fact. The core structure of this model entails the notion that decisions are externally influenced. Basically, decisions are made with interactions involving one or more individuals; this means that decisions are not compelled internally, but socially. Central decision-making strategies used under this model include negotiating, consensus-seeking, and arbitrating.

With the understanding that this model is social in nature, the role of culture would intertwine nicely in this theory. Unfortunately, culture is vaguely mentioned, and apparently no attempt has been made to deal with this variable more thoroughly in this model.

Collaborative Model

Davis (1997) criticized the existent rational model by asserting that in the current professional world, a model based on a group's perspective would be superior to one founded on an individual's perspective. Davis deemed his decision-making strategy a collaborative ethics model based on the values of cooperation and inclusion. This relational approach utilizes a sequence of four steps: (1) identifying the parties who would be involved in the dilemma; (2) defining the various viewpoints of the parties involved; (3) developing a solution that is mutually satisfactory to all the parties, based on group work focusing on expectations and goals; and (4) identifying and implementing the individual contributions that are part of the solution. However, cultural components are not systematically elaborated in this model, other than reflecting a theoretical compatibility with the collectivist values underlying multicultural counseling.

Integrative Model

A fourth type of model utilized in resolving ethical dilemmas is an integrative model that incorporates elements of both principle and virtue ethics (Tarvydas, 1998). This author described a four-stage Integrative Decision-Making Model that combines an analysis of the morals, beliefs, and experiences of the individuals involved, along with a rational analysis of the ethical principles underlying the competing courses of action. This model requires professionals to utilize reflection, balance, attention to the context, and collaboration in making decisions involving ethical dilemmas (Tarvydas, 2003).

Stage I, entitled Interpreting the Situation through Awareness and Fact Finding, requires that counselors closely examine the situation and develop an awareness of what types of situations constitute an ethical dilemma. If the counselor is not aware of the latest information in his or her field of expertise, it is his or her responsibility to gather the relevant information. This stage calls for an increase in sensitivity and awareness in the counselor's field of specialization. The fact-finding process assists the counselor in labeling a situation as an ethical dilemma, and in determining which individuals are directly affected by these types of situations. If a dilemma occurs, the counselor is not only aware of the situation, but also recognizes the parties affected and their ethical stance in the situation.

Stage II (Formulating an Ethical Decision) is no different than the typical rational decision-making model described earlier (Forrester-Miller & Davis, 1995). First, counselors review the problem specifically to determine what ethical codes, standards, principles, and institutional policies are pertinent to this type of situation. Second, after careful review and consideration of these regulations, they generate a list of potential courses of action along with the positive and negative consequences for following each course of action. Third, counselors are urged to consult with supervisors or other knowledgeable professionals to determine the most ethical course of action. Finally, the best ethical course of action is selected based on a rational analysis of the principles involved. This entails making a rational decision as to which ethical principle should supersede the other competing ethical principles in this case.

Stage III (Selecting an Action by Weighing Competing Nonmoral Values) involves analyzing the course of action from the perspective of competing personal and contextual values (e.g., institutional, team, collegial, and societal/cultural). The assumption here is that counselors and others involved in the situation may encounter "personal blind spots" or levels of prejudice that need to be addressed before affirming the final course of action selected in Step II.

In Stage IV (Planning and Executing the Selected Course of Action) the counselor determines the concrete actions that need to be taken, with consideration given to the potential obstacles for taking that course of action. During this stage, it is important to anticipate personal and contextual barriers to the effective implementation of the course of action selected (Tarvydas, 2003).

Transcultural Model

A team of researchers (Garcia, Cartwright, Winston, & Borzuchowska, 2003) published a *transcultural integrative* model as an ethical decision-making method, grounded in both ethics and multicultural psychology/counseling theory. This model is comprised of the same four stages that make up the original Tarvydas' integrative model with the addition of a cultural component under each of those stages. The first stage is Interpretation of the Situation through Awareness and Fact Finding. The cultural elements within this stage include examining one's attitudes and emotional reactions toward cultural groups; awareness of personal and client's cultural identity, acculturation, and role socialization; and gathering relevant cultural information.

Stage II involves Formulating an Ethical Decision. The cultural tasks in this stage include: ensuring that the cultural information gathered earlier was taken into consideration when defining the dilemma; examining the cultural diversity standards in the professional ethics codes and their compatibility or conflict with state laws (e.g., some state laws may discriminate against people with a different sexual orientation); using culturally appropriate strategies to have parties with differing worldviews agree on a course of action; considering the cultural implications or consequences of each course of action (e.g., some actions may pose a threat to family interdependence); consulting with experts in multicultural knowledge; and checking that the final course of action is consistent with the client's cultural worldview.

Stage III consists of Weighing Competing Values and Contextual Factors. These values and factors may impact the course of action. Cultural tasks within this stage would involve examining whether the cultural values of the professional are in conflict with those held by the client, and whether collegial, professional, institutional, or societal values that apply to the situation are consistent with the worldviews of the individual parties involved, particularly the client's.

Finally, Stage IV requires the Planning and Implementation of the Final Course of Action. Relevant cultural tasks associated with this stage would include identifying culturally relevant resources for the implementation of the plan (e.g., appropriate list of jobs; appropriate information materials); anticipating cultural biases, discrimination, stereotypes and prejudices; developing culturally appropriate countermeasures to those barriers (e.g., support groups); and identifying data collection methods and measures that are culturally appropriate. A summary of the model and stages is included in Table 13-1 on the next page. The reader should focus on the transcultural components under each stage of the model in order to be able to understand the difference with the Tarvydas' integrative model.

Evaluation of the Tarvydas Integrative Model

The author of this chapter along with a team of researchers first conducted empirical research aimed at evaluating the integrative and rational models. This was done for four reasons: (1) the rational model has been the standard model disseminated by the main professional counseling association to its members, so new models are often compared against this more established approach; (2) both models appear to be equally formalized into clearly specified and discrete steps which facilitate comparisons; (3) both models have distinct theoretical and philosophical assumptions; and (4) previous research (Garcia et al., 2003; Garcia, Forrester, & Jacob, 1998) suggests that the integrative model holds great promise for resolving complex ethical dilemmas given the broad scope of theories, philosophies, and practices that have been integrated into one model, as well as its attention to contextual variables such as culture. In addition, other researchers have stated that the rational model alone appears insufficient given the difficulty in reaching an agreement about what principle should prevail over other(s) within the context of an ethical dilemma (Jordan & Meara, 1995). This study served the purpose of not only evaluating the effectiveness of the rational approach but also determining whether an integrative model would be an improvement over this traditional model as perceived by rehabilitation professionals using this model and by experts rating the process and outcomes of each model.

A total of 69 participants out of an initial group of 81 rehabilitation professionals working in various Virginia, West Virginia, and Pennsylvania Rehabilitation Agencies volunteered to participate in this study, completing all the requirements. These professionals included vocational rehabilitation (VR) counselors (70%), and supervisors, district managers, and division administrators (30%). In terms of gender, 42% were females and 58% were males. Other descriptors included degree, years of experience working in rehabilitation, and previous training in ethics. Approximately 8% had a doctoral degree, while 70% had a master's degree, and 22% had an undergraduate degree. Regarding previous training, 82% of participants had previous training in ethics, 11% reported no previous training, and 7% described their previous training in ethics as minimal. None had received training on specific ethical resolution models.

From the 69 participants who completed the study, 18 had been originally assigned to a control group who received training later, 22 to an experimental group receiving training in the integrative ethical decision-making model, and 29 to a second experimental group who received training on a rational ethical decision-making

Table 13-1 Transcultural Integrative Model of Ethical Dilemma Resolution in Counseling*

		General	Transcultural
Step I: Interpret the Situation Through Awareness and Fact-Finding	1. Enhance sensitivity and awareness.	Determine emotional, cognitive sensitivity and awareness of needs, and welfare of the people involved.	Examine counselor attitudes and emotional reactions toward cultural groups; counselor knowledge of client's culture; counselor awareness of their own and the client's cultural identity, acculturation, and role socialization; counselor awareness of own multicultural counseling competence skills.
	2. Reflect to analyze whether a dilemma is involved.	A dilemma occurs when counselors have opposing options.	Determine whether the identification of the courses of action involved in the dilemma reflects the counselor's world-view, the client's, or both.
	3. Determine the major stakeholders.	Identify the parties who are affected and their ethical and legal relationships to the client.	Determine the meaningful parties involved based on the cultural values of the client.
	4. Engage in the fact-finding process.	Review and understand current information as well as seek new information.	Gather relevant cultural information such as immigration (history, reasons, and patterns), family values, and community relationships.
Step II: Formulate an Ethical Decision	1. Review the dilemma.	Determine whether the dilemma has changed or not in light of the new information gathered in Step I.	Ensure that the cultural information gathered in Step I was considered when reviewing the dilemma.
	2. Determine relevant ethical codes, laws, ethical principles, institution policies, and procedures.	Determine the ethics laws and practice applicable to the situation.	Examine whether the ethics code of your profession contains diversity standards; examine potential discriminatory laws, institutional policies and procedures; estimate potential conflicts between laws and ethics resulting from a cultural perspective.

Table 13-1 Transcultural Integrative Model of Ethical Dilemma Resolution in Counseling* (cont.)

	General	Transcultural
3. Generate courses of action.	List all possible and probable courses of action.	Make sure courses of action selected reflect the cultural worldview of the parties involved. Use relational method and social constructivism techniques (negotiating, consensualizing, and arbitrating) as appropriate to reach agreement on potential courses of action.''
4. Consider potential positive and negative consequences for each course of action.	List both positive and negative consequences under each of the courses of action selected.	Consider the positive and negative consequences of each course of action from within the cultural worldview of each of the parties involved. Again, consider using a relational method and social constructivism techniques to reach an agreement on analyzing consequences.
5. Conduct a consultation.	Consult with supervisors and other knowledgeable professionals.	Consult with supervisors and professionals who have pertinent multicultural expertise.
6. Select the best ethical course of action.	Based on a rational analysis of the consequences and ethical principles underlying the competing courses of action, determine the best course of action.	Based on a relational method and a cultural analysis of the consequences of each selected course of action, choose the course of action that best represents an agreement between the cultural worldview of the client and that of the other parties involved. Use social constructivism techniques to choose a course of action mutually satisfying to key parties.
	Identify counselor's nonmoral values that may interfere with the implemen-	Identify how the counselor's nonmoral values may be reflecting a culture differ-

Step II: Formulate an Ethical Decision

Table 13-1 Transcultural Integrative Model of Ethical Dilemma Resolution in Counseling* (cont.)

	General	Transcultural
Step III: Weigh Competing Values and Contextual Factors		
1. Engage in reflective recognition and analysis of personal blind spots.		
2. Consider contextual influences on values selection.	Consider contextual influences on values selection at the collegial, professional team, institutional, and societal levels.	In addition to the levels mentioned, counselors should consider values selection at the cultural level.
Step IV: Planning and Executing the Final Course of Action		
1. Develop a reasonable sequence of concrete actions.	Divide that course of action into simple sequential actions.	Identify culturally relevant resources and strategies for the implementation of the plan.
2. Anticipate personal and contextual barriers and countermeasures.	Anticipate and confront personal and contextual barriers to successful implementation of the plan of action and countermeasures.	Anticipate cultural barriers such as biases, discrimination, stereotypes, and prejudices. Develop effective and relevant culture-specific countermeasures for instance, culturally sensitive conflict resolution and support.
3. Implement, document, and evaluate the course of action.	Execute course of action as planned. Document and gather valid and reliable information and evaluate accuracy of the course of action.	Utilize a relational method and social constructivism technique to identify measures and data sources that include both universal as well culture-specific variables.

*Adapted from the Integrative Model developed by Tarvydas (1998).

**Relational model as described in A. Davis (1997), and Social Constructivism model as described by R. Cottone (2001).

model. The participants in the control group received a case scenario that they needed to solve before receiving any of the training. Assignment to groups was done randomly. For a power of .80, an alpha level of .05, a medium effect size, and an ANOVA with three groups, the estimated sample size is 52 (Cohen, 1992). The final sample size of this study exceeded that estimate.

The independent variable was type of training on ethical decision-making models received by the participants. The levels of this variable comprised training on the integrative model, training on the rational model, and no initial training. The integrated and rational training model was delivered online using software named Prometheus produced by The George Washington University.

The researchers organized the training in a total of five online sessions within a six-week format; during the first week, the participants received training on ethics theory and principles; the second week focused on key ethical issues such as confidentiality, client welfare, dual relationships, informed consent, and client diversity; and the third week included specific training on either the integrative ethical decision-making model or the rational model. Each of these first three sessions consisted of a posted lecture, posted readings, and a weekly discussion around a set of posted questions. Session Four involved solving a case scenario depicting an ethical dilemma utilizing the model learned in Session Three (see a sample case scenario in Exhibit 13-1). As resources for completing this task, the authors posted a step-by-step description of each model, making certain that trainees were only able to access the one model targeted for their group. In addition, the authors posted both the American Counseling Association (ACA) Code of Ethics and Standards of Practice and the Commission on Rehabilitation Counselor Certification (CRCC) Code of Professional Ethics. Trainees received detailed feedback about their response from the senior trainer. Session Five consisted of posting a different final case scenario that the trainees had to solve in a two-week span, utilizing the feedback they received in Session Four and the resources provided for that previous session. The senior author of this study delivered all the training, with the assistance of an assistant research professor and two doctoral students in counseling (see Exhibit 13-1).

Exhibit 13-1: Case Scenario*

Norma is a 21-year-old college student who immigrated to the United States with her parents from El Salvador when she was 2 years old. She is bicultural in the sense that she proudly identifies herself as a Latina while at the same time has learned the instrumental behaviors that allow her to be effective and successful in the host culture. She speaks English and has been able to advance educationally to the point that she will soon graduate with a bachelor's degree. Socially, she interacts with people from different cultures.

Two years ago she started dating a young Latino man about her age named Javier. They became close very quickly and started spending lots of time together. He moved to the

 continued

United States from El Salvador about one year ago, never went to college, but finished high school and learned some mechanical skills in his native country; he was able to do mechanical repair work for a while, but since he does not have his immigration papers he could not get a permanent job. Norma has been helping him and told him that since she is a citizen, she will help him get papers if they get married and has even contacted a lawyer who is involved in the case, although her parents and her relatives oppose her doing so since they think Javier can bring her down. He lives in the United States with other friends and a cousin in a shared apartment. His parents and siblings are back in El Salvador.

About two months ago, Javier had a vehicle accident and is now paraplegic. Norma told him about rehabilitation services so they went to a state VR agency and met with a rehabilitation counselor, Ms. Jones, who is African American and has been with the agency for about 10 years. Javier is unsure about his vocational goals and thinks that his best option may be to get disability and go back to his country or live with Norma, (neither of which does Norma agree with). Ms. Jones now has a problem since she does not know what route to take in this case and thinks that there may be an ethical dilemma here that she needs to solve in the best way possible.

What do you think about this case? If there is an ethical dilemma how would you go about solving it from the rehabilitation counselor's perspective? What steps would you follow?

*Adapted from Young (1996).

To maximize the effectiveness of the online training sessions, the researchers organized the training into three cohorts, with a maximum of 25 participants at a time, making sure that each cohort was balanced in the number of participants in each experimental and control condition. Participants in the control group were assigned to either the integrative or rational model in the third cohort to ensure that they received training. Their responses were only used once (as controls) for purposes of data analysis of the second dependent measure to avoid biasing the interpretation of the results, since having been exposed to the ethics scenario before the training could have biased their responses. As a result of using cohorts, the entire training period took approximately five months, with each cohort receiving five online sessions of training over six weeks.

The content, materials, and format for the five sessions were validated by using a three-step procedure: (1) reviewing of the pertinent literature and consultation with the author of the Integrative Decision-Making Model; (2) sending the lectures, materials, and format description to five national ethics experts who evaluated them using a validation questionnaire developed by the authors; and (3) testing the entire training procedure with a pilot sample of 20 doctoral rehabilitation counseling students and rehabilitation counselors working in Maryland state VR offices. This pilot sample provided feedback about the proposed training using the same questionnaire sent to the experts.

There were two dependent measures: (1) the participants' 5-point Likert rating scale of the quality of the ethical decision-making model learned through training (ranging from 1 = strongly disagree to 5 = strongly agree), and (2) the experts' 5-point Likert rating scale of the quality of the responses of participants to the final case scenario depicting an ethical dilemma (ranging from 1 = totally inadequate to 5 = excellent). The Rating Scale 1 (participants' model ratings) consisted of 14 items. Participants were asked to rate the degree to which the learned model met certain quality standards, such as whether it was easy to learn, easy to follow, and useful for professionals. Four of the items reflected aspects of self-efficacy theory: increasing self-confidence, satisfying expectations, decreasing anxiety, and increasing the belief in performing ethically.

The Rating Scale 2 (expert ratings) consisted of 17 items that addressed relevant characteristics of an ethical decision-making model, such as defining the dilemma, identifying the parties involved in the dilemma, and analyzing the legal aspects involved. The raters were asked to evaluate the extent to which each response addressed each item effectively, codifying each individual respondent's ability to apply the model to multiple aspects of the dilemma. See Table 13-2 for a complete list of the questions used in the rating scales.

The rating scales were validated by following the same three-step procedure utilized to validate the intervention: (1) development of items by the authors, based on a review of pertinent literature; (2) sending out items to the same ethics experts who reviewed the training materials; and (3) administering the scales to the pilot sample of 20 participants described earlier.

The test-retest reliability for Rating Scale 1 was .98 and the internal consistency reliability was .89. The inter-rater reliability for Rating Scale 2 across the three raters was .78 and its internal consistency reliability was .98.

The authors posted Rating Scale 1 on Prometheus, and participants could access it upon completion of the five program sessions. After rating the items, the participants submitted them electronically in a format that could be viewed by the authors only, not by the trainees. Rating Scale 2 was mailed to the three ethics experts along with a hardcopy of each of the trainee's case scenario responses. These experts were faculty members with a scholarly record focusing on ethics and/or a history of serving on professional ethics committees. The authors ensured the anonymity of the responses by deleting any identifying information about the participants. In addition, the responses did not contain any indication that could have revealed information about the existence of different experimental groups to the raters. Moreover, the raters were unaware of the nature of the study.

The analysis of the data involved descriptive and multivariate statistical procedures as described in the results section that follows. Means and standard deviations were calculated for the 13 items under Scale 1 and the 17 items under Scale 2.

Table 13-2 Measurement Questions

Rating the Ethical Dilemma Model Competency Measurement Questions (Scale 1)	Ethical Dilemma Resolution Rating Questions (Scale 2)
The ethical decision-making model is:	How well does the model used by the respondent. . .

The ethical decision-making model is:

1: Easy to follow
2: Clearly distinct from other models
3: Easy to learn
4: Useful for me as a professional
5: Inclusive of the perspective of all parties involved
6: Founded in sound theory
7: One that increases awareness of my own values and morals
8: One that increases awareness of my own ethical decision-making style
9: One that leads to feasible courses of action
10: Helpful in increasing my confidence in making appropriate ethical decisions
11: One that satisfies my expectations as a user of this model
12: Helpful in decreasing my anxiety about making ethical decisions
13: One that increases the probability that I would actually perform more ethically
14: One that includes cultural factors systematically

How well does the model used by the respondent. . .

1: Define the ethical dilemma?
2: Identify the parties involved in the dilemma?
3: Analyze the legal aspects of the dilemma?
4: Identify and analyze individual values of parties involved?
5: Identify the counselor's own values regarding the dilemma?
6: Determine the rights and responsibilities of the various parties in this dilemma?
7: Determine the different parties' involvement in the dilemma?
8: Address the emotions of the parties involved?
9: Consult with other professionals or other sources of help or information concerning the dilemma?
10: Consider professional and institutional guidelines?
11: Consider principle and virtue ethics?
12: Generate different courses of action?
13: Consider consequences (both benefits and risks) of all identified courses of action?
14: Analyze and choose most appropriate course of action for this dilemma?
15: Plan the implementation of their chosen course of action?
16: Analyze contextual influences to execution of course of action?
17: Plan to evaluate the identified course of action?

Multivariate tests (Wilk's Lambda) of between-subject effects were performed to analyze the difference between the integrative and the rational models on the model ratings by participants and among the integrative, rational, and control groups on the competency ratings by the ethics experts. In testing the latter comparison, the authors pooled together the scores by the three raters.

The results showed that all the means were above 3, indicating that the participants scored both models favorably. However, a multivariate Wilk's Lambda test showed that significant differences existed between the two groups (F = 3.812; Sig. = 001; observed power = .99).

Individual-item tests of between-subject effects showed that there were significant rating differences between the integrative and rational group on six of the scale items. Participants in the rational model provided significantly higher ratings for this model over the integrative model on seven of the items: easy to follow (.002), easy to learn (.000), useful for me as a professional (.001), founded in sound theory (.02), helpful in decreasing anxiety related to ethical decision making (.01), model leads to feasible courses of action (.002), and model satisfies the expectations of the user (.000).

The means of the combined scores by the independent raters were consistently above 3 for the integrative and rational group's responses, and below 2 for the responses of participants in the control group. A Wilk's Lambda multivariate test showed significant differences across groups (F = 5.223; Sig. = .000; observed power = 1.00). A post-hoc Tukey HSD test with an alpha level of .05 revealed significant differences between both experimental groups and the control group at a significance level of .000 across all 17 items. Even though the mean ratings for the integrative group responses appeared higher than those for the rational group in 13 of the 17 items, no significant differences between the ratings of the integrative and rational group responses were detected, except for item "consult with other professionals" in which the ratings of the integrative group were significantly higher than those of the rational group (mean difference = .84; standard error = .239; Sig. = .002).

The results of this study showed that participants rated both models of ethical decision making highly across the 13 items of the scale since the scores were well above the midpoint. However, the ratings by participants in the group trained on the rational model were significantly higher than the ratings by participants receiving training on the integrative model in seven of the items. These ratings seem to indicate that the rational model is easier to follow, easier to learn, more useful, leads to more feasible courses of action, is more anxiety-reducing, and, overall, is more satisfactory to users than the integrative model. In addition, the rational model received significantly higher ratings on theoretical foundations than the integrative model. These results also seem to indicate that the integrative model needs to be revised to make it simpler to use. This may be achieved by revising its length, sequence, steps, and feasibility of implementation. Interpretation of the results of this study indicates that users appear to prefer the linear and faster model offered by the rational approach.

The expert ratings yielded a different picture. Both models were similarly helpful in helping rehabilitation professionals resolve ethical dilemmas, and both were significantly superior to no training on a decision-making model. Looking at the items in the scale, it seems that both models lead to appropriate definition of dilemmas, identification of the parties involved and their rights and responsibilities, consideration of the legal aspects and institutional guidelines, inclusion of principle and virtue ethics, and identification and evaluation of courses of action. In addition, it seems that both models are equally responsive to the values and emotional reactions of professional users and the parties involved in a dilemma. The responses of those using the integrative model received significantly higher ratings pertaining to consultation with other professionals, which was expected by the researchers since the integrative model is founded on collaboration strategies. The fact that the results showed no significant differences between using either model in all but one of the 17 items was somewhat unexpected by the authors, even though the responses of participants using the integrative model received higher ratings than the responses of those using the rational model in most of the items.

Based on the theoretical assumptions and characteristics of each model, the authors expected that the integrative model would receive significantly higher ratings than the rational model, particularly regarding inclusion of parties involved, discussion of personal values, adherence to both principle and virtue ethics, and reaching a more appropriate course of action. This expectation was based on the premise that these variables were specific components of the integrative model. It is unlikely that these results are due to methodological limitations since participants were assigned randomly to groups, the raters were unaware of the nature and conditions of the study, the three raters had expert training in ethics, the interventions were standardized in an electronic format, and each group of participants received training exclusively on one model to avoid response contamination. Moreover, the fact that participants across groups had a similar background in ethics could not explain these results since the authors found significant differences between the two experimental groups and the control group.

Consequently, the leading interpretation of these results is that even though training on ethical decision-making models appears necessary to resolve dilemmas more effectively, there is no significant advantage in using the rational model over the integrative model (or vice versa), at least as suggested by the comparison of the two models targeted in this study. Researchers could further corroborate this conclusion by having all three groups (including the control group) receive equal training on general ethics first, and then provide specific ethical decision-making training to the experimental groups only. This design could address the comparison between general knowledge of ethics and specific knowledge about ethical resolution models more precisely. Another possible methodological modification would involve making the rating scale more specific, containing items that would lead to increased model discrimination. For instance, the inclusion of items reflecting personal, contextual, and cultural variables defined more narrowly in the feedback data could allow the results to better discriminate differences between the models.

This study provided initial evidence that training on ethical decision-making models does improve the ability of rehabilitation professionals to solve ethical dilemmas. Further research is necessary to demonstrate that the integrative model adds significantly to these skills, and to evaluate whether modifications to this model would lead to greater acceptance by users. This research appears warranted since the responses of the participants trained on the integrative model were rated significantly higher on one of the items by the expert raters. In addition, addressing some of the aforementioned methodological issues could lead to an improved research design. Nevertheless, the authors believe that the empirical methodology used in this study is a step forward in the development of strategies to test and validate ethical decision-making models.

Testing the Transcultural Integrative Model

Again, the author and a team of researchers conducted a study to test the transcultural integrative model. The purpose of this study was to evaluate the effectiveness of the transcultural integrative model by comparing it to the rational model described by Forrester-Miller and Davis (1995). There is a precedent in the use of this model as a comparison for testing other ethical decision-making models, as discussed elsewhere in this chapter. As previously mentioned, the rational model received high ratings by rehabilitation professionals across 13 selected model characteristics, and these scores were significantly higher than those received by the integrative model (Tarvydas, 1998). This new study replicated that design except that this time the rational model was compared against the transcultural ethical decision-making model described earlier.

The research question of this study was whether there was a significant difference between the participants' ratings of the rational ethical decision-making model and the participants' ratings of the transcultural ethical decision-making model. All participants used the same rating forms.

The researchers recruited participants from Virginia state VR agencies by contacting the training director of the state VR office, who posted flyers and sent electronic announcements to the professional staff working in those agencies. Target participants were professionals who would likely have experienced ethical dilemmas through the process of providing VR services to clients. A total of 60 professionals agreed to participate in this study and each received 10 CEUs towards certification in rehabilitation counseling. Most participants were master-level rehabilitation counselors (60%) and other direct service rehabilitation professionals such as vocational evaluators, rehabilitation technicians, and supervisors (40%). About 85% had master's degrees and 15% had advanced certificate or bachelor's degrees. The majority of the participants (65%) had taken an ethics course before as part of their education, and the others (35%) only had a workshop or less of previous ethics training. The gender distribution showed that about 82% of the participants were female, and identified themselves as White (76%), African American (12%), or Latina (2%). Thus, the typical participant in this study (across both groups) was a White female with a master's degree in rehabilitation counseling who had one course or less of previous ethics training, and worked in a VR agency in the Virginia Commonwealth.

Since the total number of 60 participants was too high from a pedagogical standpoint, the researchers divided the group into three cohorts of 20. Each cohort received exactly the same training. Within each cohort, the researchers assigned the participants randomly to one of two groups, one receiving training on the rational model of ethical decision-making and the other receiving training on the transcultural integrative model. Attrition was 13% ($n = 8$) and distributed about evenly across the three cohorts. The total number of participants who completed the training in each of the three cohorts was 18 for the first cohort (9 in the rational group and 9 in the transcultural group), 17 for the second cohort (9 in the rational group and 8 in the transcultural group), and 17 for the third cohort (9 in the rational group and 8 in the transcultural group).

The independent variable was type of training, with two levels: training on the transcultural model and training on the rational model of ethical decision making. The training was conducted online, using Blackboard software. The training consisted of seven online sessions lasting seven weeks. In the first four weeks, all participants received training on general ethics theory, principles, and main ethical issues concerning the counseling–client relationship; in Week Five, one group received training on the specific features of the transcultural model and the other group received training on the rational model. In Weeks 6 and 7, participants practiced the use of the model they learned by solving two case scenarios provided by the researchers and receiving feedback on how well they applied the model to each case. The training was adapted from the one utilized and validated in a previous study by Garcia, Winston, Borzuchowska, and McGuire-Kuletz (2004). At the end of the study, each participant had to rate the model they learned across the same 13 item, 5-point Likert scale Model Ratings Form validated by Garcia et al. (2004). Nine of these items refer to characteristics of the model and four to self-efficacy in using the learned model. The Alpha coefficient for the ratings of the transcultural model was .97 and .96 for the rational model.

The researchers used descriptive statistics and a multivariate test to analyze the data. For a two-group comparison, the multivariate test chosen was the Hotelling's Trace. The results showed that, generally, the means for both groups were high across all three cohorts, and the multivariate analysis (Hotelling's Trace) yielded no significant differences across groups for all cohorts ($F = 2.175$; $df = 13$; Sig = .053 for cohort 1; $F = 1.052$; $df = 13$; Sig = .588 for cohort 2, and $F = .617$; $df = 13$; Sig = .767 for cohort 3).

The main research question in this study was whether there were significant differences between a group receiving training on a rational model of ethical decision making and a group receiving training on a transcultural integrative model on the model ratings completed by participants after the training. The results of a multivariate analysis showed no group differences for all three training cohorts. The means reflected high ratings (approximately 4 out of a maximum of 5) for each model across the 13 items, which means that, in general, participants across the three cohorts viewed both models quite favorably. The finding of no differences across groups represents an improvement over previous findings that showed the rational model as better than the integrative model of ethical decision making (Garcia et al., 2003). This integrative model provided the foundation for the transcultural model evaluated in this study, but it was devoid of the cultural variables incorporated in the transcultural model. Thus, a plausible explanation for this improvement could be that the addition of cultural components made the integrative model developed by Tarvydas (1998) more useful and attractive to professionals in the VR field. From a practitioners' perspective, the finding that the transcultural model is equal to the rational model is relevant because, traditionally, the rational model has been the accepted practice. This means that the transcultural model, pending further replication studies, could be considered best practice along with the rational model. This allows professionals to choose what model to use depending on the nature of the ethical dilemma they are facing or the cultural context in which it occurs.

Still, several limitations of this study need to be addressed. Perhaps it would have been reasonable to add a no-training comparison group to investigate whether training was better than no training at all. However, the authors had ethical concerns associated with having a group that would not benefit from the study. In addition, there has been consistent evidence that training is significantly better than no training in helping professionals deal effectively with ethical dilemmas, particularly when that training includes the use of ethical decision-making models (Garcia et al., 2004).

Another limitation is statistical power. The size of the groups under each cohort was not sufficient to have at least a power of .80. The authors could have aggregated the group data from the three cohorts and compared the transcultural data to the rational data without considering their cohort. Then the size of each group would have been around 26, which is the number required to meet a power of .80 for a comparison analysis with two groups, an alpha of .05, and a large effect size. However, the authors thought that this procedure would have violated the integrity of the data since the cohorts received training at different times.

IMPLICATIONS FOR PRACTICE

Providing an extensive case illustration of the use of the transcultural model exceeds the scope of this chapter. However, a point can be made about its potential applicability in a variety of settings. Garcia et al. (1998) conducted a confirmatory factor analysis study that showed the complexity of ethical dilemmas faced by counselors working with HIV/AIDS populations. They found that counselor ratings of the dilemmas loaded onto eight categories; disclosure, family/social, legal, health, death, vocational, sexual, and counselor–client relationship issues. This study also examined demographic characteristics of counselors that could predict their ratings of the extent to which they face those dilemmas. Three predictors were found to be significant: previous training in HIV/AIDS, age, and sexual orientation. An argument can be made that the latter two variables involve aspects of culture as a source of variability. The authors of this study concluded that counselors addressing dilemmas encountered in their work with this population need to be competent in dealing with the cultural aspects involved. Moreover, Garcia et al. (1998) wrote an extensive article on why an integrative model of ethical decision making was best suited for counselors working in this setting, and suggested that cultural modifications of the integrative model (Tarvydas, 1998) were necessary. The transcultural model responded to that statement and appears particularly suited to use in HIV/AIDS counseling settings.

Herlihy and Corey (1996) examined a broader set of possible dilemmas in the practice of rehabilitation counseling that included issues related to informed consent, competence, multicultural counseling, multiple clients, working with minors, dual relationships, suicidal clients, counselor training and supervision, and the interface between law and ethics. They presented a series of case studies illustrating the nature of the dilemmas and a potential solution based on an analysis of the professional code of ethics. An argument can be made that the transcultural ethical dilemma resolution presented here could add specific tools to deal with those issues, particularly those related to multicultural counseling, competence, dual relationships, counselor training and supervision, and serving multiple clients.

Other authors have presented case examples that involve cultural factors in counseling women, women in prisons, and individuals with disabilities. Pitman (1999) described cases involving lesbian clients who faced rigid societal values and prejudices concerning their sexual desire, sexual behavior, and physical appearance. Bruns and Lesko (1999) analyzed the complexities of working with women in prisons, where they face dilemmas related to working in an oppressive, racist, and patriarchal institution, as they described it. Olkin (1999) presented dilemmas encountered by professionals working with people with disabilities. Central dimensions associated with those dilemmas include value and quality of life, morality, normality and deviance, justice, interdependence, and mortality. Again, most of these aspects imply differing cultural values and worldviews, which is the focus of a transcultural ethical model.

The studies examined here provide a nonexclusive sample of settings in which the model proposed in this article could be of benefit. Surely, additional studies will appear in the future when other researchers begin to focus more closely on this subject.

IMPLICATIONS FOR CAPACITY BUILDING

The implications for capacity building are varied. Over the last decade, there has been a trend to require professionals to receive more training in ethics. This is true of all fields in mental health, including counseling and psychology, and particularly in rehabilitation counseling. However, based on the theory and research analyzed in this chapter, the focus of such training should include more aspects of ethical decision making. This is where theory and practice merge, and the quality of our thinking and acting ethically rests to a large extent on how effectively professionals translate theory into courses of action that best address the dilemmas they encounter when working with clients from different cultural/ethnic backgrounds. Like never before, culture interacts with every aspect of our rehabilitation counseling efforts and there is a need for models that incorporate such variables systematically. By expanding training in the interface of ethics and culture, more specific guidelines could be developed to ascertain what models, for what clients, in what settings, and for what type of disability work best. Finally, more training experience and research in this topic should provide valuable information on what credentials, personal characteristics, and level of knowledge is required for professionals to be more effective in dealing with the complex ethical dilemmas of today. Clients are getting older, with multiple chronic disabilities, and representing multiple languages and cultures, which means that it is more likely that ethical dilemmas will become more frequent and difficult to address in the future. Capacity building in the colleges and universities responsible for training professionals in this subject would most certainly lead to best practices in ethical decision making.

IMPLICATIONS FOR FUTURE RESEARCH

The state of the scientific knowledge in this area of study is rather lacking. There are many models available for making ethical decisions, based on particular moral, principle, virtue, and even constructivist theories, but few of them have been submitted to empirical analysis or evaluation, so there is a lack of research designs and measures to conduct this kind of research. In addition, most of these models assume a monocultural perspective, implying that practitioners would be able to apply them to clients from all cultural backgrounds, with no specific integration of multicultural theories or methods that are readily available today.

Without question, more research needs to be conducted in this area. At the theoretical level, much can be done to develop theories that combine multicultural psychology or counseling theory with ethical theory. The models discussed so far, particularly the transcultural model, use both theories separately, making no attempt to truly integrate both theories into one that may explain or predict professionals' effectiveness in resolving ethical dilemmas. For instance, we could compare models including ethnic identity theory and ethics theory against models integrating cultural identity and ethics theory, or gender role socialization and ethics theory. In addition, other rehabilitation counseling theories such as acceptance of disability or disability identity development may play a role in predicting effective ethical dilemma resolution with clients with disabilities.

Regarding research, many more studies are needed to address issues of research type and research design. For instance, future studies would have to assess whether combining quantitative and qualitative research would best contribute to learning more about ethical decision making, culture, and disability. In terms of research design, more sophisticated experimental designs are needed to test specific elements of ethical decision-making models or to predict professional effectiveness by looking at previous experience, ethnicity, or knowledge about ethics. There is also the need to develop and validate more measures and instrumentation, particularly to measure competence, applicability and knowledge of ethical decision making.

Finally, more knowledge is needed to evaluate the translation of these models into specific ethical decision-making practices. Questions such as how, when, and what models are to be used with particular clients need to be examined by future researchers. For example, it is unclear whether practitioners need to use a model every time they face an ethical dilemma, whether only certain aspects of the model need to be used, or what type of model works best for specific ethical dilemmas. In addition, based on the empirical research described earlier in this chapter, it appears that much attention needs to be given to aspects of simplicity, linearity, and guidelines for application of these models.

REFERENCES

American Counseling Association. (2006). *Code of ethics and standards of practice*. Alexandria, VA: Author.

Baruth, L. G., & Manning, M. L. (1999). *Multicultural counseling and psychotherapy: A lifespan perspective* (2nd ed.). Upper Saddle River, NJ: Prentice Hall.

Bersoff, D. N. (1996). The virtue of principle ethics. *The Counseling Psychologist, 24*, 86–91.

Bruns, C. M., & Lesko, T. M. (1999). In the belly of the beast: Morals, ethics, and feminist psychotherapy with women in prison. In E. Kaschak & M. Hill (Eds.), *Beyond the rule book: Moral issues and dilemmas in the practice of psychotherapy* (pp. 69–85). New York: The Haworth Press.

Cohen, J. (1992). A power primer. *Psychological Bulletin, 112*, 155–159.

Cottone, R. R. (2001). A social constructivism model of ethical decision-making in counseling. *Journal of Counseling Development, 79*, 39–45.

Davis, A. H. (1997). The ethics of caring: A collaborative approach to resolving ethical dilemmas. *Journal of Applied Rehabilitation Counseling, 28*(1), 36–41.

Falvo, D. R., & Parker, R. M. (2000). Ethics in rehabilitation education and research. *Rehabilitation Counseling Bulletin, 43*(4), 197–202.

Forrester-Miller, H., & Davis, T. E. (1995). *A practitioner's guide to ethical decision-making.* Alexandria, VA: American Counseling Association.

Freeman, S. J. (2000). *Ethics: An introduction to philosophy and practice.* Belmont, CA: Wadsworth/Thomson Learning.

Garcia, J., Cartwright, B., Winston, S., & Borzuchowska, B. (2003). A transcultural integrative ethical decision-making model in counseling. *Journal of Counseling and Development, 81,* 268–276.

Garcia, J. G., Forrester, L. E., & Jacob, A. V. (1998). Ethical dilemma resolution in HIV/AIDS counseling: Why an integrative model? *International Journal of Rehabilitation and Health, 4*(3), 167–181.

Garcia, J., Winston, S., Borzuchowska, B., & McGuire-Kuletz, M. (2004). Evaluating the integrative model of ethical decision-making. *Rehabilitation Education, 18*(3), 147–164.

Herlihy, B., & Corey, G. (1996). *ACA ethical standards casebook.* Alexandria, VA: American Counseling Association.

Ibrahim, F. A., & Arredondo, P. M. (1986). Ethical standards for cross-cultural counseling: Counselor preparation, practice, assessment, and research. *Journal of Counseling and Development, 64,* 349–352.

Jordan, A. E., & Meara, N. M. (1995). Ethics and the professional practice of psychologists: The role of virtues and principles. In D. N. Bersoff (Ed.), *Ethical conflicts in psychology* (pp. 135–141). Washington, DC: American Psychological Association.

Kitchener, K. S. (1984). Intuition, critical evaluation and ethical principles: The foundation for ethical decisions in counseling psychology. *The Counseling Psychologist, 12*(3), 43–55.

LaFromboise, T. D., & Foster, S. L. (1989). Ethics in multicultural counseling. In P. B. Pedersen, J. G. Draguns, J. Lonner, & J. E. Trimble (Eds.), *Counseling across cultures* (3rd ed., pp. 115–136). Honolulu: University of Hawaii Press.

Maturana, H. R. (1980). Biology of cognition. In H. R Maturana & F. J. Varela, *Autopoiesis and cognition: The realization of the living* (pp. 5–58). Boston: Reidel.

Olkin, R. (1999). The personal, professional and political when clients have disabilities. In E. Kaschak & M. Hill (Eds.), *Beyond the rule book: Moral issues and dilemmas in the practice of psychotherapy* (pp. 87–103). New York: The Haworth Press.

Pedersen, P. E. (1997). The cultural context of the American Counseling Association code of ethics. *Journal of Counseling and Development, 76,* 23–28.

Pitman, G. E. (1999). The politics of naming and the development of morality: Implications for feminist therapists. In E. Kaschak & M. Hill (Eds.), *Beyond the rule book: Moral issues and dilemmas in the practice of psychotherapy* (pp. 21–38). New York: The Haworth Press.

Remy, G. M. (1998). Ethnic minorities and mental health: Ethical concerns in counseling immigrants and culturally diverse groups. *Trotter Review, 9,* 13–16.

Steiner, L. (1997). A feminist schema for analysis of ethical dilemmas. In F. Casmir (Ed.), *Ethics in intercultural and international communications* (pp. 59–88). Mahwah, NJ: Lawrence Erlbaum.

Tarvydas, V. M. (1998). Ethical decision making processes. In R. R. Cottone & V. M. Tarvydas (Eds.), *Ethical and professional issues in counseling* (pp. 144–155). Upper Saddle River, NJ: Prentice-Hall.

Tarvydas, V. M. (2003). Ethical decision-making processes. In R. R. Cottone & V. M. Tarvydas (Eds.), *Ethical and professional issues in counseling* (pp. 85–111). Upper Saddle River, NJ: Prentice Hall.

Welfel, E. R. (2002). *Ethics in counseling and psychotherapy: Standards, research, and emerging issues.* Pacific Grove, CA: Brooks/Cole.

Young, M. E. (1996). Case Study 2—Pressures from all sides: A rehabilitation counselor's dilemma. In B. Herlihy & G. Corey (Eds.), *ACA ethical standards casebook* (5th ed.) (pp. 156–158). Alexandria, VA: American Counseling Association.

Models to Improve Rehabilitation Services for Multicultural Populations with Disabilities

(B) MODELS FOR REHABILITATION PRACTICE

CHAPTER 14

Cultural Competence: A Review of Conceptual Frameworks

Fabricio Balcazar, PhD;
Yolanda Suarez-Balcazar, PhD;
Celestine Willis, MA;
Francisco Alvarado, MA

INTRODUCTION

Due in part to the growing diversity of the population in the United States and documented racial/ethnic disparities in health and rehabilitation outcomes, human service providers and practitioners are under increasing pressure from their professional organizations to become more culturally competent. This pressure is especially strong in the fields of health care, psychology, counseling, and rehabilitation (cf., U.S. Department of Health and Human Services [HHS], 2001; American Psychological Association [APA], 2003; Commission on Rehabilitation Counseling Certification, 2001). As a result, many professionals in these service systems see the need to clarify what is involved in providing culturally competent care. In fact, researchers and providers from multiple disciplines have proposed various skills, knowledge, and approaches that can increase *cultural competence* (CC) in systems, organizations, and programs (Goode, Sockalingam, Brown, & Jones, 2000). Although they may be helpful, these practices and interventions have not been empirically evaluated, therefore assertions about their effectiveness are often premature (Blase & Fixsen, 2003).

In this chapter we present definitions of CC, consider some key reasons for promoting CC among service providers, review CC conceptual frameworks, and finally present a synthesis model that we developed on the basis of our review of the literature. The proposed model represents an attempt to distill and integrate the literature on CC from multiple disciplines and conceptual orientations.

DEFINITIONS OF CULTURAL COMPETENCE

There is an ongoing debate among professionals about how best to define and operationalize the construct of CC and there is a lack of a universally accepted definition of the term (Bonder, Martin, & Miracle, 2004). For example, researchers have proposed terms such as *cultural sensitivity, cultural responsiveness, cultural effectiveness*, or *cultural humility*, which emphasize different aspects of the process and reflect a general lack of consensus about what CC is. Rosenjack-Burcham (2002) explained that these phrases are often used in place of CC but have greater meaning as components of CC.

It is generally agreed that the word *culture* refers to an integrated pattern of behaviors, norms, and rules that are shared by a group and involves their beliefs, values, expectations, worldviews, communication, common history, and institutions (Gladding, 2001). Culture was defined by Fiske, Kitayama, Markus, and Nisbett (1998), cited by the APA guidelines of 2003, as the "belief systems and value orientations that influence customs, norms, practices, and social institutions, including psychological processes (language, caretaking practices) and organizations (media and educational systems)" (p. 380). The implication is that every person is a cultural being and all persons have a specific cultural, ethnic, and racial heritage.

The word *competence* can denote having the capacity to function effectively as an individual and an organization within the context of the cultural beliefs, behaviors, and needs presented by consumers and their communities (Cross, Bazron, Dennis, & Isaacs, 1989). Cultural competence among providers has the potential to influence the outcomes of most interventions because it focuses on understanding the different experiences of members of diverse cultural groups; it attempts to address the barriers in communication across cultures; and it helps develop professionals' abilities to work effectively with individuals and families from various cultures (Pope-Davis & Dings, 1995).

Betancourt, Green, and Carrillo (2002) argued that a culturally competent system of care is one that acknowledges the importance of culture, includes assessments of cross-cultural relations, examination of the dynamics that result from cultural differences, expansion of cultural knowledge among providers, and has the capacity to adapt services to the needs of culturally diverse consumers. Suarez-Balcazar and Rodakowski (2007) suggested that "becoming culturally competent is an ongoing contextual, developmental, and experiential process of personal growth that results in a greater ability to adequately serve individuals who look, think, and behave in ways that are different from us" (p. 15).

Cultural competence transcends racial and ethnic backgrounds and includes all aspects of human diversity to incorporate groups that have been historically marginalized or oppressed like women, people who are gay and lesbian, and people with disabilities. In this chapter we focus our attention on CC as it relates to addressing the service needs of ethnically diverse individuals with disabilities in the United States.

REASONS FOR PROMOTING CULTURAL COMPETENCE

Cultural competence has become an essential component of professional training and development efforts in most disciplines and specialties that provide human services.

Wittman and Velde (2002) argued that service providers must acknowledge and be aware of cultural differences and recognize the influence of their own culture on their actions and thoughts. There are multiple reasons for encouraging service providers, especially within the health and disability service systems, to become more culturally competent. We focus on three reasons. *The first is the increased diversity of our nation and growth in the number of ethnically diverse individuals with disabilities.* According to the 2000 U.S. Census, after non-Latino Whites, the largest ethnic group in the United States is Latinos, followed by African Americans, while Asians—although numerically smaller—have had the fastest percentage of growth during the last 10 years. These groups represent about 30.58% of the total population, and adding other minority groups, up to 32.1% of the total U.S. population is now comprised of non-European Whites (U.S. Census Bureau, 2004). This represents more than 93 million ethnically diverse individuals who tend to concentrate in the nation's large metropolitan areas and are increasingly making their homes in suburban and rural areas as well.

The historic diversity of the United States starts before the arrival of the Europeans with millions of Native Americans who occupied the land and that today represent less than 1% of the total population. In 1619, a Dutch ship brought the first African slaves to the shores of North America and today African Americans are more than 38 million strong. Of all ethnic groups, African Americans were the only ones to arrive on these shores against their will. Throughout U.S. history, immigration has been a significant factor in the population growth, accompanied by high birth rates among some groups, particularly Latinos (U.S. Census Bureau, 2007). It is appropriate to acknowledge that Latino is not a racial category but an ethnic, linguistic, and cultural category. Latinos can be White, Native Amerindian Black, Asian or of mixed ancestry (i.e., various combinations of the main racial groups). In fact, the term "criollo" was used for many years throughout Latin America to denote those whose ancestry included at least one parent of European origin and the other from the Native Amerindian populations (Palmie, 2006).

Each year, the United States admits between 700,000 and 900,000 legal immigrants from various ethnic and racial backgrounds (Waters & Jimenez, 2005). These are the total number of people who were granted permanent residence, about half of whom are already living in the United States, legally on temporary visas (Bean & Stevens, 2003). Up to 65% of legal immigrants tend to settle in six states—California, New York, Florida, Texas, New Jersey, and Illinois (Waters & Jimenez). The resulting population diversity in these states becomes evident to anyone visiting a large metropolitan city like Los Angeles, New York, Chicago, San Francisco, Houston, or Miami. In the state of California, for example, the non-White population is now the majority. Unlike the first wave of settlers, today's immigrants and refugees are not drawn from Europe but come from diverse nations of Latin America, Asia, Africa, and the Middle East (Lee & Bean, 2004). Currently, five countries account for 40% of the immigrants to the United States—Mexico, India, the People's Republic of China, the Philippines, and Vietnam (Lee & Bean).

Table 14-1 summarizes the racial breakdown and the disability prevalence rates by racial category in the year 2000 (U.S. Census Bureau, 2003). It is important to note the large prevalence of disability among Native Americans and African Americans. The variation of disability by ethnicity has been attributed to class status and the greater exposure of poor ethnically diverse individuals to environmental hazards, dangerous occupations, and limited access to adequate healthcare services (Birenbaun, 2002).

We should also consider that among newly arrived refugees resettled in communities throughout the United States, far more have disabilities than in the past. For example, in 2003, 879 resettled refugees met the definition of having a disability and in 2006, 2600 refugees with disabilities were admitted into the United States (U.S. Committee for Refugees and Immigrants, 2008). This increase may be attributed to several factors including where the refugees are coming from and what they have been exposed to. Considering that conservative figures estimate 19% of people in the

Table 14-1 Percentage of U.S. Noninstitutionalized Population with any Disability by Race and Age

	Percentage of Total Population	Percentage with a Disability (5 to 64)	Percentage with a Disability (65 and older)
European American	67.85%	18.3%	40.4%
Latino American	13.72%	20.9%	48.5%
African American	12.76%	24.3%	52.8%
Asian American	4.10%	16.6%	40.8%
Native American and Alaska Native	0.96%	24.3%	57.6%
Native Hawaiian and other Pacific Islander	0.17%	19.0%	48.5%
Two or more races	1.48%	21.7%	51.8%
Total:		19.3%	41.9%

Source: U.S. Census Bureau (2003).

United States have a disability and the government anticipates resettling 60,000 refugees in 2009, these numbers are most likely understated.

The second reason to promote CC is *its potential to address the disparities in services for ethnically diverse individuals with disabilities*. Several scholars inside and outside of the disability field have noted some of the challenges of serving ethnically and racially diverse populations (Suarez-Balcazar et al., 2009). For example, Papado-poulos and Lees (2002) pointed out that it is increasingly difficult to be responsive to the different needs, experiences, values, and beliefs of a growing number and size of ethnically diverse groups in health research endeavors. Blase and Fixsen (2003) summarized the report of a national panel of experts reviewing evidence-based programs on CC in mental health and concluded that "there are practices and interventions that consumers and practitioners have found to be helpful in address-ing their problems and achieving their goals but for which the evidence base has not been fully established. Therefore, assertions about the effectiveness of these pro-grams are premature" (p. 17). One of the main reasons for this is that little research related to evidence-based programs has been conducted with diverse populations. For the most part, when randomized-controlled trials are conducted, assessing dif-ferences in outcomes for persons of different racial and ethnic origins or persons of various cultures has not been a focus of the research (Blase & Fixsen).

What is concerning is that one of the panels reviewing evidence in the Blase and Fixsen (2003) meeting concluded that "there is evidence that there are current ser-vices and programs that are ineffective for the problems they are intended to address, and under certain circumstances, may actually be harmful. These harmful effects can have disproportionately greater impact on persons belonging to specific racial, ethnic, and cultural groups." (p. 18). Examples of ineffective professional prac-tices include failing to listen before doing, failing to build personal relationships with the consumers, defining problems without input from the consumers, failing to com-municate (this includes problems with using interpreters or their absence in some cases), failing to ask for feedback from consumers, or failing to recognize that pro-fessionals are an integral part of the relationship.

In the field of vocational rehabilitation (VR), several studies have analyzed state VR data to assess racial and ethnic group differences in rehabilitation outcomes (e.g., Feist-Price, 1995; Herbert & Cheatham, 1988). With few exceptions (e.g., Bolton & Cooper, 1980; Wheaton, 1995; Wilson, 1999), the findings tend to show that compared to European Americans, ethnically diverse individuals are significantly less likely to be accepted for services, or be successfully rehabilitated (i.e., obtain gainful employment), and if employed, they have lower incomes (e.g., Baldwin & Smith, 1984; Capella, 2002; Olney & Kennedy, 2002; Wilson, 2002; Wilson, Harley, & Alston, 2001).

Brach and Fraserirector (2000) reviewed the CC and health disparities literature and concluded that there are several techniques that can have a significant outcome: providing appropriate interpreter services, having policies for recruiting and retaining minority staff, training, coordination of services with traditional healers, use of community health workers, utilizing culturally competent health promotion techniques, including family or community members, immersing staff into other cultures, and implementing administrative and organizational accommodations. However, the authors concluded that "health systems have little evidence about which cultural competency techniques are effective and less evidence on when and how to implement them properly" (p. 181).

The final reason for promoting CC is that *ignoring cultural differences creates and strengthens barriers and/or conflicts between groups, which may lead to continued racism, prejudice, and/or discrimination and poor outcomes* (Suarez-Balcazar, Muñoz, & Fisher, 2006). The complex fabric of social relations between various ethnic and cultural groups in American society often includes both positive acts of support and solidarity as well as incidents of discrimination and racism in communities and systems. An influential factor in maintaining many people's negative perceptions about lower socioeconomic groups—which often are overrepresented among minority populations—is what social psychologists have called the *Just World Hypothesis* (Lerner, 1980; Lipkus, Dalbert, & Siegler, 1996). According to this hypothesis, people are often eager to convince themselves that beneficiaries deserve their rewards and victims their suffering. The Just World Hypothesis means that people have a strong desire or need to believe that the world is an orderly, predictable, and just place. Therefore, in order to plan our lives or achieve our goals, we need to assume that our actions will have predictable consequences. Moreover, when we encounter evidence suggesting that the world is not just, we quickly act to restore justice by helping the victim, or we persuade ourselves that no injustice has occurred (Rubin & Peplau, 1975). Recent research (Sutton & Douglas, 2005), shows that the belief that the world is fair to the self is associated with indices of psychological health, whereas the belief that the world is fair to others is associated with harsh social attitudes. Their findings provide strong support for the distinction between perceived justice for the self and for others, and suggest that perceptions of justice are indeed the "active ingredient" responsible for their ability to predict psychological and social outcomes.

We argue that this commonly held belief contributes to perpetuating prejudice, segregation, and discrimination against poor, ethnically diverse individuals by the majority. Assuming that the world is already just also contributes to the unwillingness of many politicians to seek real solutions to the problems that afflict marginalized populations. In an effort to move beyond various definitions of CC and better understand the process, researchers have proposed a number of models that are reviewed and analyzed in the next section of this chapter.

REVIEW OF CONCEPTUAL MODELS FOR PROMOTING CULTURAL COMPETENCE

Analysis of the Current Literature

We conducted a search of databases in the social sciences (i.e., PsychINFO), education (i.e., ERIC), and health (i.e., PubMed), as well as Google Scholar for all English-language journal articles and books published from 1991–2006 using these search terms: *cultural competence models, cultural knowledge, cultural awareness, cultural competency research, multiculturalism, minorities,* and *cross-cultural services/care.* From these searches, we identified 259 peer reviewed articles and/or book chapters, excluding dissertations, technical reports, and conference presentations. Two independent reviewers examined the abstracts of these documents and identified 32 publications that refer to cultural competency models. After reviewing the full manuscripts, we identified 18 articles representing unique CC models. We excluded nine articles that offered professional guidelines for displaying culturally sensitive behaviors but did not attempt to provide a conceptual framework for explaining CC. We also excluded five articles that illustrate factors that impact cultural diversity. Table 14-2 provides a brief summary of the models, a list of the main components, their intended utilization and field of application.

There are a number of important aspects about these models of cultural competence that are worth examining. First, the models include from 3 to 12 components with considerable overlap. The most common components include: (1) *willingness to engage* (refers to having an attitude of openness or desire to interact with others who are different); (2) *cultural awareness* (developing a critical view of cultural differences, including experiences of oppression and marginalization, class differences, discrimination, racism, and becoming aware of one's cultural biases); (3) *cultural knowledge* (learning about the cultural practices of specific racial or ethnic groups and about the factors that lead to human diversity); (4) *cultural skills* (developing professional practices and behaviors designed to improve service delivery to diverse populations); and (5) *cultural practice* (experiencing other cultures and applying previous components). Thirteen of the models (72%) include awareness, knowledge, and skills as central components that lead to effective multicultural practice. Although *cultural competence desire or willingness to engage* was mentioned in five of the models, we agree that it is a necessary first step in the process of becoming culturally competent, since it cannot be forced upon any individual.

All of the models include cognitive and behavioral components, with few attending to contextual elements. The cognitive components emphasize awareness and knowledge acquisition. The behavioral components emphasize skills development—such as being able to engage culturally diverse clients in a genuine accepting manner

Table 14-2 Review of Cultural Competence Models

Author(s)/date	Model Components	Purpose	Field
Camphinha-Bacote (1999)	1) Cultural awareness 2) Cultural knowledge 3) Cultural skill 4) Cultural encounters 5) Cultural desire	It is developed for healthcare providers and healthcare organizations to use as a framework for developing and implementing culturally responsive healthcare services.	Nursing
Doorenbos and Schim (2004)	1) Cultural diversity 2) Awareness 3) Sensitivity 4) Cultural competence (this is the goal)	The model tries to achieve the goal of CC by promoting acknowledgement of cultural diversity, increasing awareness and knowledge about other cultural groups and the variations within groups, and increasing sensitivity of trainees regarding values, beliefs, and practice, particularly regarding communication skills, and use of translators when needed.	Nursing
Glockshuber (2005)	1) Cultural beliefs 2) Cultural knowledge 3) Cultural skills	The objective is to explore alternative ways for counselors to better understand how they perceived multicultural competencies.	Counseling
Harris-Davis and Haughton (2000)	Guide to developing multicultural nutrition counseling competence: 1) Multicultural nutrition counseling skills 2) Multicultural awareness 3) Multicultural food and nutrition counseling knowledge	1) Dieticians in supervisory or administrative positions can use the model to promote culticultural competence of their staff. 2) Dieticians and dietetics educators can use the model to organize self-evaluation and professional education.	Dieticians

Table 14-2 Review of Cultural Competence Models (continued)

Author(s)/date	Model Components	Purpose	Field
Hart, Hall, and Henwood (2003)	1) Equalities awareness 2) Equalities skills 3) Equalities actions 4) Equalities encounters 5) Equalities knowledge 6) Equalities analysis 7) Equalities desires	The model attempts to develop awareness of the "cultural inequalities" in healthcare professionals, emphasizing the importance of seeking equality with different cultures.	Nursing
Jezewski and Sotnik (2001, 2005)	The model has three stages: Stage 1: Identify the problem or need for brokering (identifies the issues of diversity and/or cultural differences that may cause problems in the relationship) Stage 2: Propose strategies/interventions to try out in the counseling relationship Stage 3: Examine the rehabilitation outcomes; resolution or lack of resolution of the issues	The model tries to bridge, link, and mediate between groups or persons of differing cultural backgrounds for the purpose of reducing a conflict or producing a change.	Vocational rehabilitation counseling
Kim-Godwin, Clarke, and Barton (2001)	1) Promotes cultural competence (involves critical awareness, cultural knowledge, and skills) 2) Examines the characteristics of the healthcare systems 3) Examines the health outcomes for community members from minority populations	Primarily designed to predict public health outcomes of culturally competent health care in communities. First construct of the model developed after a conceptual analysis following development and testing of a Cultural Competence Scale (CCS). The other two constructs are based on a literature review.	Nursing

Table 14-2 Review of Cultural Competence Models (continued)

Author(s)/date	Model Components	Purpose	Field
Leininger (1993)	Level I: Understanding of social structure, world view, and environment Level II: Identifying cultural values and healthcare features Level III: Understanding the healthcare systems and taxonomic classification of illnesses Level IV: Recognizing the roles, functions, and activities of health providers	The model was developed as a general guide for health professionals. This model depicts the different levels or areas of study to grasp a comprehensive view of health care with different cultures.	Nursing
McPhatter (1997)	The model has three main components and multiple factors: 1) Enlightened consciousness (reorientation of the case worker's primary worldview) 2) Grounded knowledge base (history and culture, dynamics of oppression, racism, sexism, classism, and other forms of discrimination, family structure, and functioning, etc.) 3) Cumulative skills proficiency (ability to engage in the culture of the client in a genuine, accepting manner)	The model was designed to help child welfare workers become culturally competent.	Social work

Table 14-2 Review of Cultural Competence Models (continued)

Author(s)/date	Model Components	Purpose	Field
Moffitt and Wuest (2002)	Model 1 The integration of culture: 1) Inquisitive way of being 2) Receptive way of being 3) Interactive way of being 4) Reflective way of being	The first model encourages practitioners to consider how they interact with others and examine their own behaviors.	Nursing
	Model 2 Modern knowledge model: 1) Traditional knowledge 2) Scientific knowledge 3) Examination of individual and community values	The second model emphasizes the acquisition of knowledge about other cultures.	
Papadopoulos and Lees (2002)	1) Cultural awareness 2) Cultural competence 3) Cultural knowledge 4) Cultural sensitivity	Focuses on two layers of cultural competence: culture-generic (apply to any culture) and culture-specific. The relationship between these two is dynamic.	Nursing
Poole (1998)	Cultural competence requires five components: 1) Knowledge of the context, influence of the family, and social networks 2) Skills to be able to adjust to work in cross-cultural situations 3) Adjustment in diagnosis and treatment 4) Change policy to hire staff from the target population and allow staff to engage in the target community 5) Being open to others	Attempts to allow professionals to recognize similarities and differences in the values, norms, customs, history, and institutions of diverse groups of people.	Social work and health care

Table 14-2 Review of Cultural Competence Models (continued)

Author(s)/date	Model Components	Purpose	Field
Salimbene (1999)	1) Ethnocentricity 2) Awareness and sensitivity 3) Ability to refrain from forming stereotypes 4) Acquisition of knowledge 5) Acquisition of skills	The model helps to support and improve cultural competency throughout an integrated healthcare system.	Nursing
Steenbarger (1993)	The process of multicontextual counseling has several stages: 1) Engages in the client's life context 2) The counselor facilitates new modes of experiencing, understanding, and acting 3) Helps professionals develop skills that enable them to interact effectively and sensitively with those who are different 4) Raises awareness about problems in the person-environment level 5) Attempts to modify communities so they become more supportive of desired behaviors 6) Helps community members deal with decision makers in order to help the disempowered	This model utilizes brief therapy principles in the context of multicultural counseling.	Counseling

Table 14-2 Review of Cultural Competence Models (continued)

Author(s)/date	Model Components	Purpose	Field
Sue, Arredondo, and McDavis (1992)	The dimensions of cultural competence have three components: beliefs and attitudes, knowledge, and skills. These are applied to the following guidelines. 1) Development of counselor's awareness of own assumptions, values, and biases 2) Understanding the worldview of the culturally different client 3) Developing appropriate intervention strategies and techniques	This model utilizes the guidelines proposed by the Association for Multicultural Counseling and Development to help counselors engage with consumers from diverse cultures.	Counseling
Suh (2004)	Attributes: 1) Cultural ability 2) Openness to cultural diversity 3) Cultural flexibility Antecedents: 1) Cognitive domain 2) Affective domain 3) Behavioral domain 4) Environmental domain Consequences: 1) Receiver-based variables 2) Provider-based variables 3) Health outcomes variables	This model provides a theoretical guide for developing strategies to achieve culturally competent care in nursing practice and research.	Nursing

Table 14-2 Review of Cultural Competence Models (continued)

Author(s)/date	Model Components	Purpose	Field
Wells (2000)	Cultural competence requires openness, flexibility, and ability. The model has antecedents and consequences. 1) Antecedents: Cognitive Domain: Cultural awareness and cultural knowledge Affective Domain: Cultural sensitivity Behavioral Domain: cultural skills Environmental Domain: cultural encounters 2) Consequences: Health Receiver-based variables: improved quality of life, healthcare satisfaction, and adherence to treatment HealthPprovider-based variables: personal and professional growth Health outcomes: improved quality of nursing performance; cost effective	The Cultural Development Model allows individuals and institutions to assess growth in cultural development from the cognitive through the affective phases.	Nursing

Table 14-2 Review of Cultural Competence Models (continued)

Author(s)/date	Model Components	Purpose	Field
Willis (1999)	1) Knowledge of one's own cultural affiliation: beliefs, values, and life ways 2) Knowledge of others: beliefs, values, and life ways 3) Nonthreatening/non-fear provoking interaction 4) Tolerance 5) Inclusion 6) Appreciation/ acceptance	The progression towards achievement of components is a building block approach. This conceptual framework was developed to help nurses provide culturally competent care during the perinatal period.	Nursing

(McPhatter, 1997). Only five of the models explicitly address learning about the context of the people they are trying to serve (Leininger, 1993; Poole, 1998; Steenbarger, 1993; Suh, 2004; Wells, 2000). In addition, Poole considered the need to examine organizational policies in order to allow the agencies to hire staff members (outreach) from the target community and allow staff members to engage in the community (e.g., attending evening and/or weekend events with community members and/or agency clients). This is a theme that would become a central component of the U.S. Department of Health and Human Services recommendations (HHS, 2001).

Although the main focus of all of the models is changing the behaviors of the professional practitioners and/or changing their interactions with people who are culturally different from them, only four of the models have developed assessment instruments to evaluate their models. Camphinha-Bacote (1999) developed and tested an inventory to assess the process of acquiring CC with a sample of healthcare professionals. She later replicated the study with a sample of rehabilitation professionals serving people with disabilities (Camphinha-Bacote, 2001). Doorenbos and Schim (2004) tested their model with a sample of 113 hospice employees. Harris-Davis and Haughton (2000) also evaluated their model with a sample of nutrition counselors. Finally, Kim-Godwin, Clarke, and Barton (2001) tested their model with a convenience sample of 192 nursing students. A systematic review of the studies that evaluated interventions designed to improve the CC of health professionals (Beach et al., 2004), indicated that training improves the attitudes, knowledge and skills of trainees, and that the training can impact patient satisfaction. However, no studies have evaluated patient health status outcomes resulting from CC training.

Finally, the majority of the models are in the field of nursing or health care (72%), followed by counseling (22%), and social work (6%). These are occupations that involve a great deal of direct contact between professionals and individuals from different cultural backgrounds. In fact, many professional organizations such as rehabilitation counseling (Commission on Rehabilitation Counselor Certification, 2001) and psychology (APA, 2003) have revised their code of ethics to include respect for cultural diversity as part of the professional standards for education, training, research, and practice. For example, one of the guiding principles for psychologists is to "recognize that, as cultural beings, they may hold attitudes and beliefs that can detrimentally influence their perceptions of and interactions with individuals who are ethnically and racially different from themselves" (APA, p. 382). In health care, the U.S. Office of Minority Health is promoting national standards for culturally and linguistically appropriate services in all states.

A Proposed Model of Cultural Competence

Based on our review of these CC models, we developed a synthesis model that incorporates the most common elements identified in the literature. Our model has five components (see Figure 14-1). The components reflect the iterative process (ongoing) of becoming culturally competent, which suggest that as service providers become familiar or comfortable working with a particular group of people, they may be challenged by the emergence of a different group and so on.

The first step, *willingness to engage* reflects the assumption that service providers seeking CC training must be willing to engage in the process. Feist-Price and Ford-Harris (1994) pointed out that multicultural rehabilitation counseling is especially critical for Anglo American counselors who often are poorly or inadequately trained in understanding the cultural dynamics of consumers of color. However, service providers from any race or ethnic group are likely to face similar challenges when dealing with consumers from other races and/or those who speak a different language than English. In fact, Jones (1997) argued that human beings of any race or ethnicity share both similarities and differences with each other. They are not either different or similar from each other, they are both. This assertion helps explain why service providers from one ethnic group may not necessarily attain better results with consumers from the same group.

Second, *critical awareness* reflects an understanding of our personal biases towards people who are in any way different from us, and a critical examination of our own position of privilege in society, including class differences and experiences of oppression. The process of self-reflection allows professionals to examine their personal

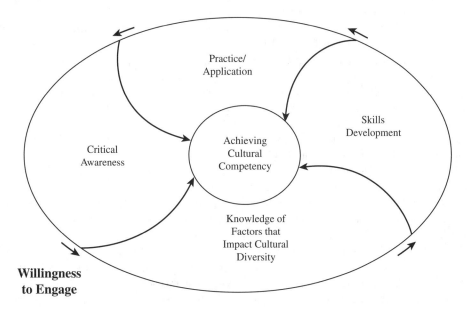

Figure 14-1 CCBMDR Cultural Competence Model

attitudes toward others, and to foster views about acceptance, inclusion, and consideration of the rights of others. Leininger (1995) argued that without cultural awareness, researchers and service providers tend to impose their beliefs, values, and patterns of behavior upon cultures other than their own, making it harder to recruit and sustain the participation of multiethnic populations in research and service use.

Third, *cultural knowledge* leads to familiarization with others' cultural characteristics, history, values, belief systems, and behaviors. Several researchers (e.g., Purnell & Paulanka, 2003) have conducted detailed reviews of the complex cultural characteristics of multiple ethnic or national groups, particularly regarding health-related practices, rituals associated with birth and death, nutritional practices, etc. This information is becoming increasingly available with the advent of the Internet. Researchers have also identified multiple factors that can influence human diversity (D'Andrea & Daniels, 1991). Sawyer et al. (1995) defined cultural knowledge as the practitioner's understanding of integrated systems of learned behavioral patterns in a cultural group including the ways in which members of this group talk, think, and behave, and their feelings, attitudes, and values. We argue that a critical way to know about others is to understand the factors that influence diversity. Based on our review of the literature, we identified several factors that are primarily responsible for determining cultural diversity—establishing our similarities and/or differences with one another. There are both observable and nonobservable factors that contribute to diversity. Any one of the *observable factors* (i.e., race/ethnicity, age, gender, disability. and attractiveness) is among the first things that people notice about a person, which may trigger differential responses. Unfortunately, many people react to others (discriminate) purely on the basis of their general appearance and fail to recognize the complexity of their humanity by ignoring the nonobservable factors. Research evidence suggests that race plays a central role in predicting poor or limited outcomes—in the case of minority groups—for employment, education, rehabilitation, and/or health outcomes, particularly when associated with other factors like low socioeconomic status, limited levels of education, and/or immigration status (e.g., Brach & Fraserirector, 2000; Feist-Price, 1995).

The *nonobservable factors* (i.e., socioeconomic status—which includes the range of income distribution; experiences of oppression—which include knowledge of rights and services and sense of entitlement; level of education; religion—which includes beliefs and values; level of acculturation—which includes language, social identity, and perceptions of time and space; having a nonvisible disability; level of community and family support; immigration status—which includes national origin, cultural identity, and family history; level of urbanicity—which includes the range of habitats from rural to urban; political involvement; and sexual orientation) reflect the complexity of the individuals that interact with a service provider in a given time. We argue that the experience of oppression, which is often related to socioeconomic status, plays a very important role in determining the individual's lack of a sense of entitlement—which may be a construct outside of their previous life experience. A history of oppression also has a negative impact on people's awareness of rights and services, because these individuals—if they are immigrants—may not expect much in the way of services provided by their government and may have had very limited rights, if any. These factors may also interact with the process of acculturation, which can change people's sense of entitlement as a function of language acquisition and their knowledge about the availability of rights and services. The factors interact with each other and can change as a function of a person's experiences. Level of education for instance, which is also related to socioeconomic status and level of urbanicity (poor people and those from rural areas often do not have access to good education) is a very important predictor of the effective interaction of the consumer with the service system (Lorence & Park, 2007).

Fourth, *skills development* refers to the ability of the professional to communicate effectively and empathically with the consumer, being able to incorporate the consumer's beliefs, values, experiences, and aspirations into the provision and planning of the services (Rosenjack-Burchum, 2002). The process requires multiple skills like problem solving (Jezewski & Sotnik, 2005); understanding the dynamics of oppression, racism, sexism, classism, and other forms of discrimination (McPhatter, 1997); understanding the complexity of the service delivery systems (Leininger, 1993; Steenbarger, 1993); increased awareness of personal biases (e.g., Doorenbos & Schim, 2004; Hart, Hall, & Henwood, 2003; Moffitt & Wuest, 2002; Papadopoulos & Lees, 2002); having knowledge of the contexts that influence the behaviors of individuals and families (Poole, 1998); and utilizing a process of questioning that recognizes the individual as the expert of his/her own experience (Anderson & Goolishan, 1992). We also argue that in order to be able to better understand and interact with their clients, service providers need to develop communication skills that would allow them to identify the nonobservable factors mentioned earlier and recognize how the external and internal factors play out in the cultural encounter.

Fifth, *practice/application* refers to the process of applying all of the previous components in a particular context. Perhaps the most difficult part of addressing CC is implementing individual and organizational practices that will improve professionals' ability to deliver care in a culturally competent way. The Office of Minority Health of the U.S. Department of Health and Human Services has proposed standards for culturally and linguistically appropriate services (CLAS) in health care (HHS, 2001). These standards are intended to influence professional practice in all health-related areas. The standards address three main areas: (1) *delivering culturally competent (CC) care* (including developing a consensus on the core cultural competencies for health providers; conducting and disseminating research to connect CC to specific health outcomes; supporting efforts to expand the pool of healthcare professionals from diverse communities; developing consensus on curricular standards for

CC training; and integrating CC into the education and training of health professionals at all levels); (2) *language access services* (including collecting and disseminating information on model programs for implementing language assistance services; supporting the financing of language assistance services at all levels of health services delivery; supporting the development of national standards for interpreter training, skills assessment, certification and code of ethics; developing national standards for the translation of health-related materials; developing standard language for key documents like consent forms, health information, and medication information; and developing an internet clearinghouse of downloadable sample translated documents); and (3) *organizational supports for CC* (including the development of a model implementation plan for CLAS, with measurable short- and long-term process goals; expanding the availability of centralized information on CLAS model programs and practices; surveying and disseminating information on model strategies to involve ethnic communities in the development and oversight of CLAS services; conducting a review of current organizational self-assessment tools and defining the organizational self-assessment process for cultural and linguistic competence; developing standard tools for measuring customer satisfaction and access to CLAS; developing standardized data sets at the federal and state levels related to the race, ethnicity, and language of consumers; developing methods to help healthcare organizations integrate race, ethnicity and language data components into their data collection processes; developing processes for maintaining culture-sensitive community profiles and needs assessments; and development reporting guidelines to help organizations share information with the public about their efforts to implement the CLAS standards). As the HHS report suggests, there are no simple solutions to the problem of improving the CC of service systems in our nation.

CONCLUSION

Cultural competence is a process of *becoming*, which represents a commitment towards multiculturalism that is manifested in a desire and obligation to learn and experience cultural diversity while at the same time remaining humbled by the vastness of human diversity (Tervalon & Murray-Garcia, 1998). Laird (1988) called this openness to cultural understanding "informed not knowing." As suggested by our literature review, the process starts with personal willingness to engage and learn about other cultures, developing a critical understanding of our personal biases, and making efforts to increase our knowledge of other cultures and the factors—external and internal—that influence diversity. CC is attained gradually and the skills involved represent the state-of-the-art in care and service delivery. As described in the HHS recommendations, the application of CC involves individual, organizational, and systemic changes. The model that we have identified here provides steps that practitioners can use to examine the complexity and uniqueness of each consumer, while allowing them to discover the ways in which the various factors interact with each other in the context of the individual's life.

Culture is always evolving and never stays the same. Likewise, the amount of knowledge necessary to understand different cultures is vast and our very being in the contemporary, interconnected world requires cultural understanding as never before. Attending to cultural variations and developing sensitivity and awareness of the cultures in our social contexts are necessary to help us achieve CC (Dickie, 2004). Becoming culturally competent is an intentional endeavor, a journey, and a lifelong process (Padilla & Brown, 1999). The development of CC means our willingness to engage in a series of practices like examining the institutional biases of traditional practices and services; being open and willing to accept individuals from other cultures; trying nontraditional interventions or changing standard procedures to fit individual needs; and challenging racist practices, discrimination, and oppression when observed.

There is still a lot of work to do, since many of the proposed models for promoting CC have not been empirically tested and validated. As suggested in the HHS (2001) report, new standards of care (CLAS) should replace the patchwork of definitions and practices we have today, while acknowledging that this is a process that is going to take years of experimentation, investment of resources, and many efforts to adapt and refine the standards themselves. Most importantly is to conduct research in the relationship between culturally competent services and consumer outcomes, in order to clarify concerns about the costs and cost-benefits of providing culturally and linguistically appropriate services to people. We all need to continue to develop a deeper knowledge and understanding of race/ethnicity, poverty, and oppression in the life experiences of diverse and disadvantaged individuals—especially ethnically diverse individuals with disabilities.

REFERENCES

American Psychological Association. (2003). Guidelines on multicultural education, training, research, practice, and organizational change for psychologists. *Journal of the American Psychological Association, 58*(5), 377–402.

Anderson, H., & Goolishan, H. (1992). The client as the expert: A not-knowing approach to therapy. In S. McNee & K. Gergen (Eds.), *Therapy as a social construction.* (pp. 25–39) London: Sage.

Baldwin, C. H., & Smith, R. T. (1984). An evaluation of the referral and rehabilitation process among the minority handicapped. *International Journal of Rehabilitation Research, 7*(3), 299–315.

Beach, M. C., Price, E., Gary, T., Bass, E., Powe, N., & Cooper, L., et al. (2004). Cultural competence: A systematic review of health care provider education interventions. *Medical Care, 43*(3), 356–373.

Bean, F. D., & Stevens, G. (2003). *America's newcomers and the dynamics of diversity.* New York: Russell Sage.

Betancourt, J. R., Green, A. R., & Carrillo, J. E. (2002). *Cultural competence in health care: Emerging frameworks and practical approaches.* New York: The Commonwealth Fund.

Birenbaum, A. (2002). Poverty, welfare reform, and disproportionate rates of disability among children. *Mental Retardation, 40*(3), 212–218.

Blase, K. A., & Fixsen, D. L. (2003, July). Evidence-based programs and cultural competence. Retrieved September 4, 2008, from the National Implementation Research Network, Luis de la Parte Florida Mental Health Institute Web site: *http://nirn.fmhi.usf.edu/resources/publications/working_paper_2a.pdf*

Bolton, B., & Cooper, P. (1980). Three views: Vocational rehabilitation of Blacks: The comment. *The Journal of Rehabilitation, 46*(2), 41, 47–49.

Bonder, B. R., Martin, L., & Miracle, A. W. (2004). Culture emergent in occupation. *American Journal of Occupational Therapy, 58,* 159–168.

Brach, C., & Fraserirector, I. (2000). Can competency reduce racial and ethnic health disparities? A review and conceptual model. *Medical Care Research and Review, 57*(1), 181–217.

Camphinha-Bacote, J. (1999). A model and instrument for addressing cultural competence in health care. *Journal of Nursing Education, 38*(5), 203–207.

Camphinha-Bacote, J. (2001). A model of practice to address cultural competence in rehabilitation nursing. *Rehabilitation Nursing, 26*(1), 8–11.

Capella, M. E. (2002). Inequities in the VR system: Do they still exist? *Rehabilitation Counseling Bulletin, 45*(3), 143–153.

Commission on Rehabilitation Counselor Certification. (2001). Code of professional ethics for rehabilitation counselors. *Journal of Applied Rehabilitation Counseling, 32*(4), 38–61.

Cross, T. L., Bazron, B. M., Dennis, K. W., & Isaacs, M. R. (1989). Towards a culturally competent system of care: Vol. 1. *A monograph on effective services for minority children who are severely disturbed.* Washington, DC: Georgetown University, Child and Adolescent Service System Program (CASSP), Technical Assistance Center.

D'Andrea, M., & Daniels, J. (1991). Exploring the different levels of multicultural counseling training in counselor education. *Journal of Counseling & Development, 70,* 78–85.

Dickie, V. (2004). Culture is tricky: A commentary on culture emergent in occupation. *American Journal of Occupational Therapy, 58,* 169–173.

Doorenbos, A. Z., & Schim, S. M. (2004). Cultural competence in hospice. *American Journal of Hospice and Palliative Care, 21*(1), 28–32.

Feist-Price, S. (1995). African Americans with disabilities and equity in vocational rehabilitation services: One state's review. *Rehabilitation Counseling Bulletin, 39,* 119–129.

Feist-Price, S., & Ford-Harris, D. (1994). Rehabilitation counseling: Issues specific to providing services to African American clients. *Journal of Rehabilitation, 60*(4), 13–19.

Fiske, A. P., Kitayama, S., Markus, H. R., & Nisbett, R. E. (1998). The cultural matrix of social psychology. In D. T. Gilbert, S. T. Fiske, & G. Lindzey (Eds.), *The handbook of social psychology* (4th ed., pp. 915–981). Boston: McGraw-Hill.

Gladding, S. T. (2001). *The counseling dictionary: Concise definitions of frequently used terms.* Upper Saddle River, NJ: Prentice Hall.

Glockshuber, E. (2005). Counsellors' self-perceived multicultural competencies model. *European Journal of Psychotherapy, Counselling & Health, 7*(4), 291–308.

Goode, T., Sockalingam, S., Brown, M., & Jones, W. (2000). *Infusing principles, content and themes related to cultural and linguistic competence into meetings and conferences.* In National Center for Cultural Competence Planning Guide. Washington, DC: U.S. Department of Health and Human Services, Office of Minority Health.

Harris-Davis, E., & Haughton, B. (2000). Model for multicultural nutrition counseling competencies. *Journal of the American Dietetic Association, 100*(10), 1178–1185.

Hart, A., Hall, V., & Henwood, F. (2003). Helping health and social care professionals to develop an 'inequalities imagination': A model for use in education and practice. *Journal of Advanced Nursing, 41*(5), 480–489.

Herbert, J. T., & Cheatham, H. E. (1988). Afrocentricity and the Black disability experience: A theoretical orientation for rehabilitation counselors. *Journal of Applied Rehabilitation Counseling, 19*(4), 50–54.

Jezewski, M. A., & Sotnik, P. (2001). *Cultural brokering: Providing culturally competent rehabilitation services to foreign-born persons.* Buffalo, NY: Center for International Rehabilitation Research Information & Exchange.

Jezewski, M., & Sotnik, S. (2005). Chapter 2: Culture and Disability Services (with a focus on culture and foreign-born characteristics). In J. Stone (Ed.), *Disability and culture. providing culturally competent services.* (pp. 15–31) Thousand Oaks, CA: Sage.

Jones, J. M. (1997). *Prejudice and racism* (2nd ed.). New York: McGraw-Hill.

Kim-Godwin, Y. S., Clarke, P. N., & Barton, L. (2001). A model for the delivery of culturally competent community care. *Journal of Advanced Nursing, 35*(6), 918–925.

Laird, J. (1998). Theorizing culture: Narrative ideas and practice principles. In M. McGoldrick (Ed.), *Re-visioning family therapy* (pp. 20–36). New York: Guilford.

Lee, J., & Bean, F. D. (2004). America's changing color lines: Immigration, race/ethnicity, and multiracial identification. *Annual Review of Sociology, 30,* 221–242.

Leininger, M. (1993). Towards conceptualization of transcultural health care systems: concepts and a model. 1976. *Journal of Transcultural Nursing, 4*(2), 32–40.

Leininger, M. (1995). *Transcultural nursing: Concepts, theories, research and practices* (2nd ed.). New York: McGraw-Hill.

Lerner, M. J. (1980). *The belief in a just world: A fundamental delusion.* New York: Plenum Press.

Lipkus, I. M., Dalbert, C., & Siegler, I. C. (1996). The importance of distinguishing the belief in a just world for self versus for others: Implications for psychological well-being. *Personality and Social Psychology Bulletin, 22*(7), 666–677.

Lorence, D., & Park, H. (2007). Study of education disparities and health information seeking behavior. *CyberPsychology & Behavior, 10*(1), 149–151.

McPhatter, A. R. (1997). Cultural competence in child welfare: What is it? How do we achieve it? What happens without it? *Child Welfare, 76*(1), 255–278.

Moffitt, P., & Wuest, J. (2002). Spirit of the drum: The development of cultural nursing praxis. *The Canadian Journal of Nursing Research, 34*(4), 107–116.

Olney, M. F., & Kennedy, J. (2002). Racial disparities in VR use and job placement rates for adults with disabilities. *Rehabilitation Counseling Bulletin, 45*(3), 177–185.

Padilla, R., & Brown, K. (1999). Culture and patient education: challenges and opportunities. *Journal of Physical Therapy Education, 13*(3), 23–30.

Palmie, S. (2006). Creolization and its discontents. *Annual Review of Anthropology, 35*, 433–456.

Papadopoulos, I., & Lees, S. (2002). Issues and innovations in nursing education: Developing culturally competent researchers. *Journal of Advanced Nursing, 37*(3), 258–264.

Poole, D. L. (1998). Politically correct or culturally competent? *Health & Social Work, 23*(3), 163–166.

Pope-Davis, D. B., & Dings, J. G. (1995). The assessment of multicultural counseling competencies. In J. C. Ponterotto, J. M. Casas, L. A. Suzuki, & C. A. Alexander (Eds.), *Handbook of multicultural counseling* (pp. 287–311). Thousand Oaks, CA: Sage.

Purnell, L. D., & Paulanka, B. J. (2003). *Transcultural Health Care: A culturally competent approach.* Philadelphia: F. A. Davis.

Rosenjack-Burcham, J. L. (2002). Cultural competence: An evalutionary perspective. *Nursing Forum, 37*(4), 5–16.

Rubin, Z., & Peplau, L. A. (1975). Who believes in a just world? *Journal of Social Issues, 31*(3), 65–89.

Salimbene, S. (1999). Cultural competence: A priority for performance improvement action. *Journal of Nursing Care Quality, 13*(3), 23–35.

Sawyer, L., Regev, H., Proctor, S., Nelson, M., Messias, D., Barnes, D., et al. (1995). Matching versus cultural competence in research: Methodological considerations. *Research in Nursing & Health, 18*(6), 557–567.

Steenbarger, B. N. (1993). A multicontextual model of counseling: Bridging brevity and diversity. *Journal of Counseling & Development, 72*, 8–15.

Suarez-Balcazar, Y., Muñoz, J., & Fisher, G. (2006). Building culturally competent community-university partnerships for occupational therapy scholarship. In G. Kielhofner (Ed.), *Scholarship in occupational therapy: Methods of inquiry for enhancing practice* (pp. 632–642). Philadelphia: F.A. Davis.

Suarez-Balcazar, Y., & Rodakowski, J. (2007, September 24). Becoming a culturally competent occupational therapy practitioner. *OT Practice*, 14–17.

Suarez-Balcazar, Y., Rodakowski, J., Balcazar, F., Taylor-Ritzler, T., Portillo, N., Willis, C., et al. (2009). Perceived levels of cultural competence among occupational therapy practitioners. *American Journal of Occupational Therapy, 63*, 496–503.

Sue, D. W., Arredondo, P., & McDavis, R. (1992). Multicultural counseling competencies/standards: A call to the profession. *Journal of Multicultural Counseling and Development, 20*, 64–88.

Suh, E. E. (2004). The model of cultural competence through an evolutionary concept analysis. *Journal of Transcultural Nursing, 15*(2), 93–102.

Sutton, R. M., & Douglas, K. M. (2005). Justice for all, or just for me? More evidence of the importance of the self-other distinction in just-world beliefs. *Personality and Individual Differences, 39*(3), 637–645.

Tervalon, M., & Murray-Garcia, J. (1998). Cultural humility versus cultural competence: A critical distinction in defining physician training outcomes in multicultural education. *Journal of Health Care for the Poor and Underserved, 9*(2), 117–125.

U.S. Census Bureau. (2003). Disability Status: 2000. Retrieved October 15, 2008, from *http://www.census.gov/prod/2003pubs/c2kbr-17.pdf*

U.S. Census Bureau, Population Division. (2004). U.S. Interim projections by age, sex, race and Hispanic origin. Retrieved September 2, 2008, from *http://www.census.gov/population/www/projections/usinterimproj/usproj2000-2050*

U.S. Census Bureau, Population Division. (2007). Population estimates: race/ethnicity. Retrieved September 2, 2008, from *http://www.census.gov/popest/national/asrh/NC-EST2007-srh.html*

U.S. Committee for Refugees and Immigrants. (2008). Meeting the challenge: Refugees with disabilities program. Retrieved September 5, 2008, from *http://www.immigrants.org/article.aspx?id=1812&subm=178&area=Participate&ssm=182*

U.S. Department of Health and Human Services, Office of Minority Health. (2001). National standards for culturally and linguistically appropriate services in health care. Retrieved September 4, 2008, from *http://www.omhrc.gov/assets/pdf/checked/finalreport.pdf*

Waters, M. C., & Jimenez, T. R. (2005). Assessing immigrant assimilation: New empirical and theoretical challenges. *Annual Review of Sociology, 31*, 105–125.

Wells, M. I. (2000). Beyond cultural competence: A model for individual and institutional cultural development. *Journal of Community Health Nursing, 17*(4), 189–199.

Wheaton, J. E. (1995). Vocational rehabilitation acceptance rate for European Americans and African Americans: Another look. *Rehabilitation Counseling Bulletin, 38*, 224–231.

Willis, W. O. (1999). Culturally competent nursing care during the perinatal period. *Journal of Perinatal and Neonatal Nursing, 13*(3), 45–59.

Wilson, K. B. (1999). Vocational rehabilitation acceptance: A tale of two races in a large Midwestern state. *Journal of Applied Rehabilitation Counseling, 30*(2), 25–31.

Wilson, K. B. (2002). Exploration of VR acceptance and ethnicity: A national investigation. *Rehabilitation Counseling Bulletin, 45*(3), 168–176.

Wilson, K. B., Harley, D. A., & Alston, R. (2001). Race as a correlate of vocational rehabilitation acceptance: Revisited. *Journal of Rehabilitation, 67*(3), 35–41.

Wittman, P., & Velde, B. P. (2002). Attaining cultural competence, critical thinking, and intellectual development: A challenge for occupational therapists. *American Journal of Occupational Therapy, 56*(4), 454–456.

CHAPTER 15

Evaluation Capacity Building: A Cultural and Contextual Framework

Yolanda Suarez-Balcazar, PhD;
Tina Taylor-Ritzler, PhD;
Edurne García-Iriarte, MS;
Christopher Keys, PhD;
Leah Kinney, MA;
Holly Rush-Ross, ScD;
Maria Restrepo-Toro, MS, CPRP;
Gloria Curtin, MA

INTRODUCTION

Community-based organizations (CBOs) in the United States provide an array of services to individuals with a variety of needs and conditions, including individuals with disabilities, to promote their independence and full participation in community life. In 1993, the U.S. government passed the Government Performance and Results Act (GPRA), which holds CBOs accountable for how they spend federal, state, and private funds to improve the lives of program recipients (Kravchuk & Schack, 1996). This pressure for accountability came at a time when vast evidence suggested disparities in the achievement of positive health, rehabilitation, and/or independent living outcomes for multicultural populations with disabilities (Black & Wells, 2007; Capella, 2002; Dziekan & Okocha, 1993; Feist-Price, 1995; Wilson, Alston, Harley, & Mitchell, 2002).

Evaluation is an essential part of the GPRA and of funders' expectations; however, many organizations have been unable to demonstrate the impact of their programs on participants, particularly on participants from multicultural backgrounds. Carman (2007) found that few organizations serving people with disabilities evaluate outcomes or measure performance. This lack of attention to evaluation is in part because these agencies have neither the knowledge nor the skills to conduct evaluations, nor the funding to evaluate their programs. Furthermore, they lack an understanding of the value of evaluation. These deficits are coupled with a difficulty in distinguishing among reporting, monitoring, and management practices and the outcome evaluation of their programs (Carman). These factors also make it challenging to conduct a culturally competent and contextually grounded program evaluation (Fawcett et al., 2003; Keys, McMahon, Sánchez, London, & Abdul-Adil, 2004; Miller, Kobayashi, & Noble, 2006; Schalock & Bonham, 2003; Suarez-Balcazar & Harper, 2003; Suarez-Balcazar, Orellana-Damacela, Portillo, Sharma, & Lanum, 2003).

While the need for evaluation has long been recognized (cf. Keys & Wener, 1980), today more than ever, CBOs experience tremendous pressure to document the impact they are making on the lives of multicultural populations and to contribute to the reduction in health and rehabilitation disparities among ethnic groups (Wilson, Harley, & Alston, 2001).

Scholars suggest the need for organizations to invest in evaluation capacity building (ECB) in order to more closely examine and pay attention to the disparity in outcomes among multicultural populations and to address the issues of program accountability and funding (Carman, 2007). The purpose of this chapter is to describe a culturally and contextually grounded framework of ECB based on a review of the literature on capacity building. In this chapter, the term "community-based organizations (CBOs)" includes not only not-for-profit organizations that serve individuals with disabilities, but also centers for independent living and vocational rehabilitation (VR) offices.

DEFINING EVALUATION CAPACITY BUILDING

Several definitions of evaluation capacity building (ECB) are available in the literature. For instance, Stockdill, Baizerman, and Compton (2002) defined ECB as "intentional work to continuously create and sustain overall organizational processes that make quality evaluation and its uses routine" (p. 14). Milstein and Cotton (2000) stated ECB is the ability to conduct an effective evaluation. For the purpose of this chapter, we will use the Stockdill et al. definition. Despite the different definitions, there is consensus among scholars that ECB is a multidimensional and complex process of organizational, networking, programmatic, and cultural activities (Nye & Glickman, 2000). For ECB to achieve its objective of making high-quality evaluations a routine practice within organizations, there is a need to foster a learning climate, provide support to staff, and allocate resources (Milstein & Cotton; Naccarella et al., 2007; Stockdill, et al.).

According to Stockdill et al. (2002), optimal ECB results in institutionalizing (making evaluation an ongoing activity in the organization) evaluation practices within organizations. In addition, ECB allows disability-related organizations to better use evaluation findings, which can be used effectively to help close the disparity in independent living and rehabilitation outcomes for multicultural populations with disabilities (Balcazar, Keys, Kaplan, & Suarez-Balcazar, 1998; Glickman & Servon, 2003; Ristau, 2001; Taut, 2007).

ECB involves a range of activities that include consultation and technical assistance provided by consultants or partners in strategic planning, staff development, logic model development, development of database systems, and data-collection methods and approaches, among others topics (Naccarella, et al., 2007; Sobeck & Agius, 2007; Suarez-Balcazar, Balcazar, Taylor-Ritzler, & García-Iriarte, 2008). As Sobeck and Agius noted, the key to these activities is to influence program and organizational effectiveness.

A review of the literature on capacity building yielded a synthesis of critical organizational and individual factors likely to influence ECB (Chaskin, 2001; Fawcett et al., 2003; Flaspohler, Duffy, Wandersman, Stillman, & Maras, 2008; Goodman et al., 1998; Sobeck & Agius, 2007; Stockdill et al., 2002). Some of the organizational factors include leadership, learning climate, and resources allocated to evaluation (Sobeck & Agius; Flaspohler et al.). Individual factors speak to staff readiness, willingness, and competencies such as skills and knowledge related to evaluation (Goodman et al.; Sobeck & Agius).

Along with these organizational and individual factors, researchers have highlighted the role of cultural factors (values, beliefs, traditions, and behavioral norms) and contextual factors (organizational policies and procedures, history of the organization within the community, etc.) in ECB (Stockdill et al., 2002). Frierson, Hood, and Hughes (2002) and Hopson (1999) posit that cultural factors, which are critical, are often ignored in ECB.

Cultural considerations in evaluation recently began taking center stage in response to the wide disparities among outcomes achieved by multicultural populations compared to White populations in the areas of health (Tervalon & Murray-García, 1998), rehabilitation, and independent living (Wilson et al., 2001). Given the importance of cultural factors in evaluation, they need to be included in ECB in order to enhance the competency of agency staff in attending to participants' pertinent values, beliefs, traditions, and norms (Frierson et al., 2002).

ECB is inextricably linked to complex organizational, individual, contextual, and cultural factors (Frierson et al., 2002). Understanding ECB within organizations requires consideration of how individual and organizational factors interact with the culture of the community (e.g., predominant language, ethnicity/race of community members) and the organization (e.g., traditions, language spoken by staff, communication style, etc.). What follows is a discourse on the importance of culture in ECB and a presentation of the framework that synthesizes the literature while considering the important role that organizational and individual factors play in ECB, placing context and culture at the center of all ECB activities.

THE ROLE OF CULTURE IN EVALUATION CAPACITY BUILDING

Humans are by definition cultural beings. Any account of human activity, including ECB, that does not place culture at the center is incomplete and potentially problematic (Keys et al., 2004). When culture is not explicitly considered, there is an implicit assumption that the dominant culture is providing the functional standard or that the capacity-building work is happening in a very homogeneous agency and/or community. Lack of attention to culture can encourage and perpetuate a lack of awareness of the importance of culture and context. If nondominant cultures are involved, it is even more essential to consider culture in order to craft ECB approaches that are appropriate to local cultural norms (cf. Keys et al.). The fact is that most CBOs that provide services to people with disabilities serve people with a wide range of disabilities, including individuals who have been marginalized because of their race/ethnicity and/or socio-economic status.

SenGupta, Hopson, and Thompson-Robinson (2004) pointed out that "culture shapes values, beliefs and worldviews" (p. 6), and evaluation is an endeavor to determine the value, merit, worth, and impact of a program. SenGupta et al. noted that social programs are infused with cultural elements related to issues that are the focus of programs. These focal issues include how the problem the programs seek to address is defined and conceptualized, how and why particular types of services are offered, and why certain approaches are used. Likewise, capacity-building activities are also infused with cultural elements that often inform which approaches are more successful with a given population (LaFrance, 2004; SenGupta et al.).

In organizations that serve individuals of diverse racial/ethnic backgrounds and ability levels, attention to cultural factors is most critical (SenGupta et al., 2004). "As American society becomes increasingly diverse racially, ethnically, and linguistically, it is important that program designers, implementers, and evaluators understand the cultural context in which these programs operate" (Frierson et al., 2002, p. 63). Cultural factors speak to the worldviews and behavioral practices of the staff, languages spoken by community residents and CBO staff, traditions of the organization, the staff's ways of learning, and belief systems that might affect the way social programs are viewed (Keys et al., 2004).

The cultures of both the organizations and the communities they serve operate within social, historical, economic, and political contexts (SenGupta et al., 2004). According to Baizerman, Compton, and Stockdill (2002), ECB is time- and space-specific and understanding the history of the organization or program and its culture is crucial for understanding ECB.

Overall, the framework presented in this chapter is intended to build the evaluation capacity of agency staff to enhance their ability to match their programs to the needs, beliefs, and cultural norms of the ethnic groups they serve, as well as to examine the impact of their programs.

THE EVALUATION CAPACITY BUILDING FRAMEWORK

The proposed framework builds on conceptualizations of ECB (Arnold, 2006; Baizerman et al., 2002; and Stockdill et al., 2002); on dimensions of community capacity building (Chaskin, 2001; Flaspohler, et al., 2008; Lord & Hutchison, 2003; Nye & Glickman, 2000; Ristau, 2001); and on two special issues in *New Directions for Evaluation*, one on ECB dedicated to conceptualization and case studies (Stockdill et al., 2002), and one issue on nonprofits and evaluation (Carman & Fredericks, 2008). The framework also draws on Bronfenbrenner's (1967) ecological work in proposing nested and interacting levels of individual, organizational, cultural, and contextual factors.

Organizational and Individual Factors

Sobeck and Agius (2007) stated that the current literature indicates a strong interaction between the organization itself and individuals within the organization. Stockdill et al. (2002) assert that ECB is a context- and culture-dependent process. Both individuals and the organization are greatly affected by context and culture. Stakeholders (e.g., staff and agency directors) bring their individual cultural characteristics, including their disability culture, to the capacity-building process. Although not much research is available that provides empirical evidence that supports the interaction and interplay between these factors (organizational and individual) and the role of culture and context in evaluation, we provide this analysis based mostly on the conceptual and practice literature available.

A visual representation of the framework is included in Figure 15-1. According to the framework, ECB is facilitated when organizational factors such as strong leadership, learning climate, resources, and support are present along with strong personal readiness and competence (knowledge and skills), and when attention is given to culture and context. In contrast, minimal evaluation capacity occurs when there is a lack of these organizational, individual, cultural, and contextual factors.

Organizational Factors

Organizational factors that provide the infrastructure for optimal capacity, thus facilitating institutionalization and mainstreaming of evaluation activities, include *leadership; learning climate; resources and support; and organizational context and culture*. The following is a discussion and synthesis of the literature on these factors.

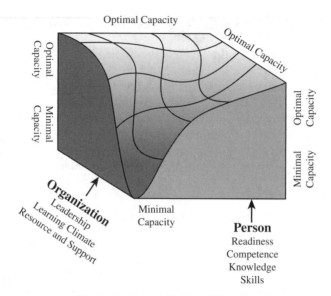

Figure 15-1 The Evaluation Capacity Building Framework

Leadership

Kettner, Moroney, and Martin (1999) and Sobeck and Agius (2007) have stated that organizational leadership and governance contribute to the effectiveness of capacity building. Effective leaders that support ECB are more likely to express, through words and actions, that evaluation is important and articulate a vision, motivate their staff, possess skills for working effectively with others, know how to bring people together, and articulate the needs of their staff (Flashpohler et al., 2008; Greenhalgh, Robert, Macfarlane, Bate, & Kyriakidou, 2004). Effective leaders are also attentive to the needs of diverse groups marked by disability, ethnicity/race, religious affiliation, and/or native language.

According to Goodman et al. (1998) and Alaimo (2008), leadership plays a key role in the sustainability and maintenance of evaluation skills over time as well as in the likelihood that evaluation findings will be used to improve programs and satisfy funders, program staff, and diverse program users. Organizational leaders committed to ECB are more likely to take ownership of the process and rally staff around the need for mainstreaming evaluation activities in their work, thereby optimizing buy-in from the staff and program recipients. Milstein, Chapel, Wetterhall, and Cotton (2002), in a study of ECB at the Centers for Disease Control and Prevention, found that leadership visibility to promote the importance of evaluation was a critical organizational factor.

Flaspohler et al. (2008) noted that to maximize ECB, the organization's leadership needs to provide staff with opportunities for participation in decision making, skills building, and personal and professional advancement. In short, leaders are essential to making evaluation part of the daily activities of the organization.

Learning Climate

An organizational climate that fosters open communication, critical self-evaluation, and new ideas, and that explores innovations is more likely to promote ECB (Greenhalgh et al., 2004; Nye & Glickman, 2000). More specifically, a learning climate involves interest in evaluating its processes for delivering and documenting services and in identifying and tracking outcomes. Cousins, Donahue, and Bloom (1996) highlighted two critical dimensions that promote learning and capacity: depth of participation by staff and other stakeholders and degree of stakeholder control over evaluation decision making. Both, those involved in the implementation of the program and those who participate in or receive the program would ultimately be the individuals reflecting on service delivery processes and outcomes and making decisions about how to evaluate and improve the program (Taut, 2007).

Overall, a culturally grounded ECB effort has to attend to people's diverse needs and their ways of meeting the needs of their constituents while fostering a key element of ECB—the presence of a climate of organizational learning (Fetterman, 2001). This includes attention to critical reflection on program goals and cultural appropriateness of practices and processes, including methods of collecting information from participants and matching services to diverse needs. When critically reflecting on these aspects of their program, the staff needs to feel that they are supported, that they have input into changes that could improve program practices, and that they contribute to organizational learning about its programs and how to evaluate them (Hoole & Patterson, 2008; Taut, 2007).

Resources and Support

Stockdill et al. (2002) assert that because ECB "is an intentional ongoing process, a wide variety of human and fiscal resources is required" (p. 21). According to the authors, several types of human and fiscal resources affect ECB, including the availability of staff, space, time, equipment (including hardware and software), and documentation systems, all of which require money.

Organizations that have access to a variety of stakeholders (e.g., staff, board members, program directors, and consumers) who are committed to culturally grounded evaluation are more likely to find and allocate the resources necessary to engage in evaluation. Given staff turnover, heavy workloads at CBOs, and current budget cuts, organizations must be creative about providing staff with the necessary support and resources so that evaluation is not seen as "one more activity or a burden" but rather as distinctly valuable and built into already existing activities and organizational culture (Fawcett et al., 2003). Andrews, Motes, Floyd, Flerx, and Fede (2005) found that technical resources influence ECB. The authors reported that small organizations struggled with old, inadequate computers, while larger organizations often struggled with software that did not fit with their program evaluation needs.

An issue related to misuse of resources, such as staff time, is that organizations often collect large amounts of data and information from participants, sometimes for funders, but often because they feel it is important or simply because it has always been collected (Stevenson, Florin, Mills, & Andrade, 2002). Unfortunately, much of the information is duplicated, never analyzed, or submitted to a funder but not used internally (L. Kinney, personal communication, June 21, 2007).

Context and Culture

Organizations are characterized by their context, meaning the organization's history, environment, type, relationship with the community, and ways in which it operates (Baizerman et al., 2002). Compton, Glover-Kudon, Smith, and Avery (2002), in a study of ECB in the American Cancer Society (ACS), assert that a fundamental factor of the process at the ACS was an understanding of the organizational context. In the case of the ACS, such context included changes in organizational forms, changes in practices, and outlining roles for staff and volunteers. Similarly, Baizerman et al. assert that ECB is a context-dependent process that needs to fit into the way the particular organization works.

Organizations are characterized by their idiosyncratic culture, meaning how they "do things," how members interact, how they greet each other, how they work together, the traditions they celebrate, the norms they follow, and the values they hold dear (Suarez-Balcazar, 2002). At the organizational level, these cultural elements influence ECB.

In all, organizational factors are essential to ECB; a supportive leader, a climate that fosters learning, adequate resources to engage in evaluation, and cultural and contextual factors can compel staff willingness to engage in evaluation and program improvements.

Individual Factors

A synthesis of the literature on capacity building (Flaspohler et al., 2008; Goodman et al., 1998) indicates that individual factors (i.e., staff attributes) that are likely to contribute to ECB include *personal readiness* (willingness and motivation), *competen-*

cies such as *knowledge and skills*, and *personal cultural and contextual factors* (cultural competence and contextual awareness). Individual factors interact with organizational factors; neither exists in isolation, and both are embedded in the contextual and cultural elements of organizations and the communities they serve (Flaspohler et al.).

Individual Readiness

Willingness and motivation to learn about evaluation are dimensions of individual readiness (Stockdill et al., 2002), which is a critical component of ECB. Although awareness is essential to readiness, staff that is aware of the need for evaluation might not necessarily be ready to support it or to engage in the process. Readiness may vary from organization to organization and from individual to individual within the same organization. According to Fawcett et al. (2003), different levels of readiness are common among staff, which leads to different interventions; some staff members need more training than others and some staff members are more committed to evaluation than others. Building on intrinsic willingness and motivation to incorporate evaluation into staff work facilitates capacity building. However, simply engaging in evaluation to be in compliance with funders or accreditation requirements without motivation may impede the sustainability of ECB efforts (Flaspohler et al., 2008). Pushing ECB through without readiness can slow down the process and it can even backfire and reduce progress later. Building readiness through culturally sensitive training, information sharing, team planning, and pilot projects, whether done by insiders (organization's leadership) or outsiders (consultants or partners), is an essential component of capacity building (Edwards, Jumper-Thurman, Plested, Oetting, & Swanson, 2000).

Individual Competence

Competence in ECB involves both *knowledge* and *skills* (Fawcett et al., 2003). *Knowledge* about evaluation includes an understanding of its value (awareness), what evaluation is, and why it is important to conduct evaluations. More specifically, it also includes understanding how to select the goals and questions of an evaluation and how to develop a logic model (Kaplan & Garrett, 2005). Moreover, it includes knowing how to select the methods or strategies that are appropriate for evaluating particular programs, what data to collect, and how to collect it (Wandersman, in press). Finally, it entails having insight into how to analyze data, how to interpret data, and how to use the results of an evaluation to both improve the program and satisfy funders or potential funders (Fawcett et al.; Suarez-Balcazar et al., 2003).

Evaluation *skills* are defined as the ability to use knowledge in the areas of program planning and evaluation to enact valuable behaviors and actions in a culturally aware manner (Livet & Wandersman, 2005). Knowledge by itself is insufficient for evaluation competence; use of evaluation skills that take into account the context and culture of the organization and the community being served, making evaluation an ongoing practice over time, demonstrates evidence of evaluation competence.

Evaluation knowledge can be built within an organization through a number of mechanisms. It can be transferred by those with existing expertise within the organization providing training and technical assistance, through partnerships with similar organizations or institutions of higher education, or through individuals who consult on evaluation issues (Fawcett et al., 1994). Building knowledge and developing skills is best seen as an ongoing process (Fawcett et al., 1996). Partners can facilitate the building of staff skills by ongoing training, troubleshooting, coaching, and involving different stakeholders in the decision-making process that affects programs (Goodman et al., 1998; Linney & Wandersman, 1996).

When it comes to data management, organizations vary in their approaches to data and data systems and their level of sophistication and experience. Often, organizations are overwhelmed with the process of documenting what they do (Nye & Glickman, 2000). Data collection in an organization is a very complicated activity, which depends on many factors, including the availability of technical skills, understanding why and how to collect information, individual competence and attitudes, cultural awareness, resource allocation, equipment, time, and organizational support, among others (Posavac & Carey, 2003). Andrews et al. (2005) engaged in ECB in an organization hosting several social programs for a working-class community. They found the evaluation coach spent a substantial amount of time helping the staff develop computer-assisted information systems, data-collection procedures, data compilation and data interpretation, and reporting.

Overall, building evaluation competencies is an ongoing process that requires staff to be ready and willing to learn new skills, new ways of thinking about the program, and new ways of tracking their outcomes. Those facilitating the ECB process need to acknowledge that different staff will have different sets of skills and knowledge about evaluation.

Individual Cultural Competence and Contextual Awareness

Cultural Competence The need for cultural competence is not limited to the CBO staff going through the ECB process; the consultants or partners brought into the organization to assist with the ECB effort must have it as well. As the staff gains evaluation capacity, they might gain an understanding of their capacity to work with the agency clients for the purpose of collecting data, obtaining feedback from program participants, and learning how to include participants in the evaluation process (Suarez-Balcazar et al., 2008). Staff needs to be sensitive and knowledgeable regarding the behavioral practices, belief systems, worldviews, and overall preferences of the community they serve in order to obtain valuable information from clients (Pope-Davis & Dings, 1995). According to Suarez-Balcazar, Harper, and Lewis (2005), for some staff the idea of collecting information or data may be inherently threatening and requires the building of mutual trust with the client population.

Contextual Awareness Organizational staff going through the process of ECB needs to know the community they serve well. This community knowledge includes coming to understand the historical aspects and the power relationships of the agency and the community. It involves becoming familiar with the geographical context and socioeconomic concerns of the community (Weiner, Trevor, & William, 2002). Information about these issues is likely to inform the types and methods of data collection for evaluation purposes (Krieger, Chen, & Ebel, 1997). Furthermore, staff needs to be aware of the context of the organization, including the organization's structure, practices, and ways of working, all of which may affect their process of gaining evaluation capacity (Stockdill et al., 2002).

Culture and context can have significant effects on ECB and need to be considered in the analysis of organizational and individual factors. The case study that follows illustrates the process of ECB with a CBO highlighting the role of cultural and contextual factors.

Evaluation Capacity Building: A Case Study

Background   For three years, the staff at the Center for Capacity Building on Minorities with Disabilities Research (CCBMDR) worked with a CBO that provides services to individuals with developmental disabilities and their families (mostly Latino) through several programs. The CBO was founded by a Latina mother of a child with a special need. She was a leader who dreamed of a community in which all members, including people with disabilities, could live, learn, work, and be fully integrated into the fabric of the community. The CBO offers a number of programs, including an acquired brain injury program, a supported employment program, and residential and day-care programs for people with disabilities, among others. The adult programs became the focus of the evaluation partnership with CCBMDR. Most members of the program staff are bilingual Latinos from diverse cultural backgrounds, and some live in the community surrounding the CBO.

The CBO staff approached CCBMDR and requested assistance in developing an evaluation plan for its adult services program to comply with requests from United Way (United Way of America, 1996). The purpose of the partnership was to build the capacity of staff in the programs for people with disabilities to evaluate the impact of their efforts.

Organizational Factors   The leaders of the CBO were very supportive of the ECB effort, in part because of pressure coming from United Way. Quite aside from the United Way pressure, leaders of the organization saw evaluation as a means to improve programs

 continued

and obtain a valuable set of skills for the staff to acquire. This view from leaders diffused among staff facilitated the capacity-building process. The leaders also showed commitment to the ECB effort by setting time aside for evaluation training and assigning staff members to work on it with the university partners. The organization also allocated resources to support evaluation by purchasing a computerized database.

The CBO's management played a key leadership role in fostering a learning climate by letting staff take time away from their typical day-to-day job tasks to attend training and receive one-on-one coaching. Furthermore, they met with staff to conduct brainstorming sessions, allowed staff to try new ways of recording information, and brought in different companies who offered the database software they were considering. To support a learning climate, the leaders invited the researchers to group sessions with staff to discuss their concerns about successfully conducting evaluations. This consultation with researchers also provided an opportunity for the staff to assess their progress in learning evaluation skills and using them in their work.

Individual Factors   To help the CBO staff develop evaluation knowledge and skills, the CCBMDR staff conducted several training sessions in evaluation. During these training sessions, CCBMDR staff introduced agency staff to the following areas: why performing evaluations is important, myths about evaluation, developing program goals, developing a program logic model, identifying outcome indicators, recording data, differentiating between outputs and outcomes, and developing an evaluation plan. These topics were covered using discussion questions, problem solving, brainstorming, critical thinking, exercises, and examples. The CCBMDR staff also reviewed the clients' case files and examined their tracking system closely. CCBMDR staff conducted four small group discussions with the CBO staff to gather their thoughts about applying their evaluation knowledge and skills to their daily work, documentation, and evaluation systems. These group discussions yielded a rich variety of strengths as well as challenges that staff encountered. After a series of one-on-one and group trainings one of the staff members demonstrated her new evaluation skills by developing her own logic model, taking control of the evaluation of her program, and training other staff members on how to develop their evaluation plans.

Cultural and Contextual Factors   Some of the cultural factors that were discussed during this ECB process included the staff beliefs and perceptions of their clients' abilities to express themselves and provide feedback. Models of capacity building and participatory research with Latinos have shown that the concepts of *empowerment and advocacy* might be foreign to some and not necessarily used in the Latino culture (Balcazar et al., 1998). CBO staff had embraced a more patronizing approach to their work with Latinos with developmental disabilities, which fostered dependency among their clients and was reinforced by parents and family members. This dependent stance is in fact considered a value by the Latino culture rather than a barrier. Through this evaluation process, the staff realized that Latinos with disabilities did not necessarily share the values of dependency held by their

↓   *continued*

family members and the CBO staff. In fact, they wanted to be more empowered and wanted programs that foster self-determination. This discovery was important for the CBO staff because it did not fit their cultural framework of the Latino individual. This value for self-determination meant changes in family values and in staff beliefs about the population they serve. The capacity-building process has assisted staff in making this shift to a more empowering stance with people with disabilities. The fact that the center staff is bilingual and bicultural facilitated the discussion of these cultural issues with the staff. Furthermore, the ECB effort helped the staff understand the role of culture in evaluation and helped them identify more authentic outcome indicators for evaluation.

Overall, this example illustrates how to work with staff and leaders to promote ECB in a culturally grounded manner. This process has not been easy or quick. It has taken time, effort, and commitment from all those involved, including the staff, the leaders, and CCB-MDR staff. Fortunately, the process has produced the desired outcomes: the mainstreaming and institutionalization of evaluation and, most importantly, the use of findings to improve programs in a way that respects the cultures of the staff and program participants.

IMPLICATIONS FOR SCIENCE AND PRACTICE

Building evaluation capacity in a culturally and contextually grounded way is a complex process that involves a number of organizational and individual factors. To mainstream evaluation practices within a CBO, a service agency, an independent living center, or a VR office, the leadership needs to demonstrate its commitment by building a culture of learning, by allocating necessary resources, and by providing staff with culturally appropriate opportunities to enhance their skills and competencies.

The value of recognizing *organizational factors* places emphasis on organizations' power to be agents of change in their communities. The organization can develop learning communities within their agency, and can allocate the necessary resources and provide infrastructure. Moreover, strong organizational leaders can support evaluation activities in a culturally competent manner that help staff understand, value, and ultimately implement evaluation. Furthermore, building evaluation capacity at the organizational level enhances use of results and innovation (Wandersman, in press).

The value of recognizing *individual factors* places emphasis on the power of CBO's staff readiness, awareness, and competence (skills and knowledge) to engage in evaluation activities. Whether an organization is committed to evaluation or not, it is really the staff that ultimately has to implement it and make it happen. Effective leadership provides culturally appropriate opportunities for staff to overcome their fears and apprehensions and facilitates readiness for, and an awareness of, evaluation.

Understanding culture and context means, in part, understanding the values, norms, belief systems, sociopolitical factors, and organizational policies that can affect evaluation and related capacity building. Organizations and individuals operate within their own cultural frameworks and sociocultural environments (SenGupta et al., 2004). Recognizing and responding to cultural issues is critical to ECB within individuals and organizations.

In terms of implications for science, research needs to be conducted to empirically validate the factors described in this chapter, which have been drawn from a synthesis of the ECB literature. Among key questions for future research are: How does ECB relate to tracking relevant independent living and rehabilitation outcomes for multicultural populations with disabilities? How can cultural dimensions of evaluation capacity and ECB itself best be measured? How does this work contribute to the conceptualization of ECB? There are many other relevant questions; however, the key is to continue this important line of research.

The implications for practice are equally important. Creating optimal, culturally competent evaluation capacity among service providers underscores the importance of tracking participants' outcomes and gains towards independent living and rehabilitation. ECB makes those providing services accountable for generating results aside from increasing their funding opportunities.

CONCLUSION

Culturally competent evaluation capacity building is critical for service providers. We do understand, however, that engaging in this process is not free of challenges and limitations, such as issues of power, limited resources, negative past experiences with evaluation, and other difficulties already well articulated by researchers in the field (see Behrens & Kelly, 2008; Fawcett et al., 1996; Suarez-Balcazar et al., 2003; Wandersman, et al., 2004). In closing, this chapter provides a synthesis of the literature on ECB suggesting a framework that recognizes the interaction between organizational and individual factors that can facilitate the building of capacity for culturally competent evaluation. An understanding of factors that promote capacity may foster attention to real outcomes and accountability among service providers.

REFERENCES

Alaimo, S. P. (2008). Nonprofits and evaluation: Managing expectations from the leader's perspective. In J. G. Carman & K. A. Fredericks (Eds.), *Nonprofits and evaluation. New Directions for Evaluation, 119*, 73–92.

Andrews, A. B., Motes, P. S., Floyd, A. G., Flerx, V. C., & Fede, A. (2005). Building evaluation capacity in community-based organizations: Reflections of an empowerment evaluation team. *Journal of Community Practice, 13*(4), 85–104.

Arnold, M. (2006). Developing evaluation capacity in extension 4-H field faculty. *American Journal of Evaluation, 27*(2), 257–269.

Baizerman, M., Compton, D. W., & Stockdill, S. H. (2002). *New directions for ECB. New Directions for Evaluation, 93*, 109–119.

Balcazar, F., Keys, C., Kaplan, D., & Suarez-Balcazar, Y. (1998). Participatory action research and people with disabilities: Principles and challenges. *Canadian Journal of Rehabilitation, 12*, 105–112.

Behrens, T. R., & Kelly, T. (2008). Paying the piper: Foundation evaluation capacity calls the tune. In J. G. Carman & K. A. Fredericks (Eds.), *Nonprofits and evaluation. New Directions for Evaluation, 119*, 37–50.

Black, R. M., & Wells, S. A. (2007). *Culture & occupation: A model of empowerment in occupational therapy.* Bethesda, MD: American Occupational Therapy Association.

Bronfenbrenner, U. (1967). The psychological costs of quality and equality in education. *Child Development, 38*(4), 909–925.

Capella, M. E. (2002). Inequities in the VR system: Do they still exist? *Rehabilitation Counseling Bulletin, 45*, 143–153.

Carman, J. G. (2007). Evaluation practice among community-based organizations: Research into the reality. *American Journal of Evaluation, 28*(1), 60–75.

Carman, J. C., & Fredericks, K. A. (Eds.) (2008). *Nonprofits and evaluation. New Directions for Evaluation, 119*, San Francisco, CA: Jossey-Bass.

Chaskin, R. J. (2001). Community capacity: A definitional framework and implications from a comprehensive community initiative. *Urban Affairs Review, 36*(3), 291–323.

Compton, D. W., Glover-Kudon, R., Smith, I. E., & Avery, E. (2002). Ongoing capacity building in the American Cancer Society (ACS) 1995-2001. In D. W. Compton, M. Baizerman, & S. H. Stockdill (Eds.), *The Art, Craft, and Science of Evaluation Capacity Building. New Directions for Evaluation, 93* (pp. 47–61). San Francisco, CA: Jossey-Bass.

Cousins, J. B., Donohue, J. J., & Bloom, G. A. (1996). Collaborative evaluation in North America: Evaluators' self-reported opinions, practices, and consequences. *Evaluation Practice, 17*(3), 207–226.

Dziekan, K. I., & Okocha, A. G. (1993). Accessibility of rehabilitation services: Comparison by racial-ethnic status. *Rehabilitation Counseling Bulletin, 36*, 183–189.

Edwards, R. W., Jumper-Thurman, P., Plested, B. A., Oetting, E. R., & Swanson, L. (2000). Community readiness: Research to practice. *Journal of Community Psychology, 28*(3), 291–307.

Fawcett, S. B., Boothroyd, R., Schultz, J. A., Fransciso, V. T., Carson V., & Bremby R. (2003). Building capacity for participatory evaluation within community initiatives. In Y. Suarez-Balcazar & G. Harper (Eds.), *Empowerment and participatory evaluation of community interventions* (pp. 21–36). Binghamton, NY: Haworth Press.

Fawcett, S. B., Paine-Andrews, A., Francisco, V. T., Schultz, J. A., Richter, K. P., Lewis, R. K., et al. (1996). Empowering community health initiatives through evaluation. In D. Fetterman, S. Kaftarian, & A. Wandersman (Eds.), *Empowerment evaluation: Knowledge and tools for self-assessment and accountability* (pp. 256–276). Thousand Oaks, CA: Sage.

Fawcett, S. B., White, G. W., Balcazar, F. E., Suarez-Balcazar, Y., Mathews, R. M., Paine-Andrews, A., et al. (1994). A contextual-behavioral model of empowerment: Case studies involving people with physical disabilities. *American Journal of Community Psychology, 22*, 471–496.

Feist-Price, S. (1995). African Americans with disabilities and equity in vocational rehabilitation services: One state's review. *Rehabilitation Counseling Bulletin, 39*, 119–129.

Fetterman, D. M. (2001). *Foundations of Empowerment Evaluation.* Thousand Oaks, CA: Sage.

Flaspohler, P., Duffy, J., Wandersman, A., Stillman, L., & Maras, M. (2008). Unpacking prevention capacity: An intersection of research-to-practice models and community-centered models. *American Journal of Community Psychology, 41*(3–4), 182–196.

Frierson, H., Hood, S., & Hughes, G. (2002). Strategies that address culturally responsive evaluation. In J. Frechtling (Ed.), *The 2002 user-friendly handbook for project evaluation* (pp. 63–72). Arlington, Va.: National Science Foundation.

Glickman, N. J., & Servon, L. J. (2003). By the numbers: Measuring community development corporations' capacity. *Journal of Planning Education and Research, 22*(3), 240–256.

Goodman, R. M., Speers, M. A., Mcleroy, K., Fawcett, S., Kegler, M., Parker, E., et al. (1998). Identifying and defining the dimensions of community capacity to provide a basis for measurement. *Health Education & Behavior, 25*(3), 258–278.

Greenhalgh, T., Robert, G., Macfarlane, F., Bate, P., & Kyriakidou, O. (2004). Diffusion of innovations in service organizations: Systematic review and recommendations. *The Milbank Quarterly, 82*(4), 581–629.

Hoole, E., & Patterson, T. E. (2008). Voices from the field: Evaluation as part of a learning culture. In J. G. Carman & K. A. Fredericks (Eds.), *Nonprofits and evaluation. New Directions for Evaluation, 119*, 93–113.

Hopson, R. K. (1999). Minority issues in evaluation revisited: Re-conceptualizing and creating opportunities for institutional change. *American Journal of Evaluation, 20*(3), 445–451.

Kaplan, S. A., & Garrett, K. E. (2005). The use of logic models by community-based initiatives. *Evaluation and Program Planning, 28*, 167–172.

Kettner, P., Moroney. R., & Martin, L. (1999). *Designing & managing programs: An effectiveness-based approach.* Thousand Oaks, CA: Sage.

Keys, C., McMahon, S., Sánchez, B., London, L., & Abdul-Adil, J. (2004). Culturally anchored research: Quandaries, guidelines, and exemplars for community psychology. In L. A. Jason, C. B. Keys, Y. Suarez-Balcazar, R. R. Taylor, & M. I. Davis (Eds.), *Participatory community research: Theories and methods in action* (pp. 177–198). Washington, DC: American Psychological Association.

Keys, C., & Wener, R. (1980). Organizational intervention issues: A four-phase approach to post-occupancy evaluation. *Environment and Behavior, 12*, 533–540.

Kravchuk, R. S., & Schack, R. W. (1996). Designing effective performance measurement systems under the Government Performance and Results Act of 1993. *Public Administration Review, 56*(4), 348–358.

Krieger, N., Chen, J. T., & Ebel, G. (1997). Can we monitor socioeconomic inequalities in health? A survey of U.S. Health Departments' data collection and reporting practices. *Public Health Reports, 112*, 481–491.

LaFrance, J. (2004). *Culturally competent evaluation in Indian country. New Directions for Evaluation, 102*, 39–50.

Linney, J., & Wandersman, A. (1996). Empowering community groups with evaluation skills: The Prevention Plus III Model. In D. Fetterman, S. Kaftarin, & A. Wandersman (Eds.), *Empowerment evaluation: Knowledge and tools for self-assessment and accountability.* Thousand Oaks, CA: Sage.

Livet, M., & Wandersman, A. (2005). Organizational functioning: Facilitating effective interventions and increasing the odds of programming success. In D. M. Fetterman & A. Wandersman (Eds.), *Empowerment evaluation principles in practice* (pp. 123–154). New York: Guilford Press.

Lord, J., & Hutchison P. (2003). Individualized support and funding: Building blocks for capacity building and inclusion. *Disability & Society, 18*(1), 71.

Miller, R. L., & Campbell, R. (2006) Taking stock of empowerment evaluation. *American Journal of Evaluation, 27*(3), 296–319.

Milstein, B., Chapel, T. J., Wetterhall, S. F., & Cotton, D. A. (2002). Building capacity for program evaluation at the Centers for Disease Control and Prevention. In D. W. Compton, M. Baizerman, & S. H. Stockdill (Eds.), *The art, craft, and science of evaluation capacity building. New Directions for Evaluation, 93*. San Francisco: Jossey-Bass.

Milstein, B., & Cotton, D., (2000). *Defining concepts for the presidential strand on building evaluation capacity*. American Evaluation Association. Retrieved December 2, 2007, from *http://www.eval.org/eval2000/public/presstrand.pdf*

Naccarella, J., Pirkis, J., Kohn, F., Morley, B., Burgess, P., & Blashki, G. (2007). Building evaluation capacity: Definitional and practical implications from an Australian case study. *Evaluation and Program Planning, 30*, 231–236.

Nye, N., & Glickman, N. J. (2000). Working together: Building capacity for community development. *Building Capacity for Community Development, 11*(1), 163–198.

Pope-Davis, D. B., & Dings, J. G. (1995). The assessment of multicultural counseling competencies. In J. C. Ponterotto, J. M. Casas, L. A. Suzuki, & C. A. Alexander (Eds.), *Handbook of multicultural counseling* (pp. 287–311). Thousand Oaks, CA: Sage.

Posavac, E. J., & Carey, R. G. (2003). *Program evaluation: Methods and case studies* (6th ed.). Upper Saddle River, NJ: Prentice Hall.

Ristau, S. (2001). Building organizational capacity in outcomes evaluation: A successful state association model. *Families in Society, 82*(6), 555–560.

Schalock, R. L., & Bonham, G. S. (2003). Measuring outcomes and managing for results. *Evaluation and Program Planning, 26*(3), 229–235.

SenGupta, S., Hopson, R., & Thompson-Robinson, M. (2004). Cultural competence in evaluation: An overview. *New Directions for Evaluation, 102*, 5–19.

Sobeck, J., & Agius, E. (2007). Organizational capacity building: Addressing a research and practice gap. *Evaluation and Program Planning, 30*, 237–246.

Stevenson, J. F., Florin, P., Mills, D. S., & Andrade, M. (2002). Building evaluation capacity in human service organizations: A case study. *Evaluation and Program Planning, 25*(3), 233–243.

Stockdill, S. H., Baizerman, M., & Compton, D. W. (2002). Toward a definition of the ECB process: A conversation with the ECB literature. *New Directions in Evaluation, 93*, 1–15.

Suarez-Balcazar, Y. (2002). Aspectos de diversidad humana en la evaluación de programas comunitarios. *Intervención Psicosocial, 11*, 167–182.

Suarez-Balcazar, Y., Balcazar, F., Taylor-Ritzler, R., & García-Iriarte, E. (2008). Capacity building and empowerment: A panacea and challenge for agency-university engagement. *Gateways: International Journal of Community Research and Engagement, 1*, 179–196.

Suarez-Balcazar, Y., & Harper, G. (2003). Community-based approaches to empowerment and participatory evaluation. *Journal of Prevention and Intervention in the Community, 26*, 1–4.

Suarez-Balcazar, Y., Harper, G. W., & Lewis, R. (2005). An interactive and contextual model of community-university collaborations for research and action. *Health Education & Behavior, 32*(1), 84–101.

Suarez-Balcazar, Y., Orellana-Damacela, L., Portillo, N., Sharma, A., & Lanum, M. (2003). Implementing an outcomes model in the participatory evaluation of community initiatives. *Journal of Prevention and Intervention in the Community, 26,* 5–20.

Taut, S. (2007). Studying self-evaluation capacity building in a large international development organization. *American Journal of Evaluation, 28*(1), 45–59.

Tervalon, M., & Murray-García, J. (1998). Cultural humility versus cultural competence: A critical distinction in defining physician training outcomes in multicultural education. *Journal of Health Care for the Poor and Underserved, 9*(2), 117–125.

United Way of America. (1996). *Measuring program outcomes: a practical approach.* Arlington, VA: United Way of America.

Wandersman, A. (in press). Program evaluation and program development. In J. Dalton, M. J. Elias, & A. Wandersman (Eds.), *Community Psychology: Linking individuals and communities.* Belmont, CA: Wadsworth.

Wandersman, A., Keener, D., Snell-Johns, J., Miller, R., Flaspohler, P., Livet-Dye, M., et al. (2004). Empowerment evaluation: Principles and action. In L. Jason, K. Keys, Y. Suarez-Balcazar, M. Davis, J. Durlak, & D. Isenberg (Eds.), *Participatory community research: Theories and methods in action* (pp. 139–156). Washington, DC: American Psychological Association.

Weiner, D., Trevor H., & William, C. (2002). Community participation and geographic information systems. In W. Craig, T. Harris, & D. Weiner (Eds.), *Community participation and geographic information systems* (pp. 3–16). London: Taylor and Francis.

Wilson, K. B., Alston, R. J., Harley, D. A., & Mitchell, N. A. (2002). Predicting VR acceptance based on race, gender, education, work status at application, and primary source of support at application. *Rehabilitation Counseling Bulletin, 45,* 132–142.

Wilson, K. B., Harley, D. A., & Alston, R. (2001). Race as a correlate of vocational rehabilitation acceptance: Revisited. *Journal of Rehabilitation, 67*(3), 35–41.

CHAPTER 16

A Systems Approach to Placement: A Culturally Sensitive Model for People with Disabilities

Madan M. Kundu, PhD, FNRCA, CRC, NCC, LRC;
Alo Dutta, PhD, CRC;
Fong Chan, PhD, CRC

INTRODUCTION

Each person has a different experience with disability based on life situations, one's access to information, services, opportunities, the environment, culture, geographic location, and the attitudes of people in one's community. But, having the chance to obtain and retain meaningful work is a crucial part of quality of life for most human beings and people with disabilities are no exception. However, in spite of the progress made as a result of the Americans with Disabilities Act of 1990, as per the recent estimates, the unemployment rate of people with severe disabilities is around 44.2% (Office of Disability Employment Policy [ODEP], 2003). In contrast, the unemployment rate of Americans in general has been hovering around 6% with variation of about 2–4% depending on economic conditions (Bureau of Labor Statistics, 2008). Among adults with disabilities, more than one-quarter live in poverty and more than 75% earn less than $20,000 annually (Bowe, 2006).

In light of this data, it is important to keep in mind that people with disabilities represent about 20% of the U.S. population and 34% of them are from racial and ethnic multicultural groups. Diverse individuals with disabilities make up a significant and important group of people who have the same healthcare, employment, and quality-of-life concerns as diverse individuals without disabilities. However, having both attributes has been termed as "double jeopardy" because of continued race-related health disparities, cultural distinctions, prejudice, discrimination, environmental and access issues, and economic barriers (Waldrop, 2003) as well as disparities associated with having a disability. Therefore, this chapter is written in an effort to identify and explain the development of a new model designed to facilitate quality job placement of ethnically diverse persons with disabilities receiving vocational rehabilitation (VR) services.

EMPLOYMENT STATUS OF PEOPLE WITH DISABILITIES

In 2002, it was reported that about 55.9% of people with disabilities aged 21–64 held some form of employment during the preceding 12 months. Those with significant disabilities were less likely to be employed than those with nonsignificant disabilities. The median wage of those with significant disabilities was $12,800 compared to $22,000 for those with nonsignificant disabilities and $25,000 for those without disabilities. Among those in the work force (full- and part-time), 12.8% of people with significant disabilities, 43.6% of those with nonsignificant disabilities, and 52.6% of those without disabilities worked full-time, year round. Employment rates varied among people with different types of disabilities and functional limitations. Approximately, 55.3% of people with difficulty seeing were employed and, if employed, their median earnings were $15,900. About 33% of those with an issue related to activities of daily living (ADL; i.e., tasks of everyday life), were employed and, if employed, had median earnings of $13,100. People with communication impairments were more likely to be employed (91%) than people with physical disabilities (56%) or psychiatric disabilities (61.6%) (Steinmetz, 2004).

Employment barriers encountered by ethnically diverse individuals with disabilities can sometimes be substantial. For example, about 63% of African Americans, 59% of Native Americans, 55% of Hispanics, and 52% of Asian Americans with disabilities are not working. For women with disabilities from culturally diverse backgrounds, the issue may be one of triple discrimination. Although barriers can occur for all people with and without disabilities, they are more persistent and pronounced for members of diverse ethnic and racial groups with disabilities (U.S. Department of Labor, 1999).

EXISTING JOB PLACEMENT MODELS

As per Berven (1979), Kundu, Schiro-Geist, and Dutta (2005), Muthard and Salomone (1969), Parker and Szymanski (1992), Rubin et al. (1984), Sink and Porter (1978), and Wilson (2002), placement is one of the fundamental functions of rehabilitation professionals in public and private agencies. Employment is typically the key to empowerment, independence, and quality of life. Therefore, understanding different approaches or models of placing people with disabilities, especially members of culturally diverse populations in jobs is essential.

The existing five approaches or models of job placement were reviewed briefly to examine their effectiveness in addressing the complexities of job placement for people with disabilities who are culturally diverse. Additionally, we considered the degree to which these approaches take into account the level of knowledge, skills, and competence required of professionals who do the placement. A Systems Approach to Placement (SAP) is proposed to combine the strengths and reduce potential limitations of current approaches by incorporating human, organizational, environmental, and cultural components. The intent is to make SAP useful for VR professionals and people with disabilities of diverse ethnicity in the process of job placement.

1. The *person-centered approach* thrives on personal responsibility and minimum counselor direction. It requires the counselor to have an optimistic attitude tempered by realism that the individual with a disability will get a suitable job (Salomone, 1971). The approach defines and redefines the essence of employment repeatedly from the job seeker's perspective (Condon, Fichera, & Dreilinger, 2003). The individual is independent, autonomous, and self-directed. The consumer sets up his/her own job interviews, acts as his/her own agent and advocate when engaging in contacts with employers. However, a person from a culturally diverse background and with severe disabilities may look up to the counselor as a knowing authority and expects the professional to be directive. Under such circumstances this approach may have limited applicability to individuals from diverse ethnic groups (Hunt, 2002).

2. The *selective approach* has been proven to be effective for individuals who need considerable professional guidance in the placement process. Heavy reliance on the rehabilitation counselor/placement specialist may be due to the severity of the disability (e.g., spinal cord injury, traumatic brain injury, mental illness, substance abuse, etc.), lack of education and prior work experience, lack of transferable skills, diverse socioeconomic/educational status, or a combination of various life factors. Some people with disabilities need more direct placement intervention, advocacy, and support for obtaining and maintaining gainful employment. The number of individuals with disabilities who seek rehabilitation services that require this type of support is higher than the number of individuals who need a person-centered placement technique (Bissonnette, 2002). An appreciable number of individuals requiring a selective placement approach are from diverse racial and ethnic backgrounds. Therefore, it is important for placement professionals to have the capability to provide aggressive and intense guidance geared to placing the person with an employer and then offering follow-up support on the job. This model also acts

as a catalyst in the identification of required job modifications and accessibility needs for better employee–job match in the long run. The characteristics of this approach make it suitable for use with people with significant disabilities from multicultural groups (Bissonnette).

3. *Self-employment* causes changes in the global marketplace such as downsizing, increase in the use of contingent and contract employees, and new ways of delivering goods and services. These changes have resulted in a significant increase in the impact of small businesses on the nation's economy. Accordingly, some people with disabilities in rural areas and other locales where jobs are scarce have created job opportunities for themselves via entrepreneurship (Silvestri, 1999). The benefits of self-employment are: (1) freedom to make their own business decisions, (2) independence to set their own goals and pace, (3) home-based and culturally relevant (e.g., traditional craft of Native American tribes) businesses reduce issues related to transportation (a large hindrance to employment of people with disabilities), and (4) continued support from SSI and SSDI when assets are within the stipulations of these programs (U.S. Department of Labor, 2008). However having a significant disability and shortage of resources may pose problems in becoming self-employed, and a large proportion of those with significant disabilities are from culturally diverse groups.

4. *Supported employment* is a unique example of the selective approach. This is an employment service for people who, because of the nature and severity of their disabilities, need ongoing support services to obtain and maintain competitive, paid jobs in an integrated setting. It does not emphasize prerequisite employability/skills, an almost nonexistent characteristic in a large number of people with disabilities, or preplacement services. Rather it focuses on post-placement training, integration, and ongoing support. These characteristics make it a viable approach for people with severe disabilities and those from diverse backgrounds (U.S. Department of Labor, 1993). Authorized by the Rehabilitation Act of 1973, its scope of services includes recruiting and matching an employee to job requirements, and training the employer and colleagues in modes of working effectively with the individual with a disability. It also may involve assisting the individual in work-related needs such as transportation, counseling, and living in the community (Kregel & Wehman, 1989; Szymanski & Parker, 1996). The provision of ongoing support services for people with severe disabilities, a category having high representation of members of multicultural groups, significantly increases the rates of employment and job retention. Supported employment encourages people to work within their communities and engage in culturally relevant social interaction. Most supported employees work at least 20 hours per week at a competitive wage (Park, Shafer, &

Drake, 1993). Generally, job-related assistance can be provided via natural support or a job coach. As per the National Council on Disability [NCD] (1997), natural supports are often preferred by people with disabilities from diverse racial and ethnic backgrounds and employment options that use natural support often allow for a better individual–job match. A job coach, on the other hand, is engaged by a placement agency to provide specialized onsite training to assist an employee with a disability to learn to perform essential activities of a job and to adjust to the work environment. This approach is appropriate for persons with mental illness or intellectual disabilities and for those who are culturally diverse (National Alliance for the Mentally Ill, 2001; National Institute of Mental Health, 1999; New Freedom Commission on Mental Health, 2003).

5. *Project with Industry* (PWI) is designed to: (1) create and expand competitive job/career opportunities for those with disabilities by involving private industry in the VR process, (2) identify competitive job opportunities and the skills needed to perform these jobs, (3) establish opportunities for job readiness and job training programs closely resembling real life situations, and (4) assist in job placement and career advancement (Eger, 1990). These programs are required to establish Business Advisory Councils (BACs) with representatives from organized labor, private industry, individuals with disabilities, state VR agencies, community representatives, and others as deemed necessary. The BACs assist in (1) identifying available jobs in the community in accordance with the prevailing and projected employment opportunities identified by the local Workforce Investment Boards (WIBs) under the purview of the Workforce Investment Act (WIA) of 1998; (2) identifying the required skill level for those jobs; and (3) recommending training/placement programs for project participants (RTI International, 2003). The concept of PWI may be helpful for placing ethnically diverse individuals with disabilities. However, it does not usually take into account culturally related skill development factors, and it is rarely applicable in geographically remote areas with limited or no businesses.

The primary goal of VR is employment outcome of consumers with disabilities. Traditional approaches like *person centered* and *selective placement* are examples of the supply-side job placement philosophy that focuses on assisting people with disabilities to get hired by selling their skills to the employer as a consumer advocate (Gandy, Martin, Hardy, & Cull, 1987; Vandergoot, 1987; Wright, 1980). *Supported employment* and the *PWI* approach are examples of the demand-side job placement philosophy that emphasizes providing services directly to employers and assisting them in addressing their human resource needs. Demand-side is less concerned with directly placing individuals with disabilities into jobs and more focused on creating a demand among employers so that people with disabilities can be recruited into the workforce. The characteristics of demand-side placement are: (1) to increase demand for people with disabilities as potential employees, (2) to provide ongoing consultation to employers in organizational and human resource development, (3) to increase the number and range of jobs that people with disabilities can perform within a specific organization, (4) to help improve the financial position and diversity need of the employer (i.e., tax incentives and assisting employers in recruiting qualified culturally diverse employees with disabilities (Gilbride & Stensrud, 1992; Gilbride, Stensrud, & Johnson, 1994; National Institute on Disability and Rehabilitation Research [NIDRR], 2005). *Self-employment* is a third way, a job creation approach that emphasizes the development of a new enterprise rather than preparing individuals for an existing one. However, the existing job placement approaches and philosophies reviewed here do not include some of the important job placement-related characteristics that can affect the labor market. Examples are academic preparation, skills, and competency of the job placement specialist, as well as cultural mores of the consumer and the professional.

The following section presents a Systems Approach to Placement model (SAP), including data related to the current validation efforts for SAP measures. This holistic model incorporates selected characteristics of the previous models and adds environmental and contextual factors, including sociocultural variables that have not been appropriately and explicitly included in the placement process before. The authors argue that SAP is a promising approach for addressing the placement needs of people with disabilities who are ethnically diverse.

A SYSTEMS APPROACH TO PLACEMENT

People with disabilities may benefit from work as much as those without disabilities (Council of Europe, 2003). The benefits from work include financial independence and security, increased self-confidence, personal growth, skill development, and greater social integration (Jordan & Enein-Donova, 2002). Traditionally, job placement is considered to be the end-state of the rehabilitation counselor–client relationship (Gandy et al., 1987; Vandergoot, 1987; Wright, 1980). However, career development, of which job placement is a part, is a lifelong process with cultural relevance and may require professional input at various stages of change (e.g., advent of a disability or change in social determinants of work). Therefore, it is imperative that the process of job placement and career development take into account all factors related to the person with a disability as a whole, including contextual variables (Kundu, et al., 2005; Wright). A Systems Approach to Placement (SAP) strives to incorporate person-organization-environment-culture specific variables in VR leading to successful and long-term career development.

Patton and McMahon (2006) propose that systems theory offers an overarching framework for addressing a number of factors in human behavior. Patton and McMahon (1999, 2006) used systems theory as a guide to redefine career counseling practice. The overarching framework provided by systems theory (McMahon & Patton, 1995; Patton & McMahon, 1997, 1999, 2006) accommodates within itself all concepts of career development described in a wide array of career theories and effectively used in service delivery. Central to the framework is the individual system which encompasses a wide variety of intrapersonal influences on career development and job placement (e.g., ethnicity, gender, personality, ability, and sexual orientation). As people do not live in a vacuum, the individual system is affected by influences that include the social and broader environmental (societal) systems. Although the influence of factors such as geographic location, disability and race interaction, and political decisions on career development is not fully explained by theoretical literature, their influence on career development and job placement may be profound.

In 1935, around the conclusion of the Hawthorne Studies, systems theory became popular in human services disciplines. Simpson and Podsakoff (1975) state that interdependence may be regarded as the defining characteristic of a system. Under this concept, for example, a social subsystem (of which family and culture are parts) is one of the subsystems that contain various independently interacting aspects of the placement process. In addition, other systems external to the placement system also function interdependently with each other. Therefore, the process of placement cannot be considered an independent construct devoid of all its components that interact and lead to their functional (e.g., counselor's academic/professional preparation) or dysfunctional (e.g., compromised counselor–consumer working alliance is secondary to culturally related expectation discrepancy between the person with a disability and the counselor) consequences. It is necessary to identify the placement process as a system consisting of two parts: 1) the internal system which is comprised of the interactional patterns of the placement process (i.e., preparation for the world of work, person with a disability's social background and cultural values, counselors' qualifications and competence, resources and reputation of the agency doing the placement), and 2) an external system that includes the labor market and geographical location of available jobs. The intersection between internal and external systems may often generate unemployment due to lack of geographic mobility (e.g., some cultures are homebound), shortage of skills needed for a certain type of job market (e.g., skilled in traditional arts and crafts not currently in demand) and/or severity and type of disability.

At this time, there is a lack of objective and culturally appropriate models of job placement that harness all of the resources/variables in the task of promoting and maintaining community integration of people with disabilities, especially those from diverse cultural backgrounds. However, it is well documented that the principal function of VR is to meaningfully place a person with a disability on a job (Kundu et al., 2005; Muthard & Salomone, 1969; Parker & Szymanski, 1992). The issues related to effectively placing a person on the job continue to pose several challenges with culture at their center. SAP offers placement professionals in human service fields a mode of ascertaining placement professionals' knowledge, skills, and competencies in providing meaningful VR services which none of the existing approaches or models consider. SAP provides a framework that incorporates selected characteristics of the existing models. It offers a systematic, objective, comprehensive, and contextually relevant approach to job placement that takes culture into account and seeks to minimize and eliminate culture and ethnic biases.

The systemic placement process is set up on a holistic foundation of human, organizational, environmental, and cultural interaction. SAP simultaneously accommodates salient characteristics of the person-centered, selective, self-employment/ entrepreneurship, supported employment, and PWI approaches. It infuses additional dimensions by identifying multiple internal characteristics of persons with disabilities and external characteristics that account for the total functioning of the placement process. Internal characteristics may include disability and need for related assistance and education, among others. External characteristics may be exemplified by social, cultural, linguistic, and religious factors, as well as sexual orientation and contextual variables—like family support or job-market conditions. Also, SAP reduces the chance of making incorrect assumptions about the job seeker's assets and limitations when evaluating the person for entry into the VR process or for a job by involving the person with a disability who belongs to a diverse racial and/or ethnic group in the service planning process. This diagnostic and therapeutic approach assists the rehabilitation counselor/placement specialist to better identify the placement-related needs that must be addressed on an individualized basis with culture in mind (Kundu et al., 2005). SAP is built to view the placement process as a system with eight constituent subsystems that play an important part in the placement process. Complex reactions and interactions of these subsystems influence the placement outcome in the long run.

SAP (see Figure 16-1) proposes the following subsystems of the placement continuum:

1. *The client subsystem*: The person with a disability as a whole and how he/she relates to the internal (e.g., interest, aptitude, and motivation) and external (e.g., transportation and child care) environment.
2. *The health subsystem*: The individual's general health as well as an assessment of his/her disabling condition(s) and needed services.

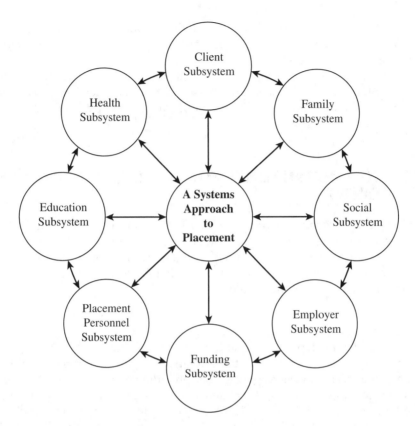

Figure 16-1 A Systems Approach to Placement

3. *The education subsystem*: Including both formal (e.g., school, college, and university training) and informal (e.g., traditional arts and crafts) training and skills enhancement (e.g., on-the-job training) needs/services received.
4. *The family subsystem*: Individual's and family members' adjustment to disability and their interactional pattern.
5. *The social subsystem*: The impact of culture, ethnicity, language, religious and social barriers, or facilitators external to the family. For example, effects of using English as a second language, effects of religion, effects of race, impact of culture—both mainstream and one's own, etc.
6. *The employer subsystem*: Consists of organizational (e.g., workplace culture), labor market forces (e.g., globalization), workers' unions, and physical ambiance (e.g., accessibility) of the workplace.

7. *The placement personnel subsystem*: Variables related to the professionals who do job placement (e.g., professional training of rehabilitation counselors and agency resources/policies).

8. *The funding subsystem*: Sources of financial aid (e.g., PELL grant, state/federal VR, SSI, and SSDI) that assist the person with disabilities in receiving needed services leading to the rehabilitation outcome of job placement.

EVALUATION INSTRUMENTS FOR A SYSTEMS APPROACH TO PLACEMENT

The following two diagnostic and therapeutic tools are designed under the SAP model to evaluate competencies of rehabilitation professionals and the needs of and services received by individuals with disabilities from diverse ethnic and racial groups. They seek to reduce cultural bias and thereby lead to successful job placement and long-term employment outcomes.

1. *SAP: Self-Assessment of Students and Counselors (SAP: SASC).* This instrument consists of 80 items belonging to the 8 subsystems of SAP. It can be used to ascertain placement-related proficiency and resulting training needs for rehabilitation counselors, placement specialists, disability managers, students in rehabilitation, and other professionals responsible for providing employment-related services. The following are the number of items in each subsystem: client (15), health (8), education (6), family (5), social (10), employer (14), placement (10), and funding (12). The level of knowledge is scored on a 5-point Likert scale where 0 = I have no knowledge or skill and 4 = I have enough knowledge or skill to train someone. The higher the average in each subsystem, the greater the level of knowledge of the rehabilitation counselor, placement specialist, disability manager, or student (Kundu et al., 2005). In an agency setting, the SAP: SASC can provide an objective evaluation of knowledge and competencies possessed by the placement personnel and strategies of developing skills enhancement leading to better placement outcomes. In an academic setting, this instrument can be administered to beginning students in rehabilitation counseling, rehabilitation services, disability studies, or disability management as a pre-test and then again at the end of their course work as a post-test. Also, it can be used as pre- and post-measure of a job development and job placement class. Thus, the SAP: SASC can be an objective measure of proficiencies acquired while pursuing a master's degree or undergraduate studies in rehabilitation and related fields.

To determine the reliability of SAP: SASC, the instrument was administered to 117 rehabilitation counselors in state/federal VR agencies in Alaska, Hawaii, Louisiana, New York, Guam, and Saipan and in Native American VR programs in Alaska, Louisiana, and Oklahoma. Cronbach alpha was calculated as a measure of internal consistency: client = 0.91, health = 0.94, education = 0.89, family = 0.92, social = 0.95, employer = 0.87, placement personnel = 0.93, and funding = 0.93.

2. *SAP: Intake Assessment and Outcome Evaluation (SAP: IAOE)*. This is an 86-item instrument belonging to the 8 subsystems of SAP. It can be used by rehabilitation professionals as a way of developing a functional Individualized Plan for Employment (IPE) and justifying the quality of their work with persons with disabilities. It supports the need for services, substantiates the decisions made by the professional, and/or documents services received. The number of items in each subsystem are as follows: client (18), health (7), education (6), family (10), social (13), employer (10), placement personnel (9), and funding (13). Items appropriate for a specific client are scored once at intake and once again at case closure. Need of services at intake are scored on a 5-point Likert scale where 1 = minimum service needed and 5 = emergency service needed. The receipt of services at outcome are scored on a 5-point Likert scale where 1 = minimum service received and 5 = emergency service received (Kundu et al., 2005).

The higher the average, the greater the need for and/or receipt of services. On the basis of the average scores at intake, services may be prioritized, a rehabilitation plan initiated, and appropriate resources allocated. At or after closure, average scores for each subsystem and the composite average of outcome can be calculated following the process mentioned above. The difference in the average intake and outcome scores (in each subsystem and composite) may vary to reflect the extent of consumer needs addressed by the placement process.

Rehabilitation counselors in state/federal agencies from Alaska, Saipan, Guam, Louisiana, Hawaii, and New York and those employed by Native American VR programs in Alaska, Louisiana and Oklahoma utilized SAP: IAOE to analyze their successful and unsuccessful cases. In terms used by the federal VR system, successful cases are assigned Status 26. These positive cases reflect that the person with a disability was determined eligible for VR services and an IPE was developed. The person received planned services and maintained employment for at least 90 days. Unsuccessful cases are assigned Status 28. These negative cases reflect that the person with a disability left the system for various reasons after IPE development. The person may have received some or all planned services, but was not employed. (Kundu et al., 2005).

To determine the efficacy of SAP: IAOE, a total of 635 completed SAP: IAOE questionnaires that assessed services received by individuals in 512 closed cases belonging to state/federal VR agencies and 123 from Native American tribal VR programs were used for these analyses. Gender was reported in 600 cases and included 332 men and 268 women; the mean age was 36.65 years. Closure status was reported for 631 cases, and included 336 Status 26 cases and 295 Status 28 cases. Race was reported for 629 cases: there were 277 Caucasian Americans, 100 African Americans, 91 Native Americans, 66 Pacific Islanders, 44 Alaska Natives, 33 Asian Americans, 8 Hispanics, and 10 classified as others with disabilities.

The following is a brief summary of some of the research questions that were asked in order to demonstrate the efficacy of the SAP: IAOE instrument in examining VR outcomes.

1. *What is the effect of VR services on employment outcomes?*

   Multivariate logistic regression analysis was computed to determine the effect of VR services on rehabilitation outcomes (employed/status 26 versus unemployed/status 28) after controlling for the effect of race, gender, age, and type of disability. VR services were measured using the SAP: IAOE. The results indicated that 53.4% of the sample obtained employment that could be predicted by the services received via their VR counselors. The omnibus test for the logistic regression model was found to be statistically significant, χ^2 (18, N = 570) = 115.52, p < 0.001, indicating that there is a significant association between the demographic covariates and VR service predictors on the one hand and employment outcomes on the other. The Negelkerke R^2 was 0.25 (medium effect size), indicating that about 25% of the variance in employment outcomes can be explained by the covariate and predictor variables. The Hosmer and Lemeshow goodness of fit test was not significant, χ^2 (8, N = 570) = 6.39, p = 0.32, indicating that the model fits the data reasonably well.

   In Step 1, the following variables were entered into the analysis: age (with age 16–34 as the reference category), gender (with men as the reference category), race (with African American as the reference category), and disability type (with substance abuse disorder as the reference category). Disability type was the only covariate found to be significant. People with visual impairments were found to be 3.62 times more likely to be employed than consumers with a substance abuse disorder (odds ratio [OR] = 3.62, 95% CI = 1.70 to 7.73). In Step 2, SAP: IAOE subsystem service outcomes total scores were entered as predictors. After controlling for the effect of age, gender, race, and disability type, four subsystems were found to be statistically significant (e.g., client, social, employer, and placement personnel). The results indicated that consumers who received employer-related services were 1.24 times (OR = 1.24;

95% CI: 1.12 to 1.38) more likely to be employed than those who did not receive this service. Likewise, consumers who received job placement services were 1.13 times (OR = 1.13; 95% CI: 1.06 to 1.21) more likely to be employed than those who did not receive job placement services. On the other hand, people with disabilities who received client support services were less likely to find employment (OR = .92; 95% CI: .87 to .97) and those who received social-related services were less likely to find employment (OR = .82; 95% CI: .72 to .94) compared with consumers who did not receive these types of services.

2. *What is the effect of race on service intensity?*

Multivariate analysis of variance (MANOVA) was used to determine the effect of race on the intensity of services received by VR consumers. The omnibus test was significant, Wilk's Lambda = 0.85, $F(12, 345) = 4.12, p < .001$. Therefore, a univariate analysis of variance (ANOVA) was computed for each dependent variable. The alpha level was divided by 8 for each pairwise comparison to control for Type I error ($\alpha = 0.05/8 = .006$). The results indicated significant differences on three of the eight SAP: IAOE subsystem factors: health, family, and social. Post-hoc comparisons using the Bonferroni procedure indicated that Native Americans received significantly more health services ($M = 4.46, SD = 3.27$) than Asian Americans ($M = 3.02, SD = 2.73$) and Caucasian Americans ($M = 3.57, SD = 3.12$). Native Americans ($M = 3.11, SD = 2.99$) also received significantly more family services than African Americans ($M = 1.92, SD = 2.80$) and Caucasian Americans ($M = 1.93, SD = 2.63$). Finally, Native Americans ($M = 1.86, SD = 2.37$) and Asian Americans ($M = 1.76, SD = 2.24$) were found to receive significantly more social services than African Americans ($M = .87, SD = 1.41$) and Caucasian Americans ($M = 1.02, SD = 1.64$). From the analysis of Research Question 1 above, it appears that receiving more social-related services is a marker for reduced odds of attaining successful employment outcomes, perhaps because of the greater need of those receiving social services.

3. *What is the effect of disability type on employment outcomes?*

A univariate analysis of variance (ANOVA) was computed to determine the effect of disability type on employment outcomes. The results indicated that there is a significant disability type effect, $F(3, 566) = 13.71, p < .01$. Post-hoc analysis using the Bonferroni procedures indicated that consumers with a sensory disability had significantly better employment outcomes ($M = .77, SD = .42$) than people with physical ($M = .56, SD = .50$), psychiatric and intellectual ($M = .40, SD = .49$), and substance abuse disabilities ($M = .46, SD = .50$). People with physical disabilities had significantly better outcomes than those with psychiatric and intellectual disabilities, and there is no difference between psychiatric and intellectual disabilities and substance abuse disabilities in terms of employment outcomes.

4. *What is the effect of race on employment outcome?*
   Race was categorized into Caucasians, African Americans, Native Americans and Alaska Natives, and Asian Americans with Pacific Islanders. One-way ANOVA was computed to determine the effect of race on employment outcomes. The results indicated that there is no significant race effect, $F(3, 607) = 0.24$, *n.s.*

DISCUSSION OF FINDINGS

VR consumers with visual impairment had a better chance of securing gainful employment than did those with physical, psychiatric, intellectual, and substance abuse disorders. This is in congruence with the findings of the U.S. Department of Education (2006) which states that VR consumers with sensory disabilities (visual and hearing) are more likely to become employed at closure as compared to their counterparts with psychiatric and intellectual impairments. Additionally, better mental/emotional health is positively related to earning greater income at successful VR case closures. The receipt of employer-related and job placement services was a good predictor of return to work. Blackwell, Leierer, Haupt, and Kampotsis (2003) found that early receipt of vocationally-related services is a good predictor of return to work for consumers with disabilities. With regard to differences in types of services received as a function of ethnicity, although a lower proportion of Native Americans obtained gainful employment after VR case closure, they received significantly more family, health, and social services than Caucasian Americans. This is partly congruent with the finding in this study that the receipt of social services was associated with reduced odds of obtaining employment because it suggests the presence of multiple problems that make employment difficult.

Additionally, there is no effect of ethnicity on employment outcome after receipt of VR services. However, it is well documented that there is significant race difference in employment outcomes for state/federal VR consumers, especially African Americans and Caucasians (Alston & Mngadi, 1992; Dutta, Gervey, Chan, Chou, & Ditchman, 2008; Kundu & Dutta, 2004; Wilson, 2002). State/federal and Native American VR consumers were also used in this study. The potentially important finding, albeit a null one, is that in this sample there is no race effect on employment outcomes. African Americans, Caucasians, Asian Americans, and Native Americans all return to work at a similar rate. As the study did not incorporate a true experimental design, a cause-and-effect relationship cannot be established between return to work and use of SAP: IAOE. However, while caution must be exercised when considering null findings, it can be pointed out that the results are consistent with a relationship between using SAP: IAOE and reduction of race effect on employment outcomes. Therefore, this issue may warrant further research using either a carefully designed case-controlled study or a true experimental study.

ADVANTAGES OF SAP: IAOE UTILIZATION

The advantages of the SAP instrument IAOE are as follows:

- SAP: IAOE assists in the determination of the person with a disability's service needs at intake in a culturally sensitive manner.
- SAP: IAOE facilitates preparation of a functional, culturally appropriate plan for rehabilitation or IPE in collaboration with the consumer.
- SAP: IAOE provides a means for systematic evaluation of the scope and quality of services provided by professionals to culturally diverse persons with disabilities.
- SAP: IAOE is a measure of placement accountability for the rehabilitation professional and agency.
- Data generated by SAP: IAOE may be utilized for weighted case closure, an approach to analyzing case closure not used by the current VR system that continues to serve people with significant disabilities. Closure weights may be used as difficulty norms for various client groups. Numeric weights may add value to difficult cases closed either successfully or unsuccessfully (Noble, 1973; Wallis & Bozarth, 1971; Walls & Moriarty, 1977).
- SAP: IAOE serves as an outcome evaluation assisting the agency in effective resource allocation and utilization.
- The data gathered may be used to convince funding resources of service quality and success.

UTILITY OF TWO INSTRUMENTS

These instruments can be used by rehabilitation professionals and job placement specialists in different ways. The SAP: SASC evaluates the competency level of the service provider or student and helps in designing a culturally sensitive continuing education/professional development plan to address the identified training needs. By jointly completing the SAP: IAOE with the individual at intake, the counselor can obtain an overall assessment of (1) the person's needs as a function of person-specific, agency-related, and contextual factors; and (2) the areas of strengths and weaknesses, and important placement-related characteristics of the individual with disabilities in a culturally appropriate manner. This information can facilitate the collaborative design of a viable placement plan. As the individual completes each phase of the plan, the instrument can be used to reevaluate his/her need for further services and readiness to obtain and maintain employment. The same instrument can be completed at closure (successful or unsuccessful) in an effort to identify the contribution of each subsystem to the outcome. This analysis can be an educational tool for both the counselor and the person with a disability who belongs to a diverse racial or ethnic group in better understanding future services related to job placement. Additionally, both SAP: SASC and SAP: IAOE can be used to assess the professional preparedness of the practitioner, the impact of organizational agency policies on the VR process, and the role of external/contextual variables (e.g., geographic location, attitudes toward a specific group) in facilitating or hindering service delivery/receipt. By systematically establishing the strengths and weaknesses of the practitioner and the agency, the instruments help identify training needs, best practices within the organization, cost-benefit factors for the development of placement techniques, and educators involved in the training of future counselors who will place persons with disabilities from diverse cultural backgrounds.

FUTURE DIRECTIONS

The global challenge of the 21st century is to secure decent work for 650 million people with disabilities of different racial, ethnic, and cultural backgrounds in an equitable, secure, and dignified manner. Employment is fundamental in the fight against poverty and social exclusion, as was stressed by the World Summit for Social Development in 1995 (International Labour Office [ILO], 2007). Productive employment is a basic individual right since it not only provides a wage but is also an expression of self-fulfillment and dignity. Selected criteria for productive employment; gender/race-sensitive labor policies, and wide-based entrepreneurship and asset-holding must focus on the education of people with disabilities, and members of other disadvantaged groups (O'Reilly, 2007). The underlying constructs of SAP embrace these principles with focus on the interaction among the person, organization, and environment. Therefore, the instruments developed under this model have the potential to be extensively used in employment-based training, practice, and research.

One area of research should focus on assessing the level of knowledge and skills of rehabilitation professionals who do placement using SAP: SASC and developing an appropriate training and skills enhancement agenda. Professional competencies go a long way in harnessing the resources of the community and labor market for the consumers. In an academic setting, it can be used as a pre- and post-measure of a curriculum or a class on job development and job placement. Another area of research should focus on empirical investigation by utilizing SAP: IAOE with people with disabilities from the beginning to the end of the rehabilitation process. Full implementation of SAP: IAOE is contingent upon SAP: SASC. SAP has the potential to be adapted to different languages, cultures, places, and disabilities (Williams, Dutta, Kundu, & Welch, 2008) based on local needs. As the SAP is being translated in various languages, it should be kept in mind that revised versions need to be validated locally to assess its full efficacy.

CONCLUSION

More than a decade after the authorization of the Rehabilitation Act Amendments of 1998, appropriate and gainful employment remains an unfulfilled dream for a large number of people with disabilities. Much of the high unemployment rate is not a direct result of a person's disabling conditions but how society reacts to the person and his/her disability-related accommodation needs (Shapiro, 1993). For those from diverse cultural groups, issues of racism and prejudice can compound the difficulty of finding valued employment. Employers often tend to believe that people with disabilities from diverse groups are not prepared for certain jobs. Sometimes, even rehabilitation and human services professionals have low expectations of individuals with certain types of disabilities, especially those from diverse racial and ethnic groups (Hutchinson, 1990). Therefore, it is imperative that the low expectations of society regarding the capabilities of people with disabilities from diverse backgrounds to become employed be minimized with the introduction of an innovative placement technique like SAP. SAP, in this dynamic global economy, makes prudent use of human, organizational, environmental, and cultural factors to appropriately identify culturally diverse persons' strengths/weaknesses, professional proficiency requirements, agency resources and policies, and labor market trends to promote optimal job placement of people with disabilities who are racially and ethnically diverse.

REFERENCES

Alston, R. J., & Mngadi, S. (1992). The interaction between disability status and the African American experience: Implications for rehabilitation counseling. *Journal of Applied Rehabilitation Counseling, 23,* 12–16.

Appelbaum, E. (2007). *Economic security and opportunity for working families: Testimony before the Committee on Health, Education, Labor, and Pensions.* New Brunswick, NJ: Rutgers University, Center for Women and Work, School of Management and Labor Relations.

Berven, N. (1979). The roles and functions of the rehabilitation counselor revisited. *Rehabilitation Counseling Bulletin, 23,* 84–88.

Bissonnette, D. (2002). *Beyond traditional job development.* Chatsworth, CA: Milt Wright and Associates.

Blackwell, T., Leierer, S., Haupt, S., & Kampotsis, A. (2003). Predictors of vocational rehabilitation return to work outcomes in workers compensation. *Rehabilitation Counseling Bulletin, 46*(108), 108–114.

Bowe, F. (2006). Memories of Mary. Speech to the 2005-2006 Switzer Fellows, National Institute on Disability and Rehabilitation Research. Retrieved December 2, 2007, from *http://people.hofstra.edu/faculty/frank_g_bowe/memories_of_mary.doc*

Bureau of Labor Statistics. (2008). The employment situation. Available online at *http://www.bls.gov/news.release/pdf/empsit.pdf*

Condon, C., Fichera, K., & Dreilinger, D. (2003). More than just a job: Person-centered career planning. *The Institute Brief, 12*(1). Boston: University of Massachusetts, Institute for Community Inclusion.

Council of Europe. (2003). Council resolution on eAccessibility: improving the access of the people with disabilities to the knowledged based society, SOC5 MI4 EDUC2 TELECOM1, from *http://europa.eu.int/comm/employment_social/knowledge_society/res_eacc_en.pdf*

Dutta, A., Gervey, R., Chan, F., Chou. C., & Ditchman, N. (2008). The effect of vocational rehabilitation services and personal factors on employment outcomes of people with disabilities: A national study. *Journal of Occupational Rehabilitation, 18*(4), 326–334.

Eger, J. (1990). Projects with industry. *OSERS News in Print. III*(3), 18–21.

Gandy, G., Martin, E., Hardy, R., & Cull, J. (Eds.). (1987). *Rehabilitation counseling and services.* Springfield, IL: Charles C Thomas.

Gilbride, D., & Stensrud, R. (1992). Demand-side job development: A model for the 1990s. *Journal of Rehabilitation, 58,* 34–39.

Gilbride, D., Stensrud, R., & Johnson, M. (1994). Current models of job placement and employer development: Research, competencies and educational considerations. *Rehabilitation Education, 7,* 215–239.

Habeck, R. V. (2006, September). *Improving employment results through retention.* Presentation at the ICDR National Summit: Employer Perspective on People with Disabilities, Alexandria, VA.

Hunt, P. C. (2002). *An introduction to Vietnamese cultural for rehabilitation services providers in the U.S.* Buffalo, NY: University at Buffalo, Center for International Rehabilitation Research Information Exchange.

Hutchinson, S.A. (1990) *The case study approach: Advancing nursing science through research,* London: Sage.

International Labour Office. (2007). *The inclusion of persons with disabilities in vocational training and employment.* Geneva, Switzerland: Author.

Jordan, M., & Enein-Donova, L. (2002). *Tool for inclusion. Starting with me: A guide to person centered planning for job seekers,* Boston: University of Massachusetts, Institute for Community Inclusion.

Kregel, J., & Wehman, P. (1989). Supported employment: promises deferred for persons with severe disabilities. *Journal of the Association for Persons with Severe Handicaps, 14*(4), 293–303.

Kundu, M. M., & Dutta, A. (2004). Pattern of service delivery to culturally diverse consumers in a state rehabilitation agency: A five-year study. *RehabPro, 12*(3), 51–57.

Kundu, M. M., Schiro-Geist, C., & Dutta, A. (2005). A systems approach to placement: A holistic technique. *Journal of Forensic Vocational Analysis, 8*, 23–29.

McMahon, M., & Patton, W. (1995). Development of a systems theory of career development. *Australian Journal of Career Development, 4*(2), 15–20.

Muthard, J., & Salomone, P. (1969). Roles and functions of the rehabilitation counselor. *Rehabilitation Counseling Bulletin, 13*, 81–168.

National Alliance for the Mentally Ill Board of Directors (2001). *Strategic plan for 2001–2003.* Arlington, VA: National Alliance for the Mentally Ill.

National Council on Disability. (1997). *Removing barriers to work: Action proposal for the 105th Congress and beyond.* Retrieved September 2, 2007, from *http://www.ncd.gov/ newsroom/ publications/1997/barriers.htm*

National Institute on Disability and Rehabilitation Research. (2005). *Federal Register* (pp. 17426–17427). Disability and Rehabilitation Research Projects Center Programs. Washington, D.C.: Author.

National Institute of Mental Health. (1999). *Bridging science and service: A report by the National Advisory Mental Health Council's Clinical Treatment and Services Research Workgroup.* Rockville, MD: Author.

New Freedom Commission on Mental Health. (2003). *Achieving the promise: Transforming mental health care in America.* (DHHS Publication No. SMA-03-3832). Rockville, MD: Author.

Noble, J. H. (1973). Actuarial system for weighting case closures. *Rehabilitation Record, 14*(5), 34–37.

Office of Disability Employment Policy. (2003). *Statistics on the employment rate of people with disabilities.* Washington, D.C.: Author.

O'Reilly, A. (2007). *The right to decent work of persons with disabilities.* Geneva, Switzerland: International Labour Office.

Park, H., Shafer, M. S., & Drake, L. (1993). Factors related to the working environment of employment specialists. *Journal of Rehabilitation, 59*(4), 38–43.

Parker, R., & Szymanski, E. (1992). *Rehabilitation counseling: Basics and beyond* (2nd ed.). Austin, TX: ProEd.

Patton, W., & McMahon, M. (1997). *Career development in practice: A systems theory perspective.* Sydney: New Hobsons Press.

Patton, W., & McMahon, M. (1999). *Career development and systems theory: A new relationship.* Pacific Grove, CA: Brooks/Cole.

Patton, W., & McMahon, M. (2006). The systems theory framework of career development and counseling: Connecting theory and practice. *International Journal for the Advancement of Counselling, 28*(2), 153–166.

RTI International. (2003). *Evaluation of projects with industry program.* Research Triangle Park, NC: Author.

Rubin, S., Matkin, R., Ashley, J., Beardsley, M., May, V., Ontott, K., et al. (1984). Roles and functions of certified rehabilitation counselors. *Rehabilitation Counseling Bulletin, 27*, 199–224, 238–245.

Salomone, P. R. (1971). A client-centered approach to job placement. *Vocational Guidance Quarterly, 19*(4), 266–270.

Shapiro, J. (1993). *No pity: People with disabilities forging a new civil rights movement.* New York: Times Books/Random House.

Silvestri, G. T. (1999). Considering self-employment: What to think about before starting a business. *Occupational Outlook Quarterly, 43*(2), 15–23.

Simpson, D. B., & Podsakoff, P. M. (1975). *Workshop management: A behavioral and systems approach.* Springfield, IL: Thomas Press.

Sink, J., & Porter, T. (1978). Convergence and divergence in rehabilitation counseling and vocational evaluation. *Rehabilitation Counseling Bulletin, 9,* 5–20.

Steinmetz, E. (2004). Americans with Disabilities: 2002. *Current Population Reports,* (pp. 70–107). Washington, D.C.: U.S. Census Bureau.

Szymanski, E. M., & Parker, R. M. (Eds.). (1996). *Work and disability: Issues and strategies in career development and job placement.* Austin, TX: Pro-Ed.

U.S. Department of Education. (2006). *Functional limitations of vocational rehabilitation consumers: Final report.* Washington, D.C.: Author.

U.S. Department of Labor. (1993). *High performance work practices and firm performance.* Washington, D.C.: U.S. Government Printing Office.

U.S. Department of Labor. (1999). *Presidential task force on employment of adults with disabilities: Notice of town hall meeting.* Washington, D.C.: Author.

U.S. Department of Labor. (2008). *Report of the taskforce on the aging of the American workforce.* Washington, D.C.: Department of Labor Employment and Training Administration. Retrieved December 18, 2007, from *http://www.doleta.gov/reports/FINAL_Taskforce_Report_2-11-08.pdf*

Vandergoot, D. (1987). Review of placement research literature: Implications for research and practice. *Rehabilitation Counseling Bulletin, 31,* 243–272.

Waldrop, J. (2003). Disability status: 2000. *Census 2000 Brief.* 1–12.

Wallis, J. H., & Bozarth, J. D. (1971). The development and evaluation of weighted DVR case closures. *Rehabilitation Research and Practice Review, 2*(3), 55–60.

Walls, R. T., & Moriarty, J. B. (1977). The caseload profile: An alternative to weighted closure. *Rehabilitation Literature, 38*(9), 285–291.

Williams, F., Dutta, A., Kundu, M. M., & Welch, M. (2008). Vocational rehabilitation services needs of female ex-inmates with mental illness: The perspective of a southern state. *Journal of Applied Rehabilitation Counseling, 39*(3), 25–32.

Wilson, K. B. (2002). Exploration of VR acceptance and ethnicity: A national investigation. *Rehabilitation Counseling Bulletin, 45*(3), 168–176.

Wright, G. N. (1980). *Total rehabilitation.* Boston: Little Brown.

Integrative Commentaries

CHAPTER 17

Exploring Cultural Competence: Implications for Research

Juan Carlos Arango, PhD;
Glen White, PhD;
Gary Kielhofner, PhD;
Angela Odoms-Young, PhD;
Felicia Wilkins-Turner, PhD

INTRODUCTION

The discussions of race, culture, and disability in this book raise a myriad of issues that will bear both theoretical and empirical scrutiny for some time. This chapter characterizes some of the more evocative and cogent themes presented in the previous sections of this text. Our intent is to identify areas that need further clarification and elaboration, and to note fruitful pathways for further empirical work.

With the growing diversity of our society, there is inevitable misunderstanding and conflict over values, worldviews, perceived needs, and rights of people with disabilities. These issues play out in multiple aspects of society. However, they are particularly pertinent in the context of providing rehabilitation and health services where differences of power and resources already reside between service providers and people with disabilities who are seeking services. Moreover, when several potentially disadvantaging characteristics such as poverty or literacy intersect and differentiate an individual with a disability from a service provider, the potential for misunderstanding is intensified.

UNDERSTANDING THE INFLUENCES OF CULTURE ON DISABILITY

It is clear that culture can have a pervasive influence on the understanding and experience of disability (Chapter 7 & Chapter 11). These influences include, for instance:

- How impairment is understood and whether a problem is even considered to exist within the cultural context of the person with a disability who belongs to an ethnically or racially diverse group.
- Attributions regarding source of impairment and what should be done about it.
- Expectations of what one should be able to do in the face of impairment (i.e., what a person is actually able and expected to do after the disability, such as working).
- Perceptions concerning what assessment and treatment, if any, should be applied to individuals with disabilities from diverse multicultural backgrounds.
- Expectations of family members concerning how a member with a disability should be treated within the family system, within the broader community, and within societal systems.

In these and many other ways, culture defines disability and some of the expectations about it (Chapter 7 & Chapter 11). Moreover, culture and associated factors also influence what impact an impairment has on a person's life. The lived experience and the cultural context and environment of a person with a disability allow person-culture-environment interactions that can take many different trajectories, depending upon the presence of risk or protective factors. For instance, consider persons from specific cultural groups associated with lower socioeconomic status who only have access to jobs requiring physical labor. For these persons, a physical impairment may present a greater impediment to employment than for members of a majority group where white collar jobs are more abundant. In sum, culture may influence the impact of a disability, the meaning ascribed to it, the care sought when someone incurs a disability, and the response of that person with a disability to rehabilitation services.

While there is a growing examination of how culture and disability intersect, this area is only beginning to be widely studied in rehabilitation. In fact, chapters in this volume aim to explore this intersection from research, teaching, and practical perspectives. As more is known about how culture affects disability, the likelihood of creating effective resources and services for those experiencing disability will be enhanced (Chapter 7).

UNDERSTANDING CULTURAL COMPETENCE WITHIN THE LIVED EXPERIENCE OF A DISABILITY

Given the impact of culture on disability experience, it is clear that health providers need to engage in culturally competent practices. Chapter 14 identifies useful dimensions and models of cultural competence that can increase the practitioners' or researchers' understanding and proficiency in this area. While there are emerging conceptual models and concepts of cultural competence and disability, there is a paucity of empirical studies that document the direct consequences of culturally competent services on consumer outcomes. Most research documents failures of access and differential rates of service provision and service success for disadvantaged groups (e.g., Chapter 5; Chapter 6). There is a lack of evidence concerning what happens in decision making about services and rehabilitation outcomes of people with disabilities that differ from providers in their disability experience, and race or ethnicity. Such research would provide a valuable empirical backdrop against which cultural competence models and applications could be more clearly considered. It could facilitate practitioners' movement toward cultural competence. For example, Smith and Alston (this volume) report progress emerging on employment and rehabilitation issues for multicultural women with disabilities. They identify risk factors that further marginalize this population in the work sector and suggest potential interventions to remediate them. These include hiring more multicultural mentors and counselors to reach out to multicultural women with disabilities. They also note the value for counselors that better understand the backgrounds and values for those receiving services. These issues could be recast into valuable research questions to be answered using empirical methods.

The term cultural competence may be somewhat problematic in itself. Many of the papers (e.g., Chapter 6, Chapter 8, Chapter 14, Chapter 16) underscore that human diversity is always defined as the intersection of many possible planes of difference. A nonexhaustive list would include race, ethnicity, age, gender, socioeconomic status, and differences of impairment or ability. These are fundamental human differences which shape how people understand themselves and their world on the one hand, and that shape how others perceive and react toward them on the other. Rehabilitation professionals can begin to bridge these differences by increasing their understanding of the perspectives, beliefs, values, concerns, and behaviors of those they serve. Equally important and often less well recognized, it also means being committed to try to discern how others live in the world. That is, what barriers, prejudices, and resources are likely to surround people by virtue of their public identities?

While the construct of cultural competence is complicated, it only becomes more so when trying to understand it within the lived experience of a disability. Chapter 9 noted the difficulty of being both a person with a disability and also from a non-majority racially or ethnically defined culture. Using concepts borrowed from the field of economics, they discuss " supply-side" and "demand-side" approaches to trying to enhance employment opportunities for multicultural women with disabilities; a similar approach was considered by Kundu et al. (this volume) when discussing their systems approach to rehabilitation. They argue that it is possible to tailor this framework to the specific needs of individuals with disabilities from diverse ethnic groups.

It is important to recognize that achieving cultural competence is not a linear, one-time process; rather, it is an iterative, lifelong journey (Chapter 14). People do not become "culturally competent," they become cognizant of the need to be culturally aware and vigilant in monitoring their own progress in a journey toward increasing cultural competency. Unlike other forms of competence, where a by-product is confidence, we propose that cultural competency may require that people never get too comfortable. This lack of comfort is especially valuable when seeking to act in a culturally competent manner with an individual with a disability who also belongs to a diverse ethnic or racial group. This individual may face multiple potentially marginalizing societal responses, such as ableism and racism, that arise separately and together in distinctive ways (see Chapter 3 & Chapter 5). Our own perceptions of culture may differ, but when also tied to a disability our perceptions and reactions may vary further.

Within the rehabilitation field culture may be at the center of a person's rehabilitation plan. What rehabilitation professionals may view as dysfunctional behavior or beliefs for a particular culture and disability may be viewed as very functional by those in that culture and/or those with that disability. For example, in some African gold mines the miners do not wear ear protection when they drill and use other heavy equipment when searching for gold. As a result, many are either deaf or have severe hearing loss. To the untrained practitioner or researcher, it may seem like a lack of concern to protect and preserve the ability to hear. However, to the workers in these mines, the loss of hearing is more of a status symbol that they *are* working and in the well-paid and often coveted job as gold miners (cf. Braddock & Parish, 2001). As we increase our understanding of personal, environmental, and cultural factors, we achieve small successes in learning about the cultures and the lived experience of disability of relevant others. Human difference is a dynamic part of life and those who wish to be culturally competent stay open to it.

When considering cultural competence in the context of human services, there is also an ethically-loaded question: How do professionals balance the person with a disability's culturally defined needs and perspectives with their own personal and professionally influenced values and viewpoint of the world? Moreover, how do cultural issues of those with disabilities who seek services interact with the organizational rules and guidelines with which the rehabilitation professional must comply? Is a culturally-influenced perspective always in the best interest of the person being served? How should one approach situations in which the best answer that one can generate is "not in the client's best interest"? Such questions must be pondered over and over in the context of service provision and they warrant research examination. Chapter 6 examined challenges in giving culturally appropriate care in rehabilitation settings. These settings might range from medical rehabilitation to more job-oriented rehabilitation services. In these different settings, the skills and information learned are necessary, but are they sufficient to generalize from the training setting to the home or work settings? There is some promising research in medical rehabilitation where most initial rehabilitation occurs within institutional settings that have a majority population orientation. Some of this research is aimed at better understanding the health experience of spinal cord injured patients once they returned to their home settings. For example, one southern rehabilitation center used telerehabilitation medicine to help transfer some of the rehabilitation and health maintenance process into the discharged patient's home setting (Vesmarovich, Walker, Hauber, Temkin, & Burns, 1999). Perhaps similar advanced technologies could be used in environments and cultures where individuals with disabilities from diverse cultural settings live their day-to-day lives. Such advances in technology can further extend rehabilitation practitioners' reach and their understanding of how those they serve interact in their environment and culture. It can provide for a reciprocal sense of learning for both the person with a disability and the rehabilitation professional.

TEACHING CULTURAL COMPETENCE WITHIN THE LIVED EXPERIENCE OF A DISABILITY

Given the complexity and multidimensionality of cultural competence intersecting with the lived experience of a disability, the question must be asked, "Can we really teach cultural competence in the context of disability?" While there are many models and approaches for teaching it (see Chapter 12; Chapter 13; Chapter 14), existing empirical evidence is not sufficient to answer the question. A number of challenges lie in the way of achieving better answers.

First, as implied in the earlier discussion in Chapter 14, we need to achieve better conceptual and operational definitions of cultural competency. The latter should lead to measures which can be used to empirically test the efficacy of interventions to enhance various approaches to increasing and enhancing cultural competency. For example, researchers could investigate whether changes in CC are correlated with different decisions and interactions in service provision and different consumer outcomes.

Another challenge that merits further investigation is assessing a person's readiness to learn more about being culturally competent. Studies in this potential line of research might lead to examination of other questions such as: When and under what circumstances is one ready to learn about cultural competence? How does one try to proactively prepare a person's readiness for learning about cultural competence?

How can one arrange for increased cultural competence knowledge and skills over time? What are the best approaches to generalize knowledge and skills learned in training to actual consumers in a service setting?

Answering each of the above questions will help guide researchers and practitioners toward successive approximations of cultural competence and under what conditions it is more robust or weakened. For the rehabilitation professionals and researchers, these guiding questions must also be posed within the context of a disabling condition. For example, do cultural mores and rules lessen or heighten the significance of the disability? Is the presence of a disabling condition viewed as a special gift or as a curse? (Braddock & Parish, 2001). As Clay and Seekins report in Chapter 8, it was not until Clay moved from her reservation and the cultural supports that her tribe offered her, did she realize she had a disability when entering a postsecondary education setting. Put bluntly, the White man's system has assigned disability labels to Native Americans where they had not previously existed.

CULTURAL COMPETENCY IN THE RESEARCH PROCESS

Researchers are no more immune to cultural misunderstandings than practitioners. Indeed, the way research is conceptualized, what topics are addressed, and how questions are raised and answered in research reflects the influence of a variety of ideologies and perspectives (Keys, McMahon, Sánchez, London, & Abdul-Adil, 2004). Current literature suggests that cultural factors influence a number of health and psychological measures (Chapter 4). These include, but are not limited to, neuropsychological test performance (Ardila, 2005), standardized testing performance (Kennephol, Shore, Nabors, & Hanks, 2004; Roselli & Ardila, 2003), health service usage (Wells, Golding, Hough, Burnam, & Karno, 1989), and medical and psychological treatment effectiveness (Rogler, Malgad, Costantino, & Blumenthal, 1987). Researchers must reexamine data collection measures and processes in order to ensure adequate quality and appropriateness for use in different cultures. Unfortunately, these studies often involved the participation of White populations only while at the same time the results are generalized to all people with disabilities.

Culturally competent investigators are especially needed. While cultural competence has been primarily a focus of practice and instruction, it is particularly important for scientists to be culturally competent in a way that enables them to study members of diverse cultures with disabilities (cf. Keys et al., 2004). A number of questions need to be addressed regarding culturally informed research concerning people with disabilities:

- What constitutes culturally competent researchers in the disability field?
- What would markers of successful culturally informed research look like?
- Would culturally informed research be additive or integrative in nature?
- What would training to prepare a culturally competent researcher look like?
- How could Cultural Competence training be incorporated into the terminal degree curriculum?
- What efforts should be made to prepare more researchers of color with disabilities?
- How do ethnically and/or racially diverse persons with disabilities approach issues of culture, race, and disability in their research?

Toward Cultural Competence in Research at Individual, Community, and System Levels

In recognition of these many questions yet to be fully addressed and answered concerning the development of culturally competent researchers, we suggest a series of steps to take to promote the development of cultural competence in rehabilitation research and practice. Discussions of cultural competency stress the extent to which professionals need to learn and change what they do. These steps need to occur at multiple levels ranging from the individual, community, and system.

Individual Level

Rehabilitation researchers and other professionals need to work to develop beliefs, attitudes, values, skills, and policies necessary to respond with respect and empathy to people regardless of culture, race, religion, and ethnic background. This work can be done in a manner that recognizes, affirms, and values the worth of the individual, family, and community. Evidence-based self-evaluation tools and effective cultural competency training may be two means of pursuing this aim. By conducting research at the individual level through the use of qualitative or single subject designs, investigators can gather needed data to understand these lived experiences more fully. The findings from these early, investigations could then be used to inform and conduct randomized clinical trials to test interventions that enhance cultural competency as it intersects with people from ethnically and racially diverse groups with disabilities.

Furthermore, at the individual level of analysis future research should document the impact of culturally competent rehabilitation services on employment outcomes. Although vast literature calls for culturally competent rehabilitation services, more empirical research is needed that examines the impact of culturally competent rehabilitation services on closing the disparities between people of color with disabilities and Whites with disabilities.

Community Level

Historically, discrimination has had a major impact on the lives of members of ethnically and racially diverse groups. Future research must contribute to a better grasp of how specific diverse groups of people with disabilities are affected. Additionally, research should also investigate the interactive effects of being from a diverse culture and also having a disability for creating communities of common concern. In order to exemplify the kinds of questions that need to be asked in research, we note the following two issues among Native Americans and Alaska Natives (Chapter 8).

- Of more than 560 federally recognized tribes, only 69 have established Native American vocational rehabilitation (VR) programs. What are the barriers that need to be removed to increase the number of VR programs for tribal communities?
- The Americans with Disabilities Act (ADA) is not recognized by the sovereign tribal governments. ADA was designed to address civil rights issues of Americans with disabilities. From a cultural viewpoint, how does each tribe consider and value their members with disabilities? Does the ADA, with its strong set of regulations for compliance or a similar statute, have a chance of adaptation within tribal governments?

Another area of community-oriented research needs to focus on the development and validation of rehabilitation techniques and programs within the settings in which consumers engage and live. A great deal of rehabilitation research occurs within institutional settings and with staff and facilities that tend to be oriented towards the majority population. Advanced technology can play a role in expanding research into community-based settings. As we have discussed, telerehabilitation medicine and its variants for other health providers offer interesting methods to treat individuals with disabilities living in rural areas. Living in isolated locations and having limited transportation means relying on help from family members. Recent advances have used personal digital assistants (PDAs) to determine the types and frequency of activities that people with disabilities are engaged in using a momentary sample technique (Seekins, Ipsen, & Arnold, 2007). A variation of this technology might be used with those from different cultures to determine the effects of different interventions in providing equal opportunities and access to rehabilitation services as majority populations receive.

System Level

Policies encouraging involvement of underrepresented groups in health research have been in place at the National Institutes of Health (NIH) since the mid-1980s (Roth, Pinn, Hartmuller, Bates, & Fanning, 2000). In 1994, the NIH issued guidelines on inclusion of women and members of ethnically and racially diverse groups as participants in clinical research projects (NIH, 1994). Despite these mandates, to date, women and minorities participate in health research at very low rates. This relative lack of participation may result, among other things, from: 1) lack of availability and accessibility to health services; 2) language barriers; 3) mistrust; 4) lack of healthcare insurance; 5) low income; 6) lack of transportation; and/or 7) lack of knowledge and information regarding health care. Research is needed to further understand systemic barriers and to evaluate the effectiveness of organizational and system-wide efforts to increase underrepresented groups in the ranks of rehabilitation researchers (see Chapter 6).

CONCLUSION

This chapter explored a number of areas that need to be addressed in research as it pertains to the intersection of race, culture, and disability, and its relationship to cultural competence. We conclude here with some observations for future directions of disability and rehabilitation research. We encourage research studies of the next decade to go beyond the study of race, culture, and disability and take into consideration other important variables that are often influenced by race and ethnicity; these include, but are not limited to, the following: acculturation, spirituality/religion, motivation, beliefs, attitudes, locus of control, coping, socioeconomic status, quality of education, language barriers, and mistrust. Moreover, rehabilitation variables must also be examined in order to provide an accurate picture of rehabilitation access, intervention, and outcomes for ethnically diverse populations. For example, what is the impact of the timing between the onset of a disability and the beginning of rehabilitation? Interdisciplinary research will be needed to address the unique concerns specific to diverse individuals with disabilities. Multicenter studies should inform clinical practice because they are more likely to be representative of the diverse population in the United States. Given the sensitivity of conducting research in the context of culture and disability, it will be critical for researchers to obtain social validation of the goals, procedures, and outcomes of their research as viewed from the potential end-users and beneficiaries (White, Nary, & Froehlich, 2001; White, Suchowierska, & Campbell, 2004). This process will help ensure that our investigations are both rigorous and relevant to the field of rehabilitation and disability research.

REFERENCES

Ardila, A. (2005). Cultural values underlying psychometric cognitive testing. *Neuropsychology Review, 15*, 185–195.

Braddock, D., & Parish, S. (2001). An institutional history of disability. In G. L. Albrecht, K. D. Seelman, & M. Bury (Eds.). *Handbook of disability studies* (pp. 11–68). Thousand Oaks, CA: Sage.

Kennephol, S., Shore, D., Nabors, N., & Hanks, R. (2004). African American acculturation and neuropsychological test performance following traumatic brain injury. *Journal of the International Neuropsychological Society, 10*, 566–577.

Keys, C., McMahon, S., Sánchez, B., London, L., & Abdul-Adil, J. (2004). Culturally anchored research: Quandaries, guidelines, and exemplars for community psychology. In L. A. Jason, C. B. Keys, Y. Suarez-Balcazar, R. R. Taylor, & M. I. Davis (Eds.). *Participatory community research: Theories and methods in action* (pp. 177–198). Washington, D.C.: American Psychological Association.

National Institutes of Health. (1994). NIH guidelines on the inclusion of women and minorities as subjects in clinical research. *NIH Guide for Grants and Contracts, 23*(11).

Rogler, L. H., Malgad, R. G., Costantino, G., & Blumenthal, R. (1987). What do culturally sensitive mental health services mean? The case of Hispanics. *The American Journal of Psychiatry, 42*, 565–570.

Roselli, M., & Ardila, A. (2003). The impact of culture and education on non-verbal neuropsychological measurements: a critical review. *Brain and Cognition, 52*, 326–333.

Roth, C., Pinn, V. W., Hartmuller, V. W., Bates A., & Fanning L. (2000). *Monitoring adherence to the NIH policy and the inclusion of women and minorities as subjects in clinical research. Comprehensive Report (Fiscal Year 1997 & 1998 Tracking Data)*. Washington, D.C.: National Institutes of Health.

Seekins, T., Ipsen, C., & Arnold, N. L. (2007). Using ecological momentary assessment to measure participation: A preliminary study. *Rehabilitation Psychology, 52*(3), 319–330.

Vesmarovich, S., Walker, T., Hauber, R. P., Temkin, A., & Burns, R. (1999). Use of telerehabilitation to manage pressure ulcers in persons with spinal cord injuries. *Advances in Wound Care, 12*(5), 264–269.

Wells, K. B., Golding, J. M., Hough, R. L., Burnam, M. A., & Karno, M. (1989). Acculturation and the probability of use of health services by Mexican Americans. *Health Services Research, 24*, 237–257.

White, G. W., Nary, D. E., & Froehlich, A. K. (2001). Consumers as collaborators in research and action. *Journal of Prevention and Intervention in the Community, 21*, 15–34.

White, G. W., Suchowierska, M., & Campbell, M. (2004). Strategies for a systematic implementation of participatory action research in community research. *Archives of Physical Medicine and Rehabilitation, 85*, S3–S12.

CHAPTER 18

Implications for Practice in Rehabilitation

Teresa Garate, M.Ed;
Jim Charlton, BA;
Rene Luna, BA;
Orville Townsend, MA

INTRODUCTION

Understanding the intersection of race, culture, and disability from a practitioner's perspective is both challenging and critical to any discussion of rehabilitation research and practice. If the ultimate goal of the field of rehabilitation is to support the development of individuals with disabilities to achieve the maximum level of independence and self-determination possible, then the community of practitioners working in this area can no longer ignore the intersection of race, culture, and disability as defining factors. The understanding of these factors must guide the rehabilitation plan designed to support success among direct service recipients; that is, success as defined by the individuals with disabilities themselves.

This chapter presents the perspectives of three different groups of practitioners: (a) vocational rehabilitation (VR) professionals, (b) independent living advocates, and (c) special educators. The process of rehabilitation requires support from multiple service providers and multiple approaches that represent different but related perspectives contributing equally to the area of rehabilitation practice. Research supports the importance of rehabilitation in promoting the successful attainment of personal, professional, and educational goals for individuals with disabilities (Capella, 2002; Fullerton & Tossi, 2001). Thus, from the practitioner's perspective we recognize the interdependence of employment, education, and independent living and the service delivery models designed to support individuals in their pursuit of positive outcomes.

While the discussion on client-centered planning and services is not new to the field of rehabilitation, there is limited research on evidence-based practice that takes into account the intersection of race, culture, and disability in the development of effective practice and service delivery models (Geenen, Powers, & Lopez-Vasquez,

2005). This void significantly impacts the development of individual plans for employment that are mindful of cultural and racial influences. However, it is critical to keep in mind that most values related to the rehabilitation system and the independent living movement have been influenced by White middle-class beliefs.

The challenges to rehabilitation professionals are considerable. This does not just have to do with paucity of jobs; the potentially drawn-out recession; or the lack of funding in the area. It has much to do, first, with how people with disabilities are situated in the world today—their marginalization and degradation. Secondly, it has to do with how paradoxical and confounding disability is as a social phenomenon. Thirdly, the challenge is further complicated when the impact of culture is added, when one examines how disability and culture intersect, and when we include race in the equation. As practitioners we acknowledge that attention to and discussion of culture, race, and racism is not only relevant and meaningful, but also difficult and necessary. Further, it should be emphasized that race and culture mean different things to different people. For the purpose of this chapter, by culture we mean "the realm of the symbolic—that amorphous web of values, belief, assumptions, and ideals that we internalize by being members of certain groups in a certain place at a certain time. It is within the realm we call culture that we get our bearings in life; it is there that we ingest the notions of what is good, bad, just, natural, desirable, and possible" (NACLA, 1994, p. 15).

The impression of culture on beliefs and mythology, traditions and rituals, institutions and doctrines, has individual and social implications. Culture exerts a profound influence on the way in which people think and about what they think (Balcazar et al., this volume). Race, of course, exerts just as much, if not more influence on the way people think and feel (Wilson & Senices, this volume). Our approach to race and its intersection with disability must be a cautious one. We view race as socially constructed (Fujiura & Drazen, this volume). Just as disability has little to do with impairment, race has little to do with skin pigmentation. Both have more to do with how people of color with disabilities live in society informed by cultural dimensions that are constantly changing. Many other critical factors—class, gender, geography, family values, and religion impact this intersection.

As noted throughout this book, evidence suggests that clients from diverse racial backgrounds have experienced discrimination and differential treatment in the rehabilitation system and in general in the community. This differential treatment has contributed in part, to the disparity in rehabilitation outcomes between White and non-White individuals with disabilities. The National Council on Disability (2008) and the United States Department of Labor, Office of Disability Employment Policy (ODEP, 2005) report that non-White individuals with disabilities have significantly lower rates of employment than White individuals with disabilities. Moreover, research evidence suggests that individuals from multiethnic backgrounds experience greater challenges in other areas of adult life, including education and independent living (Geenen, Powers, Vazquez, & Bersani, 2003; National Council on Disability, 2008).

We know from existing literature that several factors (i.e., ethnicity, race, income, education) influence the opportunities of people with disabilities to obtain positive life outcomes such as employment, independent living, and accessing post-secondary education (Geenen et al., 2003; McDonald, Keys, & Balcazar, 2007; Wagner, Newman, Cameto, Garza, & Levine, 2005). Consequently, for a practitioner seeking to have an impact on diverse people with disabilities, it becomes critical to be culturally competent. By having a basic understanding of the interaction between culture and disability experience, a practitioner will be better prepared to support his/her client's attainment of meaningful and positive outcomes. Practitioners who consider themselves to be culturally competent are aware of the important role that culture plays in rehabilitation outcomes and the need to provide culturally competent services while addressing the needs of diverse populations with disabilities and promoting their empowerment. In this chapter we discuss culture and disability and attempt to recognize race as a function of culture but not as the ultimate determining factor that has the greatest impact on a client's experience.

The gap that exists in the attainment of rehabilitation and independent living outcomes between individuals with disabilities who are White and those who are non-White has practitioners and researchers alike considering the impact of cultural competence (Geenen et al., 2003; Moore, Feist-Price, & Alston, 2002; Simon, 2001; Wagner et al., 2005; Wilson, Alston, Harley, & Mitchell, 2002). In some fields more than others, the issues of cultural competence (CC) are more readily considered. For example, in VR there is a considerable amount of research recognizing the importance of attending to culture and race and considering the types of support systems needed by diverse clients (Alston, 1994; Wilson, Edwards, Alston, Harley, & Doughty, 2001).

As practitioners grapple with CC, they must also understand that the goal is not to understand or embrace every single culture, but rather to understand the key role that culture plays in rehabilitation and to be ready to embrace an approach to rehabilitation that is open to changes and to diversity, and is flexible enough to meet the needs of diverse populations (Jacobson, 2004; Purnell & Paulanka, 2003). Practitioners who recognize that this is paramount in "sorting out" such complicated influences as race and culture are in a better place to assess the rehabilitation and independent living needs of multicultural populations with disabilities and promote their empowerment and participation in society.

The following sections highlight the reflections about race, culture, and disability from the perspective of three critical groups of practitioners: a rehabilitation counselor, independent living advocates, and a special educator. Forging a strong partnership among these three fields is necessary to begin to affect systemic change in the rehabilitation arena.

REFLECTIONS OF THREE CRITICAL PRACTITIONER GROUPS

Vocational Rehabilitation Counselor

Reflecting upon the experiences of people with disabilities and other traditionally marginalized groups, such as multicultural populations, evidence suggests that these groups of individuals have faced similar experiences of discrimination and differential treatment that have, in part, contributed to poor rehabilitation outcomes. As such, evidence suggests that individuals with disabilities and individuals from ethnic minority groups often encounter roadblocks when attempting to enter employment (Wilson, 2005; Chapter 5). Disadvantages reported in employment and access to services are often the result of negative attitudes, lack of knowledge about consumer's needs and about the accommodations necessary to obtain employment, as well as other systemic complex factors (Chapter 9). Although there are similarities among ethnic groups, there are also differences in the issues they experience when facing the VR system. For instance, Latinos are more likely to experience language barriers. Some individuals might experience both ethnic minority status and disability which forces VR counselors to recognize the influences of culture and disability together, and not separately.

Individuals with disabilities often experience multiple obstacles in striving to achieve the attainment of personal goals related to employment (see Chapter 8; Chapter 9). It is not uncommon for prospective employers to focus on what the individual limitations are and arrive at the conclusion that the individual will not be able to perform the essential functions of certain job positions. Similarly, an employer may also have preconceived notions regarding a specific ethnic group or cultural group. As rehabilitation counselors, we need to recognize the bias of potential employers and work to facilitate the entry into careers for consumers that foster a positive intersection of disability and culture.

Is the role of the rehabilitation counselors to educate the employer or to educate the consumer to better understand how individual goals and personal experiences are tainted by the presence of multiple factors? In order to address this question it is important that we shift our focus to the term *"ability"* instead of *"disability."* Based on history and past challenges that individuals with disabilities have experienced while attempting to enter the work force, it is evident that more effort needs to be directed at changing the attitudes of stakeholders. Education is a key ingredient and it is essential that employers understand the importance of focusing on the necessary accommodations and how to maximize the performance of people with disabilities given their abilities and not their deficits. Employers also need to understand what abilities mean to each individual employee with a disability, and its context within the life of the individual.

The rehabilitation counselor is more often than not at the center of the individual with a disability's life. In fact, if the rehabilitation counselor does not understand the intersection of disability and culture among their consumers, they will not be able to support their empowerment process, resulting in limited or failed rehabilitation outcomes. Unfortunately, the consumer–rehabilitation counselor interaction often results in the imposition of the professional's own cultural values and biases (Alston & Hampton, 2000; Wilson et al., 2002).

How do we move to a healthier recognition of the intersection between race, culture, and disability? One way is to have a greater understanding of the commonalities among marginalized groups, specifically in their attempts to enter the workforce. Practitioners in rehabilitation should understand that their clients are complex individuals and must take into account all the factors in the rehabilitation process in order to provide counseling that is empowering and meets the specific needs of each client.

Additionally, the new generation of rehabilitation counselors should examine how their professional preparation influences their ability to meet the needs of an increasingly diverse consumer population within a global context. There are general issues to consider: First, we must focus on how well we equip new professionals with the tools that are needed to have an effective foundation to launch from. Next, we must focus on what needs to be learned in order to provide ongoing services to individuals with disabilities from various cultures (as defined by ethnicity, class, gender, geography, etc.). We have to accept the fact that this means changing systems, policies, and models of practice that have dominated the rehabilitation field for many years but are no longer effective. Professional preparation programs need to emphasize the development of active listening and observational skills and the building of cultural competency (Chapter 11).

Unfortunately, stereotypes are still prevalent in the rehabilitation system. As such, counselors often see all Latinos as a large group that share similar cultural and ethnic characteristics. Latinos are marked by important differences depending on the country of origin, level of education, social class, and often skin color. Several authors (see Chapter 5) have concluded that White Latinos have privileges similar to those enjoyed by White Americans in the United States based on skin color. Furthermore, evidence clearly suggests that when several demographic variables are controlled, one's skin color is a salient feature for being discriminated against in the United States—thus the complexity of racism and its influence on all aspects of life.

Rehabilitation counselors cannot assume all individuals from the same ethnic group are dealing with the same life experiences. Counselors need to be well-trained and culturally competent to address the need of diverse consumers.

Independent Living Advocates

The Independent Living (IL) philosophy emerged as a rejection of the prevailing medical model of disability which focuses on cure and rehabilitation of the individual. IL proponents sought to organize people with disabilities by emphasizing key principles such as "consumer" control, personal choice, participation, peer support, self-help, and civil rights. Furthermore, disability rights activists sought to unite people with diverse disabilities in recognition of the common experiences of societal discrimination and oppression. In essence, an independent living movement emerged which has focused on the process of empowering people with disabilities and fostering self-determination. Centers for independent living (CILs) in the United States have led much of the work in creating greater accessibility within society for people with disabilities (White, Nary, & Froehlich, 2001).

IL advocates attempt to equip individuals with disabilities to be self-advocates in achieving IL goals such as employment, independent housing, and other life goals which rehabilitation professionals ought to see as useful partners in their work. While many rehabilitation counselors do not particularly focus on consumer empowerment or on teaching their consumers how to advocate for themselves, IL advocates can be ideal partners in this process. Unfortunately, the link between CILs and the rehabilitation arena is limited and inconsistent across the United States (National Council on Independent Living [NCIL], 2008) and might be a missed opportunity to promote greater understanding of cultural competent issues among consumers and service providers alike. Although from a philosophical perspective the IL movement has not been in favor of the rehabilitation movement, which is mostly guided by the medical model, representatives from both fields have begun working together to make a change (NCIL). The work to link IL programs and the rehabilitation services has just recently begun having the potential to provide greater support to the increasingly diverse consumer base.

An observable shortcoming of CILs and the IL movement in general is the limited participation of individuals from culturally diverse backgrounds. That is, CILs and advocates have had to grapple with many of the challenges that rehabilitation services and professionals have confronted regarding race and culture. As stated throughout this volume some of those challenges are related to the lack of outreach to people with disabilities from multicultural backgrounds. This shortfall has actually informed, to some degree, the relevance and need for CC among IL advocates.

In order to address the intersect of race, culture, and disability, we need to recognize that IL advocates are critical agents of change that can promote the empowerment process of individuals with disabilities regardless of their race and culture. However, in order to do that, they need CC training. We need to address the fact that very little training is provided to IL advocates on cultural competency and on how to best advocate for the needs of multicultural populations. Although many practitioners working in this field are themselves individuals with disabilities, it does not mean that they are competent to address the needs of multicultural populations. The individual practitioner with a disability may be able to relate to the individual consumer at a unique, disability level but may need support in understanding the cultural influences that have to be taken into account in the process of promoting independence among racial and ethnically diverse populations.

Cultural differences exist among ethnic groups in their conceptions and views regarding employment, participation, and community integration. CILs need to engage in a process of understanding what independence means to each individual given their own personal experience and cultural values. CILs must formulate recruitment of staff based on a perspective of building organizational and individual cultural competency. CILs must network and outreach based on this perspective as well and recognize that the concept of independence is also "socially constructed." Independence is situated in the context of culture and varying from one historical point to another, from one country to another. For example, a Latino individual with a disability may understand independence as rooted in a family arrangement while another person with a disability may understand such an arrangement as an interdependent or even dependent arrangement. Understanding this will facilitate the determination of appropriate supports and services for the greater number of consumers.

As IL advocates, we must recognize the need for additional research in the area of empowerment for people with disabilities from diverse racial and cultural backgrounds. Research on the perspectives of diverse individuals with disabilities and advocates can inform future practice.

Often resources within the IL community are used to provide direct services to a small group of consumers. Aligning resources that can be used to inform the community at large, including stakeholders may have a greater impact and result in the sustainability of change, thereby attracting more diverse groups into the IL movement. Finally, understanding how the bridge can be forged between IL programs and the rehabilitation system may help improve outcomes for people of color with disabilities. Increasing the integration and participation of people with disabilities into the fabric of society may mean rethinking how we provide services and how we can move towards integration. We must not necessarily impose the values of the IL movement on every client (i.e., empowerment, advocacy, and independence), but rather we must engage in the process of understanding what independence means to each individual given their own personal experiences and cultural values.

Special Educator

Teachers, whether in special education or general education, have a unique opportunity to influence the lives of individuals with disabilities, especially those born with a disability or those who have acquired it at an early age. However, rarely is the education community engaged in a discussion of rehabilitation research and practice. Some might argue that this is because of the pressure to educate and meet the demands of accountability within schools since the passage of the Individuals with Disabilities Education Act (IDEA; U.S. Department of Education, 1997; 2004) and No Child Left Behind (NCLB; U.S. Department of Education, 2001). This, however, is not necessarily the case, as rehabilitation issues have been in existence long before these two mandates were in effect. More accurately, we propose that it is because the fields of education, independent living, and rehabilitation rarely intersect or even recognize the importance of each other's contributions to creating holistic approaches to meet the needs of individuals with a disability.

Special educators focus on the individual students with a disability and on meeting the demands of their individualized education plan (IEP). One limitation of this focus is that the IEP does not require school systems to address employment, independent living, education, or community integration until the student is sixteen years old. A second limitation is that "cultural" considerations are only examined as a general question in the IEP process once and are rarely incorporated throughout the entire planning effort. A third limitation is that the IEP is rarely aligned with the student's individual plan for employment (IPE) or considered in such a development. The transition planning process from middle school to high school for students with an IEP is often completed by individuals with little to no understanding of rehabilitation issues, support services, or of how culture should be considered in the development of these plans (Valenzula & Martin, 2005).

In fact, when we examine education in general in the United States, we see that there are achievement gaps between White students and students from multicultural backgrounds, particularly African Americans and Latinos (U.S. Department of Education, 2001). For students with disabilities, the discrepancies in student progress are even more disturbing (Wagner et al., 2005). For each of the ethnic subgroups, the gap between those individuals with and those without disabilities is actually growing larger. Unfortunately, the response from government officials has been to continue to create more accountability measures without appropriate dialogue about the need to include CC into the educational system. Although educators recognize the differences in outcomes achieved by various cultural groups, they do not necessarily address culturally competent educational practices as a way to try to close the gaps.

Professionals in other fields such as health care, however, are addressing these disparities, in part, with more culturally competent outreach, services, and dissemination efforts (Beach et al., 2005; Taylor & Lurie, 2004).

Hiring African American teachers to teach in highly African American schools is not necessarily the answer to achieving CC; a practice that is often done in public school systems. If that practice was effective, then we should focus efforts on training individuals with disabilities to become special education teachers so they can stand in front of youth with disabilities as their teachers. This does not mean that it is not important for students to be surrounded by individuals they can relate to. However, relating to someone because of personal experience is only the first step in understanding the importance of cultural competency and recognizing that students are complex individuals marked by contextual and cultural factors.

One important step to begin to address cultural competency in the educational system is to examine teachers preparation programs. To be able to address the specific needs of their multicultural population, teachers need training, preparation, and ongoing support. Similarly, having a better understanding of how special education teachers understand the process of disability identity among their students and the importance of this disability identity within the context of rehabilitation may improve the type of supports that are provided to youth with disabilities.

Any discussion of rehabilitation must include a basic understanding of the role of transition planning for youth with disabilities. While mandates for transition have been in place for over a decade (Lehman, Clark, Bullis, Rinkin, & Castellanos, 2004), it was not until recently that the federal government started requiring state education agencies to report on these services and to link them to student outcomes after graduation to be used for school accountability. This is the right step towards improving overall services to young people with disabilities and eventually adults with disabilities. However, little to no guidance is given to school systems to recognize the intersection of disability and culture in the planning and service delivery and provision of educational supports. As such, we run the risk of once again missing an opportunity to achieve systemic change that not only recognizes cultural differences but also uses them to individualize supports.

Similar to the field of IL, students with disabilities also often identify themselves differently, as individuals with a disability, depending on the type of disability they have. For example, students with physical disabilities may identify with other students with physical disabilities more easily than they do with students with learning disabilities. While this is not surprising, teachers are not currently equipped to facilitate the development of self-identify of their students who may or may not choose to identify themselves as having a disability. This has grave implications for how a young adult will fair within the rehabilitation arena, given that if they are to access supports for attaining life goals, they must first identify themselves as individuals with a disability, which is surely influenced by their experiences of acceptance and respect or stigma and marginalization within their communities. To facilitate the transition of students with disabilities into the rehabilitation system and for IL programming, teachers need to be able to assist students in developing disability identity, identify their needs and strengths, and prepare them for integration and participation in the community.

Beyond educators involved in the K–12 education system, there are also educators within higher education. These individuals, often overlooked in this dialogue, can play a critical role, especially in facilitating the transition for individuals with invisible disabilities who recognize the importance of identifying with their disability in order to seek the necessary resources and support systems needed to become successful adult learners (Gregg, 2007). Adult educators, with appropriate information and training, may be able to guide or mentor adults with disabilities to understand themselves, their strengths and challenges, and access services and supports from practitioners and related service providers.

Education in general has strong links to cultural factors. As we discuss various groups, whether they are identified by gender, race, class, or ethnicity, the concept of education is influenced by all. How is it then that little has been done to examine the role of education in promoting more effective rehabilitation and IL practices? Despite the fact that at the federal level the Office of Special Education Programs–(OSEP; which oversees national policy in special education) and the Office of Rehabilitation Services Administration—(RSA; which oversees the VR services in the country), sit within the same organizational structure, there has been little progress to achieve systemic change that could trickle down to the day-to-day functioning of special education teachers. Without this clear link, we will continue to miss the opportunity to influence the greatest number of individuals with disabilities that are accessing the VR system.

CONCLUSION AND RECOMMENDATIONS

We have discussed the challenges and juxtapositions of three service delivery systems (VR, IL, and special education) that need to be considered in the discussion of race, culture, and disability. All three service delivery systems are important to consider when discussing rehabilitation options for culturally diverse individuals. This has given us an opportunity to discuss the challenges of each field. We recognize that there has been work done in this area, as reflected within the chapters included in this book; however, further research needs to be conducted. Future work should focus on improving the relationship and collaboration between the three practitioner-based fields to emphasize the critical need of identifying consumers as culturally complex individuals.

In addition, we recommend that practitioners, regardless of their area of expertise, begin to incorporate concrete practices that address the cultural needs of their consumers. Special education must begin to require teacher preparation and professional development that helps teachers and administrators understand the roles of race and culture in providing education and support. Additionally, educators should also be addressing transition-related supports that are in line with the individual's experience and beliefs and can facilitate entrance into the VR system and the CILs.

IL advocates must continue to work on the policy level to promote legislation, policy, and practice related to disability to address the needs of multicultural populations with all types of disabilities. In other words, the disability rights movement must move from a predominantly White and physical disability perspective to one that addresses the needs of all people with disabilities, particularly multicultural populations. A current example of federal policy that is recognizing the importance of culture and race is the NCLB, which holds schools accountable for specific ethnic subgroups. However, this is only a starting point and recommendations for improvements need to be in place in order to ensure that all people with disabilities have the potential to obtain positive outcomes.

Over the last two decades, those in the VR field have started to understand the importance of viewing consumers as complex cultural individuals. As a result, we now have state VR systems trying to provide professional development for their counselors in this area. The fields of special education and IL have not done enough to provide this type of support to its workforce. We recommend that the state systems examine the complex diversity of their client groups and mandate that existing teachers, IL advocates, and counselors become prepared in understanding CC. The systems should also commit to hiring professionals trained in the area of CC and/or mandate ongoing CC trainings.

Though most of the recommendations focus on the practitioners, it is also important that individuals with disabilities themselves become increasingly aware of their strengths, needs, and cultural perspectives thereby becoming empowered consumers able to advocate for themselves.

REFERENCES

Alston, R. J. (1994). Family functioning as a correlate of disability adjustment for African Americans. *Rehabilitation Counseling Bulletin, 37*(4), 277–289.

Alston, R. J., & Hampton, J. L. (2000). Science and engineering as viable career choices for students with disabilities: A survey of parents and teachers. *Rehabilitation Counseling Bulletin, 43*(3), 158–164.

Beach, M. C., Price, E. G., Gary, T. L., Robinson, K. A., Gozu, A., Palacio, A., et al. (2005). Cultural competence: A systematic review of health care provider educational interventions. *Medical Care, 43*(4), 356–373.

Capella, M. E. (2002). Inequities in the VR system: Do they still exist? *Rehabilitation Counseling Bulletin, 45*, 143–153.

Fullerton, H. N., & Tossi, M. (2001). Labor force projections to 2010: Steady growth and changing composition. *Monthly Labor Review Online, 124.* Retrieved May 13, 2007, from *www.bls.gov/opub/mlr/2001/11/art2exchhtm*

Geenen, S. J., Powers, L. E., & Lopez-Vasquez, A. (2005). Barriers against and strategies for promoting the involvement of culturally diverse parents in school based transition planning. *Journal for Vocational Special Needs Education, 27*(3), 4–14.

Geenen, S., Powers, L., Vasquez, A. L., & Bersani, H. (2003). Understanding and promoting the transition of minority adolescents. *Career Development for Exceptional Individuals, 26*(1), 27–46.

Gregg, N. (2007). Underserved and unprepared: postsecondary learning disabilities. *Learning Disabilities Research & Practice, 22*(4), 219–228.

Jacobson, E. (2004). An introduction to Haitian culture for rehabilitation service providers. In J. H. Stone (Ed.), *Culture and disability: Providing culturally competent services* (pp. 139–159). New York: Sage.

Lehman, C. M., Clark, H. B., Bullis, M., Rinkin, J., & Castellanos, L. A. (2004). Transition from school to adult life: Empowering youth through community ownership and accountability. *Journal of Child and Family Studies 11*(1), 127–141.

McDonald, K. E., Keys, C. B., & Balcazar, F. E. (2007). Disability, race/ethnicity and gender: Themes of cultural oppression, acts of individual resistance. *American Journal of Community Psychology, 39*(1), 145–161.

Moore, C. L., Feist-Price, S., & Alston, R. J. (2002). VR services for persons with severe/profound mental retardation: Does race matter? *Rehabilitation Counseling Bulletin, 45*(3), 162–167.

National Council on Disability. (2008, April). *Keeping track: National disability status in programs performing indicators.* Retrieved April 26, 2008, from *http://www.ncd.gov/newsroom/publications/2008/indicators_report.html*

North American Congress on Latin America. (1994, September/October). The political uses of culture. *North American Congress on Latin America, 28(2)*, 15.

National Council on Independent Living. (2008). *Rehabilitation Act and independent living funding.* Retrieved November 3, 2008, from *www.ncil.org/news.html*

Purnell, L. D., & Paulanka, B. J. (2003). *Transcultural healthcare: A culturally competent approach.* Philadelphia: F.A. Davis.

Simon, M. (2001). Beyond broken promises: Reflections on eliminating barriers to the success of minority youth with disabilities. *Journal of the Association for Persons with Severe Handicaps, 26*(3), 200–203.

Taylor, S. L., & Lurie, N. (2004). The role of culturally competent communication in reducing ethnic and racial healthcare disparities. *The American Journal of Managed Care, 10*, SP1–SP4.

U.S. Department of Education. (1997). *IDEA 1997.* Retrieved November 4, 2008 from *http://www.ed.gov/offices/OSERS/Policy/IDEA/index.html*

U.S. Department of Education. (2001). *No Child Left Behind Act.* Retrieved November 4, 2008, from *http://www.ed.gov/policy/elsec/guid/states/index.html#nclb*

U.S. Department of Education. (2004). *IDEA 2004.* Retrieved November 4, 2008, from *http://idea.ed.gov/*

U.S. Department of Labor, Office of Disability Employment Policy. (2005). *Disability employment rate.* Retrieved November 3, 2008, from *http://www.dol.gov/odep/categories/research/rate.html*

Valenzula, R. L., & Martin, J. E. (2005). Self-directed IEP. *Career Development for Exceptional Individuals, 28*(1), 4–14.

Wagner, M., Newman, L., Cameto, R., Garza, N., & Levine, P. (2005). *After high school: A first look at the postschool experiences of youth with disabilities* Report from the National Longitudinal Transition Study-2 (NLTS2). Menlo Park, CA: SRI International.

White, G. W., Nary, D. E., & Froehlich, A. K. (2001). Consumers as collaborators in research and action. *People with Disabilities: Empowerment and Community Action.* In C. B. Keys, & P. W. Downik (Eds.). *People with disabilities: Empowerment and community action* (pp. 15–34). Binghamton, NY: Haworth Press.

Wilson, K. B. (2005). Vocational rehabilitation closure statutes in the U.S.: Generalizing to the Hispanic ethnicity. *Journal of Applied Rehabilitation Counseling, 36*(2), 4–11.

Wilson, K. B., Alston, R. J., Harley, D. A., & Mitchell, N. A. (2002). Predicting VR acceptance based on race, gender, education, work status at application, and primary source of support at application. *Rehabilitation Counseling Bulletin, 45*(3), 132–142.

Wilson, K. B., Edwards, D. W, Jr., Alston, R. J., Harley, D. A., & Doughty, J. D. (2001). Vocational rehabilitation and the dilemma of race in rural communities: Sociopolitical realities and myths from the past. *Journal of Rural Community Psychology, 2,* 55–81.

CHAPTER 19

Implications for Training and Educating Future Generations of Rehabilitation Practitioners and Researchers

Juleen Rodakowski, MS, OTR/L;
Erin Kelly, PhD;
Yanling Li Gould, MS, MA

INTRODUCTION

As graduate students and recent graduates moving into clinical practice and research positions, we come to this commentary with a foundation of knowledge in the theoretical and practical discourses surrounding race, culture, and disability and a continued interest in moving our thinking forward. In this commentary we seek to react to the first three sections of this book from our perspectives as new professionals. We will discuss how the information presented in this volume is likely to impact our future work, as well as explore implications for both future research and training future scholars. As students and researchers from university- and community-based settings, we offer a diverse voice, representing a variety of ethnicities, cultures, disability statuses, ages, socioeconomic statuses, and levels of graduate training. Coming from such diverse backgrounds resulted in stimulating conversations throughout the writing of this chapter.

At present, there is a dearth of literature addressing the intersection of race, culture, and disability; however, the work presented in this volume summarizes some of what has been done and presents new frameworks/models to advance disability and rehabilitation training and practice. From this work, we have attempted to summarize potential areas that could improve the understanding of race, culture, and disability. We have grouped our ideas into recommendations that we wish to highlight as important in terms of future attempts to elucidate the intersection of race, culture, and disability. These include:

- Developing a historical and interdisciplinary perspective related to the science of race, culture, and disability

- Recognizing the continuum of research methods in exploring race, culture, and disability
- Exploring the nature of disparities in outcomes for multicultural populations with disabilities
- Examining larger contextual factors, such as socioeconomic status, and their relevant impact on individuals
- Encouraging critical comparisons of conceptual models
- Bridging the gap between science and practice through both good science and effective collaborations
- Educating people about race, culture, and disability from a multifaceted approach

NATURE OF SCIENTIFIC RESEARCH AT THE NEXUS OF RACE, CULTURE, AND DISABILITY

Developing a Historical and Interdisciplinary Perspective Related to the Science of Race, Culture, and Disability

As a critical tool for heading into the future, it is important for researchers and practitioners to have some perspective of the breadth of the fields related to the study of race, culture, and disability and, specifically, of the research being conducted in these fields. Incorporating a historical perspective can broaden this understanding. Fujiura and Drazen (Chapter 2) note the difficulty of addressing challenges related to living at the intersection of race, culture, and disability. As they noted, perspective can be gained by increasing awareness of past research findings as well as the epistemological basis of research questions and the methodologies that studies incorporate. In Chapter 3, Gill and Cross offer a historical perspective by discussing the origins of the racial-cultural identity and disability identity movements, and discuss how Black identity theory has impacted disability identity theory. Recognition of the continued relevance of key issues and explicit intersections of theoretical frameworks can drive the field forward.

Included in developing a perspective that grasps the intersection between race, culture, and disability is a need for increasing the conduct of and appreciation for interdisciplinary work. Researchers, based on their skill sets, tend to cite literature from their fields of study without examining how other bodies of work can contribute to current thinking and methodological formulation. To improve the impact of the research conducted, researchers could partner with others in various fields outside of their own, to gain a potentially different perspective. Alternatively, researchers could consider alternative approaches to their work by reviewing the epistemological bases of research identified in Chapter 2. With a broadened point of view, we can critically examine existing research from multiple sides, offering different perspectives and generating new knowledge or discussion.

Recognizing the Continuum of Research Methods in Exploring Race, Culture, and Disability

Related to developing a perspective on the intersection of race, culture, and disability is the need to encourage work that spans the research methodology continuum, from quantitative to qualitative methodology. Quantitative and qualitative research methodologies each have their specific place in science, providing valuable perspectives on how race, culture, and disability contextually interact, although a truly comprehensive approach includes mixed methodology (Patton, 2002). As explained in Chapter 2, a variety of approaches are necessary for the area of research surrounding race, culture, and disability to advance, as each approach has its own merits. Quantitative research can provide a broad stroke of understanding in terms of key relationships between variables and qualitative research can allow for a rich exploration of the context and help explain how and why these relationships may exist (Patton). Because both approaches have strengths and limitations that offset each other, incorporating a mixed methods approach may allow us to be more sensitive to capturing people's experiences relating to disability, race, and culture, producing better results in terms of quality and scope. However, Chapter 3 pointed out the need for future studies to assess whether combining quantitative and qualitative research actually best contributes to learning more about race, culture, and disability.

In addition, when addressing race, culture, and disability in research, lessons from previous research should be taken into consideration. For example, Kitchin (2000) suggested that disability research should involve people with disabilities beyond the subject source and should be a collaborative effort between people with and people without disabilities, including those in academics and those in the community, through consultation and partnerships. The model of inclusivity (Kitchin), the emancipatory model (Barnes, 1992), and the participation action research model (Zarb, 1992) have been found to be effective models for collaboration for researchers and research participants; all three models involve a shift of power in the research in favor of active involvement of research participants. These models are committed to an equality-based, democratic, genuine partnership between people with disabilities and academic researchers with and without disabilities.

In conjunction with using models that are effective for collaboration, it is important to acknowledge that sample selection strategies can greatly impact research outcomes. Traditionally, people with disabilities have largely been excluded from disability discourse and thus excluded from academic and institutional research. As a result, the views of people with disabilities are often misrepresented and misinterpreted. Some individuals with disabilities are worried that research currently being undertaken is conducted in such a manner that is not representative of their views, their experiences, or their knowledge. In order to aid in the evaluation of research quality and interpretation of research findings, all forms of research should carefully consider and describe their study samples. Qualitative approaches may attend to this issue by allowing for comprehensive descriptions of the current environment and relationships between research participants and investigators, although both qualitative and quantitative explorations have a responsibility to present a thorough understanding of how culture affects disability experiences. Researchers need to be cognizant of their studies representing experiences of people with disabilities from all angles, including, but not limited to, the following: the physical environment, the social environment, the cultural and contextual environments, the socioeconomic context, and the ethnic backgrounds and disability cultures of the participants. Although we understand that not every study can represent every angle, it is important to recognize and be clear about the angle your study is representing.

Exploring the Nature of Disparities in Outcomes for Multicultural Populations with Disabilities

A growing body of research describes the nature of disparities in outcomes for multicultural populations (Olney & Kennedy, 2002; Wilson, 2002; Wilson, Harley, & Alston, 2001). Despite the fact that understanding of how disability, race, and culture impact disparities is still emerging, the authors throughout this volume demonstrated the breadth of disparities. Examples include:

- Chapter 5 describes how colorism affects multicultural populations. In their research, they have begun to prioritize race or color as a primary variable affecting outcomes among ethnic minorities in vocational rehabilitation. Their chapter demonstrates that Black Latinos with disabilities have similar negative outcomes and experiences to African Americans with disabilities in accessing Vocational Rehabilitation (VR) services.
- Chapter 6 reviews literature demonstrating the higher incidence of disability and chronic disease faced by African Americans, compounded by their lack of access to quality medical care.
- Chapter 8 presents the lack of infrastructure for Native Americans with disabilities living on reservations and in Alaska Native villages.
- Chapter 9 discusses the employment challenges faced by minority women with disabilities, whose multiple minority statuses only increase their chances of

being unemployed. In Chapter 10, it was noted that Asian Pacific Americans (APA) are severely underserved in the VR system.

- Chapter 7 recognized that racial and ethnic minorities have less access to psychiatric services and that the quality and efficacy of their care are inferior to that received by White people. Such disparities are caused to a larger extent by different cultural views of mental illness, different ways of seeking help, and different attitudes towards psychotropic medication.

Complicating such disparities are challenges created by some common psychological assessments used to determine potential clients' eligibility for receiving VR services. Chapter 4 reported that the standardization samples of the Wechsler Adult Intelligence Test, Minnesota Multiphasic Personality Inventory, Rorschach Inkblot Test, and Beck Depression Inventory tended to lack adequate racial/ethnic minority representation, especially Asian Americans and Native Americans. Practitioners must be cautious in interpreting these test results and take into consideration such sociocultural variables as linguistic differences, the social situation of the test and potential distrust of environment, and a contextual match between cognitive performance and sociocultural experiences.

The evidence presented here and throughout this volume begins to provide an understanding of the disparities facing multicultural populations with disabilities, and begins to form a foundation for this body of research. However, more research is needed to understand how race, culture, and disability status interact to affect outcomes related to vocational rehabilitation, medical rehabilitation, and independent living. A growing body of well-conducted research will provide a clearer path for effectively managing the factors that impact positive outcomes in multicultural populations with disabilities.

Examining Larger Contextual Factors, Such as Socioeconomic Status, and their Relevant Impact on Individuals

How race, culture, and disability intersect for an individual can become complicated, and at different times different aspects of race, culture, and disability might take precedence in terms of an individual's identity. While the research in this volume is based on theoretical and empirical work in its attention to the intersection of race, culture, and disability, future research should strive to better understand the various context(s) surrounding individual participants and groups of individuals. Some of these various contextual factors that should be considered are the socioeconomic status of the individuals, the educational opportunities of the individuals, their access to health care, the quality of the health care, family dynamics, ethnic backgrounds, level of acculturation and immigration status in the case of individuals with disabilities coming from countries outside the United States, and historical period of time. An important aspect of conducting research within race, culture, and disability, is developing the cultural competence needed to fully appreciate the many ecological contexts from which people originate and in which they live (see Chapter 14). Following from this, larger contextual factors and their potential for facilitating and inhibiting success need to be better understood, particularly in terms of developing points of intervention for fostering independent living and positive rehabilitation outcomes in individuals with disabilities. Socioeconomic status (SES) is one of those factors that impacts ethnic minorities with disabilities. Ethnic minorities and individuals with disabilities may face particular SES challenges; understanding these challenges, especially the challenges associated with poverty, and associated experiences of oppression is key to both creating accurate representations of participants' life conditions as well as making positive change. As suggested in Chapter 6, beginning to track disparities as part of a model systems database that would gather longitudinal data may lead to a better understanding of these larger contextual factors.

Models to Improve Rehabilitation Services for Multicultural Populations with Disabilities

Conceptual models, generally speaking, expand upon a theoretical construct, allowing a framework for logic. Models, related to the intersection of race, culture, and disability, are constructed to enable reasoning, driving practice, research, and education.

As young scholars and practitioners, we appreciate a number of elements of the conceptual models that have been laid out in this volume. First, as we develop an understanding of current philosophies of research and practice, we appreciate when models are relevant to their intended recipients. For example, Chapter 15 provides a model for building the capacity of organizations to conduct evaluations of programs for people with disabilities. Chapter 12 laid out a model for rehabilitation counselors that is straightforward and can be easily integrated into counselors' individual philosophies. Chapter 13 and Chapter 16 also suggest the need for empirically evaluating various models for making ethical decisions. Research in this area will facilitate evidence-based practice in ethics as it relates to multicultural populations.

We also appreciate critical comparisons that are made between frameworks and in particular work that points out essential components missing from one model to the next, as noted in Chapter 14. Explicitly stating similarities and differences between cultural competence models allows for a greater understanding of what a new model has to offer. Synthesizing the existing models, from our perspective, includes noting the context from where the models were developed, if and how the models were empiri-cally tested, populations that the models were tested with, and components that the models include. This translates to an appreciation for how models are used in practice and in future research endeavors. In addition, empirically testing models, such as por-trayed in Chapter 14, is beneficial from the standpoint of being user-friendly and pro-viding evidence that it was rated as thorough by independent reviewers.

Overall, as a future direction, we would like to encourage more collaborations and more interdisciplinary work in order to allow best practices to emerge. We would also like to promote more critical examination of each other's research work while continuing to demonstrate professional respect. We believe and think that critically examining others' work is what will lead to higher-quality research. With such a syn-thesis and critical appraisal, similar to what the compilation of this volume is allow-ing, the field can move forward most effectively.

Bridging the Gap between Science and Practice

A number of implications for future research, practice, and training can be taken from this text. Overall, the process of conducting research should be culturally appropriate, meaning future research should examine rehabilitation and indepen-dent living outcomes and use culturally-relevant tools. Utilizing culturally sensitive and appropriate measurement tools will allow for valid findings that can be more readily applicable to practice. Further, evaluating common outcomes across studies can facilitate comparisons of research conducted with a variety of groups, increasing overall generalization of findings. As a whole, culturally sensitive outcome measures will lead to stronger findings from research.

This volume has several implications for improving practice. An aspect of practice that could be directly impacted is the cultural competence (CC) of practitioners; in other words improve the quality of care and services delivered to people with dis-abilities who are individuals and families from various cultural backgrounds. One of the most commonly accepted definitions for CC in the healthcare field was devel-oped by Campinha-Bacote (1999), in the nursing profession. Within this definition, CC is demonstrated when the practitioner, specifically a nurse, understands and appreciates differences in health beliefs and behaviors that may be culturally deter-mined, recognizes and respects variations that occur within cultural groups, and is able to adjust his/her practice to provide effective interventions for people from var-ious cultures. Chapter 12 suggests a three-factor model for rehabilitation that involves counselors assessing a consumer's developmental stage, cultural identification, and optimal adjustment. This model offers suggestions for being more culturally appro-priate while still allowing for counselors to incorporate their individual style.

Throughout the development of models like this, research can concretely facilitate effective practice by evaluating specific models. Particular approaches to or adaptations of service delivery that are demonstrated as effective can then be offered as best practices (see Chapter 6 for a good example). In this way, evidence-based practice can truly be useful for improving outcomes for people with disabilities from a variety of cultural backgrounds.

Educating People about Race, Culture, and Disability from a Multifaceted Approach

Specifically in education, there is a need to develop culturally competent curricula for university programs; such curricula can serve as exemplars for various programs to follow. Chapter 11 provides potential educational approaches for CC training in the fields of physical therapy, occupational therapy, speech therapy, and rehabilitation counseling. Expanding our thinking in order to better understand the intersection of race, culture, and disability has specific implications for graduate training. As the science and practice related to race, culture, and disability improves, it is important that we ensure that our graduate educational programs explicitly attend to issues of race, culture, and disability, share the scientific evidence that is amassing in this area, and also train students to engage in culturally competent research and practice. We suggest that the commitment to training students to become culturally competent be integrated throughout graduate education. Best practices would include requiring students to participate in a course that focuses on racism/cultural competence/self-awareness, as suggested in Chapter 14, and would require entire curricula to incorporate race, culture, and disability throughout. A graduate-level class focused on understanding the impact of culture could allow for much needed self-reflection of students' own culture, increased knowledge of various cultures, and allow for the development of culturally competent skills. Consistent with best practices, Chapter 11, for example, focus on training and CC throughout the curricula of several disciplines to fully realize a commitment to developing culturally competent scholars and practitioners. Complementarily, Chapter 12 shows how culture can be woven into a counseling course and Chapter 13 shows how culture can be woven into a training course on ethics to help improve rehabilitation professionals' ability to solve ethical dilemmas.

In terms of implications for training professionals in the classroom and beyond, it is first important to understand that scholars and practitioners cannot be called upon to have knowledge of all of the cultures they will encounter; this is an impossible task. However, what is necessary is teaching individuals the appropriate questions to ask and providing them with skills to be continually reflective about their own and others' cultures and how these issues are impacted by context. Equally important is simply raising awareness of the need for an appreciation of cultural diversity. These skills need to be presented throughout and beyond one's education; they are truly a lifelong lesson. In this way, graduate training programs can provide a concrete start. One strategy that may be used includes providing vignettes, such as those seen in Chapter 11 and Chapter 13, which allow students and professionals to reflect on their awareness, knowledge, and skills. These vignettes can provide a greater understanding of the context and the meaning of being culturally competent, and can help the integration of CC throughout all curricula. Training with real-case vignettes helps scholars and practitioners translate theoretical knowledge into practical courses of action when working with clients of different cultural backgrounds.

To assist in this multifaceted approach to training, both educational and practice-oriented settings are encouraged to strive to become more diverse in race, culture, and disability by recruiting individuals from different ethnicities and cultural backgrounds. Creating opportunities for exposure and engagement with diverse groups, such as reaching out to disability and multicultural communities and inviting people from different ethnic groups to give lectures or presentations about their own culture and customs, can be part of this multifaceted approach.

How, why, and when individuals acquire skills for being culturally competent will vary according to each person's research or practice; however, we believe that the key to honing competencies regarding race, culture, and disability lies in developing skills to understand the characteristics of and distinctions between different settings that require different strategies. One possible strategy for assuring that CC is integrated throughout curricula is to provide items related to CC on evaluation forms for instructors. On the other hand, for individuals who have completed their studies, they must be motivated to become culturally competent. Professional practice fields, such as occupational therapy, vocational rehabilitation, and psychology, could have requirements for ongoing Continuing Education Units (CEU) related to race, culture, and disability. In addition, research fields could have publication requirements with similar stipulations; conducting and publishing specific race, culture, and disability evidence-based outcomes research is one important incentive of proving the effectiveness of incorporating CC in professional practices.

Finally, in addition to formal instruction, informal education about CC should also be facilitated by educational and professional organizations. Within educational settings and places of employment, allowing safe space for the full expression of ideas, thoughts, and attitudes will allow people to develop skills necessary to becoming culturally competent scholars or practitioners. There is no beginning or ending points to CC; people need to be taught appropriate skills and should obtain knowledge about cultures throughout their entire lifespan. Not only should this knowledge be about other individuals and cultures; but it should also be about their own culture. Being aware of your own culture is a beginning step to becoming more culturally competent. It is equally important for a White, Protestant male and a Latina female with a disability to be able to describe and reflect on their cultures.

CONCLUSION

Using scholarly work to challenge our ideas of cultural competence is important for both researchers and practitioners. Empowering individuals in need is a skill that the growing body of research on race, culture, and disability will assist practitioners to develop. Yet being aware of differences in what is culturally accepted and needed may come into conflict with what one researcher or practitioner may regard as best practice. Thus, a balance between empowerment and rescue-based mentalities needs to be respected and understood on the part of practitioners and researchers. The delicacy of the practitioner–client relationship needs to be considered as does how much we may be imposing our own values on others.

Our commentary on this volume as graduate students and recent graduates directed our attention toward a number of important considerations for future endeavors—among which were the expansion of research, practice, and education in regards to race, culture, and disability. Developing our creative skills in planning research that focuses on community and practice concerns and working through existing barriers to providing settings for dialogue will ultimately facilitate our own development in better articulating and addressing the critical issues in race, culture, and disability. As we impact the trajectory of our various fields, we look forward to a future that continues to be marked by thoughtful consideration of issues concerning researchers' training and increasing creative solutions to complex challenges, and we look forward to making our own contributions to this critical focus of study and practice.

REFERENCES

Barnes, C. (1992). Qualitative research: valuable or irrelevant? *Disability, Handicap & Society,* *7*(2) 115–124.

Campinha-Bacote, J. (1999). A model and instrument for addressing cultural competence in health care. *Journal of Nursing Education, 38*(5), 203–207.

Kitchin, R. (2000). The researched opinions on research: Disabled people and disability research. *Disability and Society, 15*(1), 25–47.

Olney, M. F., & Kennedy, J. (2002). Racial disparities in VR use and job placements rates for adults with disabilities, *Rehabilitation Counseling Bulletin, 45*(3), 177–189.

Patton, M. Q. (2002). *Qualitative Research and Evaluation Methods* (3rd ed). Thousand Oaks, CA: Sage.

Wilson, K. B. (2002). Exploration of VR acceptance and ethnicity: A national investigation. *Rehabilitation Counseling Bulletin, 45*(3), 168–176.

Wilson, K. B., Harley, D. A., & Alston, R. J. (2001). Race as a correlate of vocational rehabilitation acceptance: Revisited. *The Journal of Rehabilitation, 67*, 35–41.

Zarb, G. (1992). On the Road to Damascus: first steps towards changing the relations of disability research production. *Disability, Handicap &Society, 7*(2), 125–138.

CHAPTER 20

Conclusion: How Race, Culture, and Disability Intersect: Pragmatic and Generative Perspectives

Christopher B. Keys, PhD

INTRODUCTION

The editors and contributors to this book consider that human diversity merits attention from scientists, instructors, students, and practitioners in rehabilitation. In this view, scientists develop theory about the nature of the intersections of race, culture, and disability. Researchers study the critical psychological, social, and rehabilitation dimensions in that intersection. Instructors create, implement, and evaluate methods for engaging students in thinking about human diversity. They consider how students' views of race, culture, and disability affect their interactions with members of groups different from themselves and their provision of rehabilitation services to these individuals. Students seek opportunities to study culture and diversity, to reflect on their own cultural roots and its impact on themselves and others, and to learn from and work with those from different backgrounds. Practitioners develop cultural competence (CC) and see serving a multiethnic populace with a variety of disabilities as an opportunity to learn and serve in a profound and humbling way. Our purpose in this book has been to provide a state-of-the-field report of the study and professional practice occurring in the intersection of race, culture, and disability. We have sought to present the theoretical, empirical, and pedagogical perspectives of intellectual leaders in rehabilitation, disability studies, psychology, and related fields concerning this intersection.

We can consider this intersection from at least two perspectives. First, what is the pragmatic value of studying this intersection? What are the practical problems to be identified and solved and the issues to be addressed? What are the actions to be taken? This pragmatic perspective places problem solving at the center, emphasizing problem identification, problem specification, and finding and developing solutions, when feasible, that keep problems solved over time.

Second, we consider a generative perspective that seeks to frame questions of value for exploring this domain of human complexity: What are the key dimensions of the intersection of race, culture, and disability? How are they developed and what influences do they have? What is their heuristic value? This generative stance promotes a breadth of perspectives and understanding and the growth of relevant theory and research. It seeks knowledge from research without explicit benefit in the near term. Taken together, these two approaches complement one another and lead to the development of a body of science at the intersection of race, culture and disability. This research has great potential for enhancing our present understanding, our future research directions and our awareness of actions necessary to address racial disparities among people with disabilities receiving human services.

PROBLEM SOLVING IN THE INTERSECTION: A PRAGMATIC PERSPECTIVE

One useful way to reflect upon the preceding chapters is to consider them from a problem definition, identification, and problem-solving perspective. This pragmatic perspective guided our structuring of this book and seeks to make manifest the utility of our present knowledge, thereby encouraging future action and intellectual exploration in the intersection of race, culture, and disability. The key problems defined, identified, and documented are disparities in services for people with disabilities related to race and/or ethnicity. This is the primary problem identified in this volume and in the race, culture, and disability literature more generally. These disparities primarily are taken to mean that there is less access to services, shorter duration of services, less variety of services available, and less successful service outcomes for members of diverse racial and ethnic groups with disabilities than for members of the dominant White culture with similar disabilities (Chapter 6, Chapters 9 and 10).

Disparities also exist in the development, testing, and use of assessment resources (Chapter 4). Some psychological tests have been normed with samples that include members of some diverse ethnic and racial groups (e.g., African American and Latino). Measures that have been normed on samples that include all multicultural groups are very few to nonexistent. Tests, that are normed on any particular racial or ethnic group so as to better capture the diversity within each cultural group, are also quite rare.

Other factors like socioeconomic class, gender, and cultural practices may enter into consideration of the meaning of these disparities. Often, these factors are related to and result from racism, sexism, and/or ableism that are part of the mainstream culture. Some argue that these disparities are not solely the result of societal prejudice and discrimination but result from the behavior and qualities of the members of diverse ethnic and racial groups with disabilities. That theoretical possibility may merit further study, although the tendency to blame the victim inappropriately is ever-present in this formulation (Ryan, 1970). In fact, mainstream society has much more economic, social, and political power and cultural influence than do people with disabilities, especially those who are also members of diverse racial and ethnic groups. Therefore, it seems altogether appropriate to consider what the contributions of mainstream society are to the current disparities as a major point of departure.

The disparities members of diverse racial and ethnic groups with disabilities encounter need to be addressed so that they can have more equitable access to, assessment by, and treatment from rehabilitation services. In turn, reducing and eliminating these disparities is expected to lead to more equitable positive treatment outcomes for diverse racial and ethnic group members with disabilities. A key focus for increasing equity is enhancing the CC of service providers. Balcazar, Suarez-Balcazar, Willis, and Alvarado (Chapter 14) insightfully review most of the conceptual frameworks for exploring CC that have been developed in the last four decades. Lewis and Shamburger (Chapter 12) describe an innovative approach to enhance rehabilitation students' CC. Cook, Razzano, and Jonikas (Chapter 7) suggest some valuable content for cultural competency training with professionals and students concerning mental health issues in particular. Matteliano and Stone (Chapter 11), among others, have developed valuable resources on CC teaching concerning many immigrant groups for educators and practitioners. Garcia (Chapter 13) demonstrates that in areas often not considered in thinking about CC such as ethical decision making, culture and diversity are important considerations for those seeking to be fully competent. Kundu, Dutta, and Chan (Chapter 16) illustrate how to incorporate CC into rehabilitation activities such as job placement. Arango, White, Kielhofner, Odoms-Young, and Watkins-Turner (Chapter 17) highlight the development of CC as the main problem-solving message of this book. They emphasize the importance for all individuals, including members of diverse groups, to enhance one's own CC and to continue to do so over time. This enhancement may increase both understanding of other cultures and learning to provide services to members of those cultures. Balcazar et al.'s (Chapter 14) synthesis model of CC indicates the many dimensions of culture that are relevant. We have focused more on culture as defined by race and ethnicity in this book as has much of the scientific literature on culture. As our understanding of the culture increases, it also may lead to greater knowledge and appreciation of both disability culture and the intersection of culture, race, and disability and thus more effective service provision (Chapter 3). Thereby, generative knowledge of culture over time may have pragmatic value for rehabilitation services.

Although noted, less attention is paid in this volume to how to enhance the racial and disability diversity of those providing services, educating future professionals, and conducting rehabilitation research. Distinct progress has been made during the last generation in recruiting and educating members of diverse racial and ethnic groups and individuals with disabilities to become rehabilitation counselors, educators, and researchers. Having more diverse cohorts of rehabilitation and disability studies professionals helps bring the diversity of our nation and the world into the rehabilitation profession. It makes diversity part of the air we breathe and an issue whose relevance is palpable every day. Without the diverse talent that has developed to date, this book would not have been possible. Having a more diverse professional population in rehabilitation provides models for those who are from diverse groups and have disabilities. It can educate and engage Whites that are experienced in mentoring more diverse talent and in providing other forms of support. Building on the progress to date, the field of rehabilitation has much to do to develop more multicultural talent, especially professionals who both have disabilities and are members of diverse racial and ethnic groups. Benefits realized to date are not permanent and need to be sustained and enhanced.

Another issue of note concerns levels of analyses and operation. Most of the work about solving the problem of disparities has focused on the CC of rehabilitation counselors, other practitioners, and researchers and how to train these individuals. However, problems at larger levels of analysis than the individual or the dyad also contribute to the persistence of disparities in service provision and need to be identified and addressed. Clay, Seekins, and Castillo (Chapter 8) identify larger systemic factors that limit the development of Native American service provision. Smith and Alston (Chapter 9) examine the multiple disadvantages affecting minority women with disabilities. Hasnain and Leung (Chapter 10) consider the limited supports and services available to Asian/Pacific Americans with disabilities in this country. Kundu et al. (Chapter 16) articulate how to build a cultural dimension into services for job placement using a systemic approach. Suarez-Balcazar et al. (Chapter 15) focus on building agencies' evaluation capacity to assess services for members of diverse racial and ethnic groups with disabilities in a culturally competent manner. These efforts broaden our thinking to include program, organizational, community, and larger scale factors as we consider the causes, mechanisms, and solutions of disparities and other issues of diversity that affect individuals, agencies, and tribes.

In brief, this volume, like most theory and research in the nascent area of race, culture, and disability, has emphasized the service disparities between members of different ethnic and racial groups with disabilities. Disability has been a defining feature of those involved and the disparities examined have been those among racial and ethnic groups. Disparities among those with different disabilities from diverse ethnic and racial groups have received little if any attention. In the future, issues to explore include: How are individuals with different disabilities treated within racial and ethnic groups? In the mainstream there is a hierarchy of disability that privileges those with sensory and mobility impairments and disadvantages those with cognitive and emotional disabilities. Does this hierarchy operate in other racial and ethnic groups? What is the impact of having dual statuses of a disability and a racial minority in the United States? What are the organizational and community dimensions of race, culture, and disability and how can we best understand them? How do mainstream societies' norms, policies, and systems affect those with disabilities from diverse racial and ethnic groups constructively and destructively? We know much less about these areas of the intersection and in the future we hope to know more.

KEY DIMENSIONS OF THE INTERSECTION: A GENERATIVE PERSPECTIVE

A second perspective seeks to explore the intersection of race, culture, and disability, which has two crucial dimensions— historical and intersectional. Fujiura and Drazen (Chapter 2) provide a cogent review of much of the work to date and the work to be done. The definitions of race and disability have been linked historically in the early 1900s during the eugenics era (Block-Lourie, Balcazar, & Keys, 2001). Those who were disabled and those who were African American were seen as biologically different and inferior in ways that, at least at that time, justified and allowed sterilization and medical experimentation on them without their knowledge or consent. In recent decades as knowledge of biology has increased, so has awareness of the social component of our views of race and disability. As we unravel the mysteries of the genome in biology, it is equally important to increase our understanding of the social and ecological dimensions of racism and ableism, both separately and together.

In the United States, race is now recognized by many as a social construction that is used to maintain the privileged position of the dominant racial group—Caucasians. Similarly, the social model of disabilities underscores the responses of others and of society to those with physical, sensory, cognitive, and/or psychological impairments as a central aspect of disability (Longmore, 2003). As the social dimensions of race and disability become more widely recognized, our ability to consider them in their societal context with many layers of present and historical meaning increases. The rich meanings of African American identity theory and its implications for the development of disability identity can be explored constructively (Chapter 3). The role of disparities in services as a function of the race and/or ethnicity of people with disabilities garners increased attention (Hill-Briggs et al., this volume; Wilson & Senices, this volume). The contextual factors that agencies and individuals with disabilities from diverse communities face as they seek to obtain and provide rehabilitation services to people of color are considered more fully (Chapter 15).

In short, future research might include social dimensions to the study of race and disability. This will lead to more complete, accurate, and constructive ways of examining the interaction of these terms than were available in past generation. Race and disability are much less likely to be treated as rigid, biological categories that have immutable impacts on intellectual endowment (cf. Herrnstein & Murphy, 1994). Instead, racial and disability differences are now seen as disparities that may reflect shortcomings of the service system rather than of the individuals seeking services. The victims are no longer reflexively blamed (cf. Ryan, 1970). Rather, social perspectives provide a more nuanced understanding of the flexible, contextual dimensions of race, culture, and disability and of the many biological and social similarities that human beings share (cf. Bond, 2007). Notwithstanding the progress we still need to make, because our definitions are less exclusively biological, our understanding of race and disability is more complex and complete. Our intellectual capacity for addressing societal prejudices is enhanced, and our ability to address issues of disparities has grown. This book is a result of and reflects the sea change in American society's perspective on race and disability since World War II.

INTERSECTIONALITY

The intersectional quality of race, culture, and disability speaks to the importance of examining these constructs as they overlap and interact (Chapter 2). Historically, while links did exist between race and disability as targets of discrimination, researchers have generally been more focused on individual categories of difference from the mainstream (Braddock & Parish, 2001). Examining the combination of differences and their meaning did not galvanize scientists' attention or that of many others. Lack of numbers, means of connection, and resources impeded progress. Persons of diverse racial backgrounds with disabilities have not been a primary focus of the disability movement, which has historically been populated largely by middle-class White people with disabilities. Similarly, members of diverse racial and ethnic groups with disabilities have not been a focus of groups coping with racism and promoting positive ethnic and racial identity. These groups have had primarily able-bodied members of a particular race or ethnicity.

During the last decade or so, funding agencies have begun to invest in these intersections of race, gender, sexual orientation, and social class. Researchers have begun to address the complexity of individuals with multiple statuses that differ from that of the dominant White, middle-class, able-bodied, straight male (Chapter 17). Some university scholars in the humanities and the social sciences have thoughtfully examined the intersections in which different racial and ethnic groups participate, including, for example, not only race and gender but also race and social class (cf. Bond, 2007).

The contributions to this volume indicate that we are making important progress in developing relevant theory, research, pedagogy, and practice concerning the intersection of race, culture, and disability, yet we clearly have more ground to cover. For example, Gill and Cross (Chapter 3) introduce a rich vein of identity theory that has been invaluable in clarifying developmental pathways and the factors that influence them for African Americans and for people with disabilities considered separately. As they suggest, future work will beneficially consider the identity development of members of diverse racial and ethnic groups with disabilities. More generally, race and disability are combined empirically in a number of studies (McMahon, Parnes, Keys, & Viola, 2008; Taylor-Ritzler, Balcazar, Keys, Hayes, & Garate-Serafini, 2001). However, the development of theory to account for similarities and differences between various racial groups with disabilities that clearly explains the reality and impact of living in the intersection, remains to be done. For example, color plays a role in the disability community such that darker skin seems to be associated with poorer service access and rehabilitation outcomes in disparity research (Chapter 5). That is, racism leads to less support for persons of darker skin color with disabilities.

On the other hand, the disability aspects of the intersection have been less explored. How does ableism operate for members of diverse racial and ethnic groups? Once we acknowledge that matters of race and disability have important social dimensions that intersect, then generative research questions regarding both mainstream and diverse cultures quickly arise. How does mainstream society treat people with disabilities who have different accents, skin colors, and backgrounds? What are the manifestations of prejudicial attitudes and discriminatory actions toward those members of diverse racial and ethnic groups with disabilities? How are they in accord with the norms of dominant society?

There is also little theoretical or empirical work that captures the meaning of being exposed to both racism and ableism together and separately over time. How do the cultures of those who are targets of racism and ableism develop, support their members, and help them respond? How do different cultures respond to differences in disability, race, and ethnicity? At the supraindividual level what happens when two different cultures interact, such as African American culture and disability culture? These kinds of cultural issues are central to understanding race, culture, and disability. For example, different cultures, including those of Native Americans, Latinos, Caucasians, or African peoples, respond very differently to strong emotional displays (Chapter 7). These kinds of differences may emerge from generative research. They also underscore the pragmatic importance for American rehabilitation service providers to be familiar with the cultures of immigrants to the

United States (Chapter 10; Chapter 11) and the diverse cultures in this country (Chapter 14).

In the future, Watts (1993) has noted that multiple forms of research will be necessary to examine diversity in its full complexity. For example, to date, research concerning race, culture, and disability has been more comparative of groups and quantitative in method. This approach has been effective in identifying disparities between Whites and other racial and ethnic groups in rehabilitation services. Now, we also need qualitative research to conduct in-depth ethnographic studies of the lives of people who are members of diverse racial and ethnic groups with a variety of disabilities (Chapter 19). These studies can usefully explore race, culture, and disability, and racism, prejudice, and ableism separately and/or together. How do they influence daily lives, personal activities, psychological well-being, and opportunities to participate and be fully engaged in families and communities? We need participants of different cultures and races with a variety of disabilities to give voice to their experiences of living in the intersection of race, culture, and disability. We need to examine the impact of ableism and racism in depth and with the focus yielded by good qualitative interviewing and ethnographic research (cf. Jason et al., 2004). Thereby, we can ground future theory and research more fully in the lived experience of people with disabilities who are members of diverse racial and ethnic groups (cf. Keys, McMahon, Sanchez, London, & Abdul-Adil, 2004).

In closing, as described through the chapters of this book, the authors ask that we make more explicit the role and value of race, culture, and disability not only separately but also jointly at all levels of the rehabilitation process and more generally in society. A challenge for the future is to develop a more complete account of how race, culture, and disability are taken into consideration by rehabilitation service systems and other contexts of importance (Chapter 18). Also, how do intervention programs promote the CC of their staff and student trainees? For these efforts, generative and pragmatic research of many kinds will be needed. Generative research will cast a broad net of intellectual curiosity and will focus our understanding on the concerns affecting people in rehabilitation specifically. Taken together, these perspectives may yield synergies that enable us to both study and act on the findings concerning the intersection of race, culture, and disability. These findings may have both direct benefit and enhance our understanding. It is hoped that they help lead us to a place where, to paraphrase and build on the words of Maya Angelou, we can have the compassion to see through complexion and impairment to our common humanity, the respect to value our differences, and the courage to create a more just society.

REFERENCES

Block-Lourie, P., Balcazar, F., & Keys, C. (2001). From pathology to power: Rethinking race, poverty, and disability. *Journal of Disability Policy Studies, 12*, 18–27.

Bond, M. (2007). *Workplace chemistry: Promoting diversity through organizational change.* Lebanon, NH: University Press of New England.

Braddock, D. L., & Parish, S. (2001). An institutional history of disability. In G. L. Albrecht, K. D. Seelman, & M. Bury (Eds), *Handbook of disability studies.* (pp. 11–68) Thousand Oaks, CA: Sage.

Herrnstein, R., & Murphy, C. (1994). *The bell curve: Intelligence and class structure in American life.* New York: Free Press.

Jason, L., Keys, C., Suarez-Balcazar, Y., Taylor, R., Davis, M., Durlak, J., et al. (2004). *Participatory community research: Theories and methods in action.* Washington, DC: American Psychological Association.

Keys, C., McMahon, S., Sánchez, B., London, L., & Abdul-Adil, J. (2004). Culturally anchored research: Quandaries, guidelines, and exemplars for community psychology. In L. Jason, C. Keys, Y. Suarez-Balcazar, R. Taylor, M. Davis, J. Durlak, et al. (Eds.), *Participatory community research: Theories and methods in action.* Washington DC: American Psychological Association.

Longmore, P. K. (2003). *Why I burned my book and other essays on disability.* (pp. 174–198) Philadelphia: Temple University Press.

McMahon, S., Parnes, A., Keys, C., & Viola, J. (2008). School belonging among low-income urban youth with disabilities: Testing a theoretical model. *Psychology in the Schools, 45,* 387–401.

Ryan, W. (1970). *Blaming the victim.* New York: Vintage.

Taylor-Ritzler, T., Balcazar, F., Keys, C., Hayes, E., & Garate-Serafini, T. (2001). Promoting attainment of transition related goals among low-income ethnic minority students with disabilities. *Career Development for Exceptional Individuals, 24,* 147–167.

Watts, R. (1993). Paradigms of diversity. In R. Watts, E. Trickett, & D. Birman (Eds.), *Human Diversity.* (pp. 230–243) San Francisco: Jossey-Bass.

Index